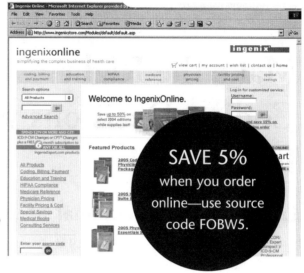
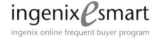

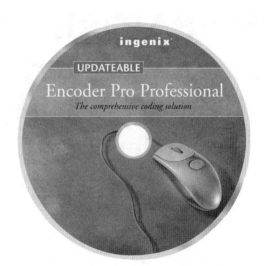

ICD-9-CM code changes happen every year— understand why and how those changes affect the way you code!

2005 ICD-9-CM Changes: An Insider's View

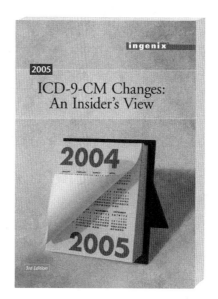

Item No.: 6372   **$59.95**

Available: September 2004   ISBN: 1-56337-593-1

Changes made each year to the ICD-9-CM classification system impact reporting and reimbursement for medical services. *ICD-9-CM Changes: An Insider's View* not only provides specific ICD-9-CM changes, but also explains the rationale behind the changes and the impact they will have on your coding practices.

- **Understand why new codes are created and why other codes are revised.** In-depth knowledge of what the code changes are and why they occurred is essential for correct coding application and use.

- **Recognize the impact of code changes both past and present.** The coding history shows how conditions were previously coded and how such changes impact current coding and reporting practices.

- **Prevent "under coding" or "over coding."** Clinical presentation and treatment information provides clarification on various procedures to help coders make precise selections for optimal reimbursement.

- **Know what terminology included in a medical record is essential.** Common clinical terminology for diagnoses and procedures related to the new codes is used so that you know when the new codes apply.

- **View changes to all three volumes of ICD-9-CM.** Annotations provide the official document of all changes with clarification of changes, including text deletions, not discussed in detail elsewhere in the book.

- **Confirm coding selection for new codes with illustrations.** Illustrations visually convey the clinical complexities associated with various code changes.

- **Gain practical guidance on how to apply new codes.** Coding scenarios demonstrate the application of new codes.

100% Money Back Guarantee:
If our merchandise* ever fails to meet your expectations, please contact our Customer Service Department toll-free at 1.800.INGENIX (464.3649), option 1, for an immediate response. *Software: Credit will be granted for unopened packages only.

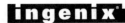

Master the Skills Needed to Be an Effective Coder!

2005 Ingenix Coding Lab: Physician Offices

Item No.: 5789   **$74.95**

Available: December 2004   ISBN: 1-56337-634-2

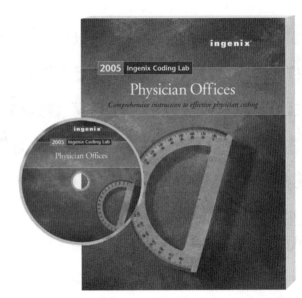

This comprehensive education module helps beginning to intermediate coders in the physician office or the classroom. Designed to allow the user to understand and master the skills needed to be effective coder, this module includes a CD that includes a student workbook with chapter quizzes and a free 3-month demo to *EncoderPRO*. It builds on the basics learned in *Ingenix Coding Lab: Medical Billing Basics*.

- **New!—Become more familiar with ICD-9-CM and CPT® coding to help you code more accurately and confidently on the job.** ICD-9-CM and CPT® chapter layouts follow actual code books.

- **Learn the foundation of coding and billing.** Broad overview of coding, payers, and the reimbursement process for the entry-level coder or billing professional.

- **Help ensure fast and accurate facility reimbursement.** Examples of complex coding scenarios are presented.

- **Test your coding knowledge.** Chapter quizzes available on the Student Guide CD to ensure students retain the most pertinent information.

- **Allows an instructor to better tutor and challenge students.** Teacher's Guide on CD is the answer key to chapter quizzes and also provides challenge exercises not found in the book.

- **Three-Month *EncoderPRO* demo included on Student CD.** *EncoderPRO* look-up includes the latest CPT®, HCPCS, and ICD-9-CM codes.

- **Earn CEUs from AAPC.** Earn 5 CEUs awarded by AAPC.

100% Money Back Guarantee:
If our merchandise* ever fails to meet your expectations, please contact our Customer Service Department toll-free at 1.800.INGENIX (464.3649), option 1, for an immediate response.
*Software: Credit will be granted for unopened packages only.

CPT is a registered trademark of the American Medical Association.

SAVE 5% when you order at www.ingenixonline.com (reference source code FOBW5)

or call toll-free 1.800.INGENIX (464.3649), option 1.

Also available from your medical bookstore or distributor.

FOBA5

Master the Skills Needed to Be an Effective Coder!

2005 Ingenix Coding Lab: Facilities and Ancillary Services

Item No.: 5790   **$99.95**

Available: December 2004   ISBN: 1-56337-635-0

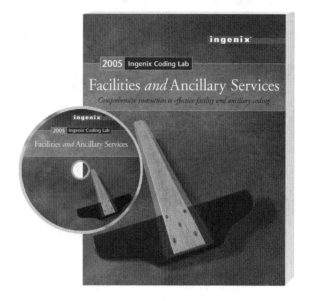

This comprehensive education module helps advanced coders in the facility billing office or the classroom. Designed to allow the user to understand and master the skills needed to be an effective coder, this module includes a CD that contains a student workbook with chapter quizzes and a free 3-month demo to *EncoderPRO*. It builds on the basics learned in *Ingenix Coding Lab: Medical Billing Basics.*

- **NEW!—Learn the intricacies of HCPCS coding through real-life coding examples in the book and on CD.** New and improved HCPCS chapter included.

- **NEW!—Become more familiar with ICD-9-CM and CPT® coding to help you code more accurately and confidently on the job.** ICD-9-CM and CPT® chapter layouts follow actual code books.

- **Learn the foundation of coding and billing.** Broad overview of coding, payers, and the reimbursement process for the entry-level coder or billing professional.

- **Help ensure fast and accurate facility reimbursement.** Examples of complex coding scenarios are presented.

- **Test your coding knowledge.** Chapter quizzes available on the Student Guide CD to ensure students retain the most pertinent information.

- **Allows an instructor to better tutor and challenge students.** Teacher's Guide on CD is the answer key to chapter quizzes and also provides challenge exercises not found in the book.

- **Three-Month *Encoder PRO* demo included on Student CD.** *EncoderPRO* look-up includes the latest CPT®, HCPCS, and ICD-9-CM codes.

- **Earn CEUs from AAPC.** Earn 5 CEUs awarded by AAPC.

SAVE 5% when you order at www.ingenixonline.com (reference source code FOBW5)

or call toll-free 1.800.INGENIX (464.3649), option 1.

Also available from your medical bookstore or distributor.

Learn to Code Easily and Accurately from Your Physician's Operative Report

2005 Ingenix Coding Lab: Coding from the Operative Report

Item No.: 5971   **$84.95**

Available: December 2004   ISBN: 1-56337-632-6

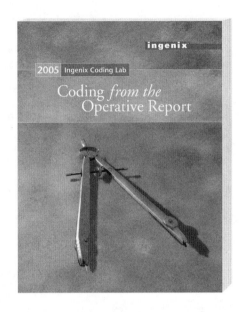

This inexpensive manual provides instruction on attaining the proper information from physicians' documentation. Beginning with a discussion of operative reports and their importance to the coding process, this book includes examples of operative reports and operative notes, information needed to successfully and accurately code, specialty-specific scenarios, and the CPT® chapter in which each service falls.

- **New!—Get real world examples of operative reports for every specialty to help you know how to handle common challenges and mistakes.** Operative reports added for every specialty.

- **Use this in concert with other Ingenix publications and software for consistent, accurate training to prepare for certification exams.** Part of the Ingenix Coding Lab series.

- **Provides and easy-to-use format for every experience level.** For use in the classroom or in the office setting to train new and existing employees.

- **Helps the end-user interpret common cryptic shortcuts, abbreviations and nomenclature used by physicians.** Includes definitions, key points, tips and glossaries.

- **Guidance through the entire operative report interpretation, abstracting and coding process.** Includes scenarios for CPT®, I-9, HCPCS, DRG and more.

- **Earn CEUs from AAPC.** Earn up to 5 CEUs awarded by AAPC.

Add Modifiers Right the First Time!

2005 Ingenix Coding Lab: Understanding Modifiers

Item No.: 3989 **$84.95**

Available: December 2004 ISBN: 1-56337-637-7

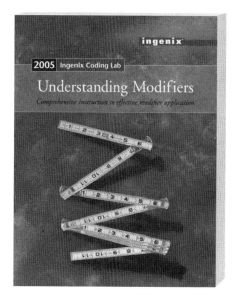

The most comprehensive resource for HCPCS Level II and CPT® modifiers on the market. This best-selling guide gives you the tools you need to apply modifiers accurately and avoid payment delays and denials.

- **New!—Helps coders understand most commonly missed HCPCS modifier errors.** Includes a new look at HCPCS modifiers and new clinical examples.

- **Designed with aspiring coders needs in mind to help them understand the key concepts that will be required on coding certification exams.** This is another training module in the Ingenix Coding Lab line that will help you prepare for AHIMA and AAPC credentialing exams

- **Contains all new and changed CPT® and HCPCS Level II modifier information.** Fully updated for 2005.

- **Choose the correct modifier when more than one could apply.** Decision-tree flow charts guide you.

- **Search the web with prior knowledge of where modifier information exists.** Supplies all of the up-to-date links a coder needs to find accurate modifier information online.

- **Helps reduce claim denials by giving correctly used modifiers.** Real-life clinical examples are provided.

- **Earn CEUs from AAPC.** Earn 4 CEUs awarded by AAPC.

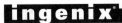

Correctly Document Specific Level of E/M Services the First Time!

2005 Ingenix Coding Lab: Understanding E/M Coding

Item No.: 3214   **$84.95**

Available: December 2004   ISBN: 1-56337-638-5

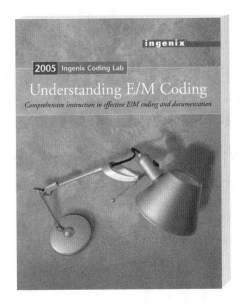

This comprehensive guide to CMS's evaluation and management (E/M) guidelines provides instructions for correctly documenting to a specific level of E/M service. Charts and templates provide excellent tools for auditing current practices and making any needed corrections. Real-world case scenarios work to help the user grasp documentation requirements.

- **Compare your coding trends with national figures.** Use the E/M profiler to help identify coding issues.

- **Helps prevent claim denials.** Self-audit forms, including the official CMS auditing form, help ensure that the documentation supports the level of E/M service coded.

- **See the impact of stricter guidelines on your practice.** 1995, 1997, and 2000 E/M guidelines included. These guidelines prepare the user for the transition to the stricter documentation requirements ahead.

- **Training help for your staff.** Real-life clinical case studies updated for 2005. Case studies illustrate how to apply the guidelines in everyday situations.

- **Earn CEUs from AAPC.** Earn 5 CEUs awarded by AAPC.

100% Money Back Guarantee:
If our merchandise* ever fails to meet your expectations, please contact our Customer Service Department toll-free at 1.800.INGENIX (464.3649), option 1, for an immediate response.
*Software: Credit will be granted for unopened packages only.

SAVE 5% when you order at www.ingenixonline.com (reference source code FOBW5)

or call toll-free 1.800.INGENIX (464.3649), option 1.

Also available from your medical bookstore or distributor.

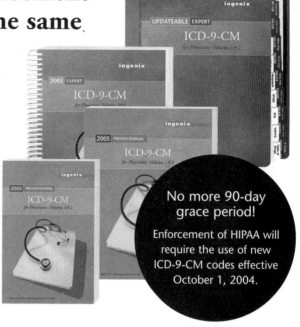

Four simple ways to place an order.

Call

1.800.ingenix (464.3649), option 1. Mention source code FOBA5 when ordering.

Mail

PO Box 27116
Salt Lake City, UT 84127-0116
With payment and/or purchase order.

Fax

801.982.4033
With credit card information and/or purchase order.

Click

www.ingenixonline.com
Save 5% when you order online today—use source code FOBW5.

ingenix *e*smart
ingenix online frequent buyer program

GET REWARDS FOR SHOPPING ONLINE!
To find out more, visit IngenixOnline.com

E-Smart program available only to Ingenix customers who are not part of Medallion, Gold Medallion or Partner Accounts programs. You must be registered at Ingenix Online to have your online purchases tracked for rewards purposes. Shipping charges and taxes still apply and cannot be used for rewards. Offer valid online only.

100% Money Back Guarantee

If our merchandise* ever fails to meet your expectations, please contact our Customer Service Department toll-free at 1.800.ingenix (464.3649), option 1 for an immediate response.

*Software: Credit will be granted for unopened packages only.

Customer Service Hours

7:00 am - 5:00 pm Mountain Time
9:00 am - 7:00 pm Eastern Time

Shipping and Handling

no. of items	fee
1	$10.95
2-4	$12.95
5-7	$14.95
8-10	$19.95
11+	Call

---

ingenix

Order Form

Information

Customer No. _____ Contact No. _____

Source Code _____

Contact Name _____

Title _____ Specialty _____

Company _____

Street Address _____
NO PO BOXES, PLEASE

City _____ State _____ Zip _____

Telephone ( ) _____ Fax ( ) _____
IN CASE WE HAVE QUESTIONS ABOUT YOUR ORDER

E-mail _____ @ _____
REQUIRED FOR ORDER CONFIRMATION AND SELECT PRODUCT DELIVERY.

Ingenix respects your right to privacy. We will not sell or rent your e-mail address or fax number to anyone outside Ingenix and its business partners. If you would like to remove your name from Ingenix promotion, please call 1.800.ingenix (464.3649), option 1.

Product

Item No.	Qty	Description	Price	Total

Subtotal _____

UT, OH, & VA residents, please add applicable Sales tax _____

(See chart on the left) Shipping & handling charges _____
All foreign orders, please call for shipping costs

Total _____

Payment

○ Please bill my credit card ○ MasterCard ○ VISA ○ Amex ○ Discover

Card No. | | | | | | | | | | | | | | | | Expires | |
MONTH YEAR

Signature _____

○ Check enclosed, made payable to: Ingenix, Inc. ○ Please bill my office

Purchase Order No. _____
ATTACH COPY OF PURCHASE ORDER

FOBA5

ingenix®

Ingenix Coding Lab:
Medical Billing Basics

2005
3rd edition

Notice

Ingenix Coding Lab: Medical Billing Basics is designed to be an accurate and authoritative source regarding coding and every reasonable effort has been made to ensure accuracy and completeness of the content. However, Ingenix, Inc. makes no guarantee, warranty, or representation that this publication is accurate, complete, or without errors. It is understood that Ingenix, Inc. is not rendering any legal or other professional services or advice in this publication and that Ingenix, Inc. bears no liability for any results or consequences that may arise from the use of this book. Please address all correspondence to:

Ingenix, Inc.
2525 Lake Park Blvd
Salt Lake City, UT 84120

American Medical Association Notice

Continuing Education Units for AAPC Certified Members

This publication has prior approval by the American Academy of Professional Coders for continuing education units. Granting of prior approval in no way constitutes endorsement by AAPC of the publication content nor the publisher. Instructions to submit CEUs are available within the "Preapproved CEU Vendor List" file at www.aapc.com/education/CEUs/ceus.html.

Acknowledgments

Anne Petrie, *Product Manager*
Sheri Poe Bernard, CPC, *Director, Essential Regulatory Products*
Lynn Speirs, *Senior Director, Publishing Services Group*
Karen Schmidt, BSN, *Technical Director*
Nannette Orme, CPC, *Technical Editor*
Deborah C. Hall, CPC, *Technical Editor*
Regina Heppes, *Copy Editor*
Stacy Perry, *Desktop Publishing Manager*

About the technical editors

Deborah C. Hall, CPC

Ms. Hall is a Senior Clinical/Technical Editor for Ingenix. Ms. Hall has more than 20 years of experience in the health care field. Her experience includes 10 years as office manager for large multispecialty medical practices. Ms. Hall has written several multispecialty newsletters and coding and reimbursement manuals, and served as a health care consultant. She has taught seminars on CPT/HCPCS and ICD-9-CM coding and physician fee schedules.

Nannette Orme, CPC

Ms. Orme has more than 10 years of experience in the health care profession. She has extensive background in CPT/HCPCS and ICD-9-CM coding. She recently served several years as a consultant with PricewaterhouseCoopers. Her areas of expertise include physician audits and education, compliance and HIPAA legislation, litigation support for Medicare self-disclosure cases, hospital chargemaster maintenance, and emergency department coding. Ms. Orme has presented at national professional conferences and contributed articles for several professional publications. She is a member of the American Academy of Professional Coders (AAPC) and the Utah Medical Group Management Association (UMGMA).

Contents

Introduction

WELCOME TO THE CAREER OF MEDICAL CODING

The fact that you are holding this book and reading this text is indication that you are actively considering training to be a medical coder. Rest assured that you are on the right track. This product, *Ingenix Coding Lab: Medical Billing Basics,* is an initiation into the field of medical coding. The chapters in this book are designed to introduce and train newcomers in a comprehensive and structured manner.

And when we say you are on the right track, it is because there are wrong ways to enter the coding business. For example, you have avoided, we hope, the career promises advertised almost everywhere: "Earn $$$ a month doing medical billing from home." These promotions push coding and billing software and equipment on unwitting participants. Only rarely do those subscribers succeed in this extremely important and competitive professional arena.

You should know that medical coding and billing offers meaningful and satisfying employment to people in all areas of the United States today. And yes, some work from home. Others work for more centralized clearinghouses that take in outsourced work. But probably many more work in offices, clinics, hospitals, and other alternative health care settings. This growing area of health care is professionally demanding, yet personally and financially rewarding. And like any work within the health care environment, a significant amount of training and education is required to succeed.

THE NATURE OF MEDICAL CODING

What is medical coding and how does its role fit into the larger picture of health care? Medical codes are part of health care information management (HIM), which includes medical records, billing and reimbursement, data quality management, and in larger facilities, morbidity and mortality registries, and statistics. Simply put, once the diagnoses have been made, the medical services provided, and supplies, drugs, and equipment prescribed, medical codes become the elements of communication. Computers everywhere in the industry are programmed to recognize and process the codes. Billing and reimbursement are tied to the codes. Inventory, statistics, and research are all compiled and analyzed by codes. To the ordinary citizen, a procedure may be described as "gallbladder surgery." To the clinician it is a "cholecystectomy." But to a coder or computer the *Physicians' Current Procedural Terminology* (CPT) procedure code is 47600.

The selection and assignment of the correct codes to describe the clinical work or medical products is the job of coders. It is an important process and the reimbursement amount depends on a single coding decision. Consequently, efficient and accurate translation of services and products into medical codes is a clear financial advantage to any health care setting. It is this economic incentive that drives much of the growth and success of the medical coding profession.

 KEY POINT

The selection and assignment of the correct codes to describe the clinical work or medical products is the job of coders. It is an important process and many thousands of dollars may ride on a single coding decision.

As you will learn in these chapters, there are three general code sets. CPT codes report the medical services and procedures. The ICD-9-CM code set reports the illnesses, injuries, and other reasons a patient might see a physician. The HCPCS Level II codes report medical equipment, supplies, certain drugs, and some procedures. Within each of these systems are major subsets and categories of codes, which are also addressed in this book.

The entry level coder must have a working knowledge of the various code sets, the types of services and products they report, and the rules and regulations that govern proper assignment. You will understand how these codes work together after completing this first step of training. Many people who train in basic medical coding continue their education. Those wishing to develop additional coding skills progress to the second product in the series, *Ingenix Coding Lab: Physician Offices.* This is a more advanced training program designed to assist medical coders in physician settings to improve their skills and obtain credentials and certification. A third level, *Ingenix Coding Lab: Hospital and Ancillary Facilities,* is tailored to experienced medical coders wishing to learn specialized aspects unique to hospital outpatient clinical settings.

The Ingenix Coding Lab training program is designed to assist students and coders to gain and/or improve medical coding skills. Ingenix does not offer certification of its own, rather, this training program prepares the user to sit for open certification examinations in medical coding. The Ingenix Coding Lab series includes material beyond the scope of the medical coding examinations. Select topics in administration, finance, legal and regulatory aspects, and reimbursement are also addressed in this training. Ingenix has a long history serving the medical coding field as an innovative leader in development of educational books, manuals, coding software, and on-site consulting.

CODING AND THE FINANCIAL PICTURE

Medical coding and billing functions are a component of medicine's significant overhead, or cost of doing business. Not surprisingly, many of those closest to the clinical functions of health care feel that all adjunct aspects of medicine should, at best, work to improve delivery of care and, at worst, not interfere with clinical duties. Unfortunately, for many practitioners the nonclinical side of health care is perceived as the enemy—a maddening distraction to the practice of good medicine. And the myriad of rules and policies surrounding coding, billing, and reimbursement are a source of frustration to many health care providers. Some choose simply to ignore coding. But the accurate selection and assignment of codes is a part of good, modern medical practices. Many physicians recognize this and the coding staff usually find clinicians to be friendly and helpful. And since assignment of codes is so instrumental to proper reimbursement of services, procedures, and supplies, coders always have the support of the physician business office, practice administrator, or financial officer.

The federal government, too, has raised the professional bar for coders. As the developer of certain code sets, and the generator of rules and regulations for coding, the government offers coders a broader workload, greater responsibilities, and of course, changing regulations with demanding rules. Facility accreditation agencies also place high demands on medical coding standards. Perhaps most significantly, though, the clinical aspect of medicine grows increasingly complex each year as new procedures and technologies are introduced.

SUPPORTING ORGANIZATIONS

The elements just discussed are components of the foundation of medical coding as a profession. The coder can be aided by one of many organizations that serve medical coding and the associated area of billing and reimbursement.

AHIMA

Perhaps chief among these is the American Health Information Management Association (AHIMA). This is the professional organization for the field of health care information and AHIMA is the sponsoring agency for several levels of medical coding accreditation.

As the sponsoring agency, AHIMA maintains a council on certification that oversees the testing and credentialing process for the various levels in health information and medical coding. Of particular interest to entry-level coders is the Certified Coding Associate (CCA) certificate. To sit for the CCA examination, candidates must hold the equivalent of a high school diploma and have either six-months experience in coding or have completed a formal training program such as *Ingenix Coding Lab: Medical Billing Basics*.

AHIMA offers two advanced coding certifications: Certified Coding Specialist-Physician Services (CCS-P) for physician-based services and Certified Coding Specialist (CCS) for hospital inpatient and outpatient services.

AHIMA also features state chapters to support coding and health information professionals. The association also publishes a monthly magazine with an extensive classified advertising section for job seekers.

Provisional membership in AHIMA is a required to earn and hold the CCA credential.

AAPC

Another major supporting agency is the American Academy of Professional Coders (AAPC), a membership organization that trains and certifies medical coders. The AAPC offers testing and certification (known as Certified Professional Coder, or CPC), as well as a newsletter and a network of local chapters. The organization divides its credentialing into physician-based and hospital-based certification. Certification through AAPC is generally accepted nationwide. The organization offers an apprentice level certification for those who pass the CPC exam but who have not yet met field experience requirements.

AAPC also offers several specialty coding certifications depending upon coder competency and interest. The CPC is for physician services and the Certified Professional Coder-Hospital (CPC-H) is available for hospital services.

Membership in AAPC is a requisite to earn and hold a credential.

Other Accreditation Agencies

Most medical coding training programs prepare students for eventual certification through the two organizations just mentioned. Please note that AHIMA does not certify or endorse any training programs, including this one, as official preparation for its examinations. It is not required to take a specific course to take the certification examinations offered by AHIMA or AAPC, although AAPC offers courses through instructors they have certified to teach their curriculum.

 FOR MORE INFO

American Health Information Management Association (AHIMA) certification program can be contacted at: 223 N. Michigan Ave., Suite 2150, Chicago, IL 60601-5800 or through the website www.ahima.org. The organization offers an introductory level exam to qualify as a Certified Coding Associate (CCA).

 FOR MORE INFO

The American Academy of Professional Coders (AAPC) is located at 309 West 700 South, Salt Lake City UT 84101 (www.aapc.com). The organization offers an apprentice certification as a Certified Professional Coder (CPC) for students who have passed the examination but who have not yet met the requisite work experience.

The Medical Management Institute's Registered Medical Coder (RMC) certification program is perhaps the best known of the other accreditations. Training is administered through the Association of Registered Medical Coders. Training for the RMC is structured through a proprietary program; however, those wishing to study independently can still test for the RMC.

Some organizations offer certification only to students who have completed a house proprietary training program, which essentially locks-in clients to both training and certification. Quality notwithstanding, these programs are not widely recognized. A number of colleges and universities offer certificates upon completion of their medical coding programs as well. This type of certification may prove valuable within a local job market; however, these types of certification are not generally accepted nationwide.

AHA

Mention should also be made to several other organizations that play important roles in coding. The American Hospital Association (AHA) has a section that specializes in information issues surrounding facilities. The AHA is a supporting organization for medical coding and has been instrumental in developing codes that meet the needs of facilities and outpatient clinics.

As one of the cooperating parties who approve final coding advice, the AHA established the AHA central office, which coordinates two services: the central office on ICD-9-CM and the central office on HCPCS.

AHA's central office on ICD-9-CM serves as representatives and advocates regarding national classification and data issues. In addition, the central office on ICD-9-CM provides a supplemental quarterly coding advice publication titled the *AHA Coding Clinic for ICD-9-CM*. Published since 1984, coding clinic provides a question and answer format for topics related to correct ICD-9-CM diagnosis and procedure coding and guidelines related to sequencing of principal diagnosis and procedure for inpatient coding. One of the central offices' objectives is to serve as the authoritative source of coding/classification information.

Federal Agencies

The federal agency, the Centers for Medicare and Medicaid Services (CMS), is another important player in the world of medical coding. This agency is organized within the Department of Health and Human Services and is charged with developing and maintaining codes, in addition to its major role in the legislation and regulation arena. The National Centers for Health Statistics (NCHS) also has a role in code development and rulemaking. Together these organizations have developed official guidelines and policies for facility coding. The American Medical Association and CMS have also worked together to develop guidelines for assignment of certain code sets.

Additionally, the Office of Inspector General (OIG) is the branch that investigates allegations of wrongdoing. The OIG works with and on behalf of CMS to conduct audits and investigations as detailed in an annual OIG work plan. The OIG's 2005 work plan can be found in appendix C of this book.

MGMA

As with any profession, membership with organizations is important. It is not uncommon for those who are responsible for the coding portion of a physician practice, to also be accountable for the day-to-day financial operations. An organization that can play a helpful role with this aspect of professional

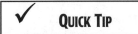

✓ QUICK TIP

As with any profession, there are organizations available to help coders. Membership in these organizations may provide information and a network of resources.

responsibilities is the Medical Group Management Association (MGMA). One of the organization's main obligations is to assist members through information, education, networking and advocacy. MGMA can be a helpful resource for obtaining regulatory information, even that which pertains to coding.

OPPORTUNITIES IN CODING

All of this may seem a bit confusing at this point, but professional coders come to know these entities as key in the arena of medical coding development. Coders are also interested in careers, jobs, and opportunities. There is a shortage of professional medical coders and opportunities are available to enter the field.

Coders with basic training have a variety of options. Working in a health care setting during, or immediately upon completion of basic training, is probably optimal because on-the-job training is so valuable. Be prepared to travel closer to major health centers to improve employment opportunities. You may also look to coding centers that process outsourced material. Clinics and even small private practices can also prove a way to gain coding experience.

Immediately advancing your training is also an option, even if it means accepting provisional certification pending more field experience. Surveys show that credentials improve job prospects and salaries. Some choose to pursue formal educational degrees in the clinical or managerial sides of health care to augment training in coding.

Wherever your coding career path takes you, successful training will make the journey more interesting, more rewarding, and a more memorable experience.

 KEY POINT

Coders with basic training have a variety of options.

Chapter 1: Medical Terminology

INTRODUCTION

Medicine uses its own language and much of the terminology refers to anatomy, or what is known as anatomical nomenclature. Anatomical terms stem from Latin, Greek, and occasionally Arabic. Learning Latin and Greek might seem a daunting task, but in fact many English words derive from these languages and will not be totally unfamiliar.

The origin of words can sometimes be traced to colorful descriptive images, which can aid the learning process. For example, the word muscle is a diminutive of the Latin word, *mus,* or mouse, probably because of the physical resemblance of certain muscles moving under the skin to the movements of a mouse under a carpet. The word *ileum* is derived from a Latin verb meaning to coil or twist. (The ileum comprises most of the small intestine, which lies coiled within the abdomen.)

Although conformity to standards is emphasized, medical terminology is not without change. Terminology becomes outdated and meanings evolve. More precise terms for individual conditions are used today. In spite of strict adherence to accepted terminology, advancements in medicine have introduced new words into the language. Acronyms, such as the word *laser* (light amplification by stimulated emission of radiation), are becoming more common. Human immunodeficiency virus is known everywhere as HIV. These types of words and acronyms for the most part lie outside the scope of this tutorial.

There is debate over the use of eponyms, the association of a name to an anatomical structure or, perhaps more commonly, to a disease or surgical procedure. Eponyms are often (although not always) named for the person to first describe the structure or disease, or to perform a given type of surgery. The suspensory muscle of the duodenum, an area of small intestine just beyond the stomach, is known almost universally as the ligament of Treitz. Wenzel Treitz was a 19th century Austrian physician and the eponym is somewhat easier said than *musculus suspensorius duodeni.* However, use of eponyms should be avoided where possible and, therefore, will not be discussed further in this chapter.

HISTORY

The search to put words to the parts of the human body goes back centuries. At least one book was written on medical nomenclature by the first century A.D. The predominance of Greek and Latin words is attributed to the early work of Hippocrates, Aristotle, and later Galen, a Greek physician who practiced in Rome and wrote in Latin. All of the influential early anatomy books were published in either Greek or Latin. And until the early 20th century anatomy lectures in medical schools were delivered in Latin.

 OBJECTIVES

In this chapter, you will learn:
- To identify how medical terms have evolved
- How to divide words into component parts
- The meaning of the component parts
- To identify the body systems
- About eponyms, homonyms, and synonyms
- Health care acronyms and abbreviations

 DEFINITIONS

Purpura. Latin for purple. Purpura is a genus of marine snails, some species of which furnish a purple dye. In medicine purpura refers to multiple pinpoint hemorrhages and accumulation of blood under the skin. Bleeding into the skin produces red-purple discoloration of the skin.

 KEY POINT

Most dictionaries abbreviate the origin of words (etymologies) and display them in boldface square brackets preceding the definition. Some dictionaries add the English translation. *Example:* Aorta [L.;Gr. *Aorte*]

DEFINITIONS

Eponym. A name of a drug, structure, disease, or procedure based on or derived from the name of a person. *Example:* Parkinson's disease.

Homonym. One of two or more words spelled and pronounced alike but different in meaning.

Synonym. One of two or more words or expressions of the same language that have the same, or nearly the same, meaning but which are spelled differently.

CODING AXIOM

When you are uncertain about the spelling of a word, it is better to look it up in the dictionary or check another resource. If a term is misspelled, assignment of a wrong diagnosis or procedure code could result.

DEFINITIONS

Anatomy (*ana*, up; *-tomy*, process of cutting). The science of body structures and relationships among structures.

Dissection (*dis*, apart; *-section*, act of cutting). Separating by cutting apart tissue.

Gross (French: *gros*, large): Macroscopic, as in "gross pathology", the study of tissue changes without magnification by microscope.

Macroscopic (*macro*, large; *-scopy*, instrument to examine or view). Of a size to be examined by the human eye.

Magnetic resonance imaging (MRI). A study that uses strong magnets and radio waves to form a sharp image of internal structures.

X-ray. Images of the bones and internal organs. X-rays work by sending small amounts of radiation through the body, leaving a shadow-like image of internal structures.

The adaptation of Greek words to Latin introduced new words, changed pronunciation of others, and gave rise to more convention. Classic Latin as written during Roman times had no letters *j, u,* or *w.* This expansion of the alphabet was introduced much later. And many terms have been anglicized, or modernized in some fashion to better suit the needs of English speaking Americans. Still, many words used by Hippocrates continue to serve the medical community well today.

A limited glossary is included in the appendixes.

SPELLING

The correct spelling of a word is critical. Two or more words may sound alike but be spelled differently and have different meanings. For example:

> hidro: sweat
> vs
> hydro: water

> dysphagia: difficulty swallowing
> vs
> dysphasia: difficulty in using language due to injury or disease

These words are pronounced the same and spelled the same, except for one letter, but their meanings differ. Other examples are:

> ostial: an opening
> vs
> osteal: bony

> viscous: sticky
> vs
> viscus: hollow multi-layered walled organ

> ileum: part of the small intestine
> vs
> ilium: part of the pelvis (hip bone)

INTRODUCTION TO HUMAN ANATOMY

Anatomy is a discipline, the field of biological science that addresses the structure and function of the human body. And although much has been learned from the dissection of cadavers, dead bodies, anatomy is ultimately the study of the living human body.

The study of anatomy is the cornerstone in the foundation of medicine. An understanding of anatomy is also essential to ensure correct code assignment.

Organization

The structure of the human body falls into the following four categories:

Cells. The basic unit of living things.

Tissues. Groups of similar cells that work to perform similar tasks.

Organs. Two or more kinds of tissue that together perform special body functions.

Systems. Groups, usually of organs, that work together to perform complex body functions.

Macroscopic anatomical study is traditionally divided into the following body systems. To assist the user, the editors have organized the systems as they appear in the *Physicians' Current Procedural Terminology* (CPT) code book, which contains codes for surgical procedures.

Integumentary system. Skin, sweat glands, sebaceous (oil) glands, hair, and nails. The medical field for the integumentary system is known as dermatology, although other specialties also address this system. The integumentary section (five-digit CPT codes beginning with 10040) reports procedures performed on the skin, nails, and breasts, including repair of lacerations, removal of lesions, and reconstruction.

Skeletal system. Bones and cartilage.

Articular system. Joints and ligaments.

Muscular system. Body tissues that primarily move bones and joints. The medical field for the musculoskeletal system is known as orthopedics. The medical field that addresses disorders of collagen and cartilaginous joints is called rheumatology. The musculoskeletal system of CPT comprises five-digit codes beginning with 20000. Procedures on bone, muscles, tendons, soft tissues, cartilage, and joints, as well as fracture care, and casting are reported by this range.

Respiratory system. The nose, pharynx, larynx, trachea, bronchus (bronchial tubes), and lungs. The medical field for the respiratory system is pulmonology, although internists and ear, nose, and throat (ENT) physicians also treat within this system. The respiratory section of CPT begins with code 30000 and includes procedures on the nose, sinuses, larynx, trachea, bronchi, lungs, and pleura.

Cardiovascular or circulatory system. The heart, blood vessels, and lymphatics (immune system) and blood (hematology). The cardiovascular medical specialties include cardiology, hematology, and internal medicine. The medical field for the immune system is immunology. The CPT cardiovascular system begins with 33010 and reports procedures to the heart, pericardium, arteries, and veins. The codes to report procedures on the hemic and lymphatic systems follow.

Gastrointestinal or digestive system. The tubular lining from the mouth to the anus (mouth, pharynx, esophagus, stomach, small intestine, large intestine, liver, and anus) and its associated glands, such as the gallbladder. The medical fields that treats disorders of the gastrointestinal or digestive system include gastroenterology and proctology, as well as oral and maxillofacial surgery, and internal medicine. The CPT codes that report procedures to this system begin with 40490. Procedures to the lips, soft and hard tissues of the mouth, esophagus, stomach, intestines, and anus are reported by this range. Procedures to salivary glands, tonsils, the liver, gallbladder, and pancreas also fall into this range.

Urinary system. Kidneys, bladder and passages of urinary excretion. This body system is serviced primarily by urologists and nephrologists. The CPT codes for procedures on this system begin with 50010. Procedures on the kidney, bladder, and urethra are reported by this range of codes.

Reproductive system. Genitalia and associated structures. The medical specialty for the male reproductive system includes urology and endocrinology. The CPT range for the male reproductive system begins with 54000 and includes procedures on the penis, testes, scrotum, spermatic cord and seminal vesicles, and prostate. The female reproductive system is treated by obstetrician/gynecologists and endocrinologists. The CPT codes begin with 56405. Procedures to the vulva, perineum, vagina, cervix,

---

 DEFINITIONS

Articular (Latin: *articulare*). Relating to a joint or the involvement of joints.

Cytology (*cyt/o*, cell + -ology, study of). The study of cells, including their origin, structure, functions, and pathology.

Histology (*histos*, tissue + *logos*, science). A branch of science specializing in the microscopic study of tissues. There are four basic types of tissue: Epithelial (*epi*, upon or over) is found throughout the body and makes up the covering of external and internal surfaces. Connective tissue is the most widespread in the human body. It forms bones, cartilage, tendons, and ligaments. Muscle and nerve tissues are the remaining basic types and are further categorized.

Integument. A covering.

Muscle tissue. There are three types of muscle tissue: smooth, skeletal, and striated. The types are categorized as voluntary (under conscious control of the individual) and involuntary (little or no control over movement).

Nervous tissue. Specialized tissue that conducts nerve impulses. The brain, spinal cord, and nerves throughout the body.

 QUICK TIP

Anatomical references are made with the understanding that the body is in the position known as the anatomical position, which means standing erect with focus outward. The position is somewhat unnatural in that the great toes are directed straight forward and the palms of the hand face outward. All directional references are based on the anatomical position.

---

uterus, and the ovaries and ducts are reported by these codes. Maternity and delivery codes follow.

Endocrine system. Secretory glands (thyroid gland, parathyroid glands, pituitary gland, testes, ovaries, adrenal glands, pancreas, pineal gland, thymus gland, and the placenta during pregnancy). The specialties here are chiefly endocrinology and internal medicine. The code range begins at 60000 and includes procedures to the thyroid, parathyroid, thymus, and adrenal glands.

Nervous system. The brain, spinal cord, nerves, and ganglia. The medical field for the nervous system is called neurology. The CPT nervous system begins with 61000 and reports procedures to the brain, spinal cord, nerves, and ganglia.

Eye and ocular adnexa. The cornea, iris, ciliary body, choroids, retina, optic nerve, macula and the large retinal blood vessels. The specialty in this body area is ophthalmology. The code range begins at 65091 and reports procedures within the eyeball, anterior segment, iris, ciliary body, lens, posterior segment, ocular adnexa, eyelids, conjunctiva, and lacrimal system.

Auditory system. Includes the outer (external), middle, and inner ear. The specialists in this body area are ENT and otolaryngology. The code range begins at 69000 and reports procedures within external, middle, inner, temporal bone, and middle fossa.

Organizational Differences

Many anatomy texts combine skeletal and muscular systems into the musculoskeletal system. Many do not distinguish the articular system (relating to a joint or the involvement of joints). Male and female reproductive systems are commonly isolated, and separate classifications for embryology, obstetrics, and neonatology are also often seen. Similarly, the anatomy of the eye may be separated from its classification within the nervous system. The organization of the surgery section of the CPT code book has its own conventions. The editors have tried to present the anatomical systems according to their appearance in the CPT code book.

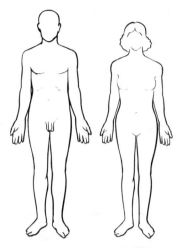

The anatomical position

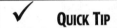

QUICK TIP

Coders should have easy access to a medical dictionary and anatomy book. Looking up unfamiliar words for meaning and spelling, as well as identification of body system helps in assigning the correct codes for procedures and diagnoses.

Rule of Nines for Burns

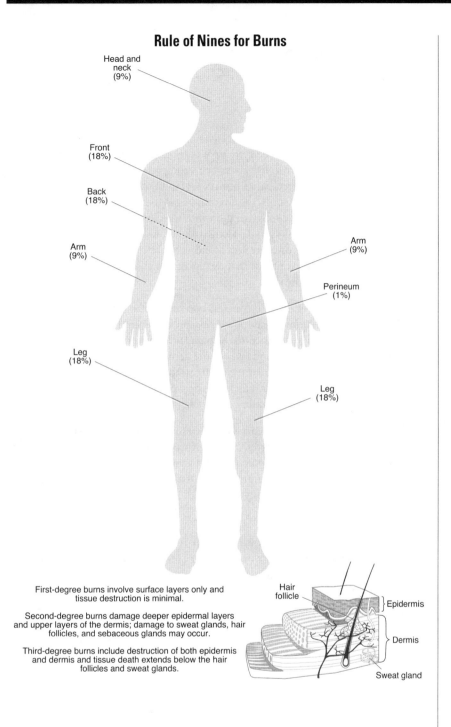

Head and neck (9%)

Front (18%)

Back (18%)

Arm (9%)

Arm (9%)

Perineum (1%)

Leg (18%)

Leg (18%)

First-degree burns involve surface layers only and tissue destruction is minimal.

Second-degree burns damage deeper epidermal layers and upper layers of the dermis; damage to sweat glands, hair follicles, and sebaceous glands may occur.

Third-degree burns include destruction of both epidermis and dermis and tissue death extends below the hair follicles and sweat glands.

Hair follicle

Epidermis

Dermis

Sweat gland

INTEGUMENTARY SYSTEM

The integumentary system includes the skin, subcutaneous tissue, and accessory structures, such as hair, and nails.

Anatomy of the Skin

The skin is the largest organ of the body and is composed of two principal divisions: the epidermis and dermis. The epidermal portion of the skin is avascular (without blood) and contains four to five layers depending on its location: stratum corneum, lucidum (e.g., soles of feet, palms of hand), granulosum, spinosum, and basale. The deepest layer of the epidermis, the stratum basale (also known as the stratum germinativum), has some cells that grow into the dermis from which sudoriferous (sweat) and sebaceous (oil) glands, along with hair follicles are derived. Nerve endings called tactile (Merkel's) discs are also found in the stratum basale. Nails and other specialized glands, such as those that excrete cerumen (earwax) also originate in the epidermal portion of the skin.

The dermal portion of the skin contains two layers. The papillary, or upper layer, contains papillae that interweave loops of capillaries into the dermis. The sense of touch can be partially attributed to the papillae because of the nerve endings in the upper layer of skin. The second layer of the dermis is called the reticular region. Between the cells in the reticular region are stratum basale cells from which the sweat and oil glands along with hair follicles are derived. In addition, the reticular region of the dermis gives our skin its ability to stretch.

The reticular region of the dermis is attached to a subcutaneous layer that lies beneath the skin. The subcutaneous layer, also known as the hypodermis or superficial fascia, is a sheet or wide band of adipose (fat) and areolar connective tissue in two layers. Arteries, veins, lymph, and mammary glands are between the layers, with the thickness depending on the body site.

Breast

In structure, the breast is filled with mammary glands, modified sweat glands that produce milk. In function, the breast is part of the reproductive system. In coding, breasts are associated with the skin and integumentary system based on their structure.

Nails

The nails are bony structures forming plates on the ends of the fingers and toes. There are four main portions. The exposed portion or nail body or plate is composed of keratin, the nail root is the portion hidden by the nail fold, and the nail rests on the nailbed, or matrix.

Hair

Hair is a thin, flexible shaft of cells that develop from the hair follicle found in the epidermis level of the skin. Hair is made up of the shaft, the root, and the follicle.

Burns

A burn is defined as a lesion caused by the contact of heat, fire, or chemicals. There are many types of burns including chemical burns (caused by contact with a caustic substance), radiation burns (caused by the exposure to x-ray, radium, sunlight, atomic or other radiant energy), and friction burns (caused by violent rubbing or friction such as a rope). Sunburn, which is caused by an overexposure to ultraviolet rays found in sunlight, also is considered a type of burn.

CODING AXIOM

Rule of nines. Used to calculate the percent of integumentary area burned. It is based on dividing total body surface area (TBSA) into segments based on factors of nine. For example the arms are each nine percent while the legs are 18 percent each. The rule is applied differently to children.

DEFINITIONS

Abscess. A circumscribed collection of pus.

Alopecia. Hair loss or baldness.

Cyanosis. A blue discoloration of the skin.

Dermatitis. Inflammation of the skin.

Mastitis. Inflammation and/or infection of the breast or mammary gland.

Tactile. Having or related to touch.

Burns are classified by degree. A first-degree burn shows only redness of the skin. A second-degree burn indicates some blistering. A third-degree burn is a full-thickness burn, and a deep third-degree burn includes deep necrosis of the tissues.

Integumentary System

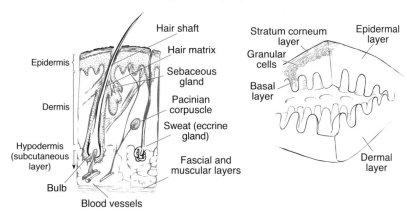

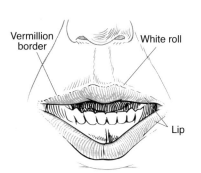

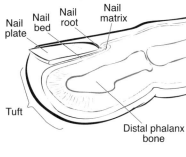

Breast

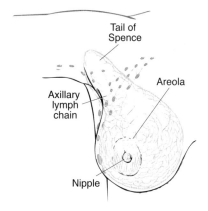

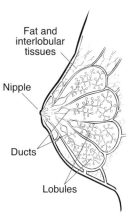

MUSCULOSKELETAL SYSTEM

The musculoskeletal system includes the soft tissue, joints, bursa, cartilage, and bones.

Anatomy of the Musculoskeletal System

Soft Tissue

The term soft tissue generally includes the deep fascia, muscles, tendons, and ligaments.

- Deep fascia lies beneath the second layer of subcutaneous tissue (hypodermis) of the integumentary system. Deep fascia in the musculoskeletal system lines extremities and holds together groups of muscles.

- There are three types of muscle tissue: skeletal, cardiac, and visceral. Muscle tissue consists of specialized cells that allow contraction to produce voluntary or involuntary movement of body parts. The term musculoskeletal in this CPT surgery subcategory refers to skeletal muscle.

Skeletal System

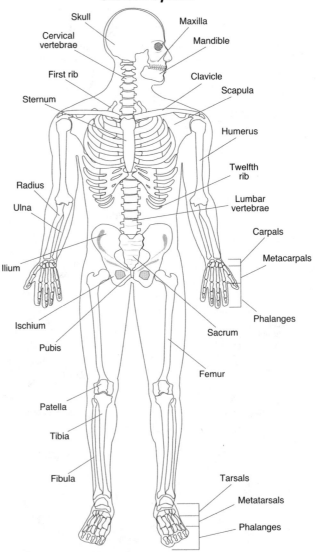

- Tendons are fibrous cords that vary in length. They are found at the ends of muscles and connect muscles to bones.
- Ligaments are bands of fibrous tissue that connect two or more bones or cartilage.

Joints

The term joint refers to the area of contact between two bones. Joints hold together bones and allow articulation (movement) between cartilage and bones. There are three structural classifications of joints: fibrous, cartilaginous, and synovial joints.

The terms "arthro" and "arthr" refer to a joint or an articulation (e.g., arthrotomy: arthro=joint, otomy=incision into).

Bursa

Bursa consists of a sac that contains synovial fluid within a synovial membrane lining. Bursae are found at friction points between tendons and muscles. They occur frequently around joints and at sites where bones are prominent, especially in areas where a tendon passes over a bone.

Cartilage

Cartilage is a type of dense connective tissue (hyaline, elastic, and fibrocartilage) that is found in joints. Hyaline cartilage is located at joints over the ends of long bones; fibrocartilage is found at other body sites, such as the pubic symphysis, intervertebral discs, menisci of the knee, and the point where the hip bones fuse anteriorly. The cartilage of the auricle of the ear is an example of elastic, or yellow, cartilage.

Bones

The types of bones that make up the skeletal system may be classified either by shape: long, short, flat, and irregular bones, or by location: sutural, and sesamoid bones. For example:

- Long bones: humerus, tibia, and femur
- Short bones: wrist and ankle
- Flat bones: sternum, scapula, and ribs
- Irregular bones: vertebra column and some facial bones
- Sutural bones: specific cranial bones
- Sesamoid bones: patella and in tendons where there is pressure (e.g., wrist)

Skull

There are 27 bones plus the mandible in the skull or cranium. The cranium is separated into two major parts: the neurocranium, the bones that encase the brain; and the viscerocranium, the facial bones or skeleton. In infants the bones of the neurocranium are still separate. The spaces between the bone margins are called fontanelles: the two most noted are the anterior fontanelle, located at the top of the head, and the posterior fontanelle. There are also anterior lateral and posterior lateral fontanelles on either side of the head. Although usually closed by the age of 2 years, the neurocranium continues to grow until mid-teenage years and in older adults may fuse without evident suture lines.

The bones of the cranial vault include frontal, occipital, parietal, and temporal bones. The facial bones include the maxilla, nasal, sphenoid, bones of the ear, and zygomatic. The mandible is part of the head, although not part of the cranium.

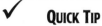

QUICK TIP

Synovial fluid not only lubricates the joint, tendon sheath, or bursa, it also provides nourishment to the avascular articular cartilage.

KEY POINT

Sesamoid bones are formed after birth, with the patella being the largest.

QUICK TIP

The bones in the ear are the smallest in the human body.

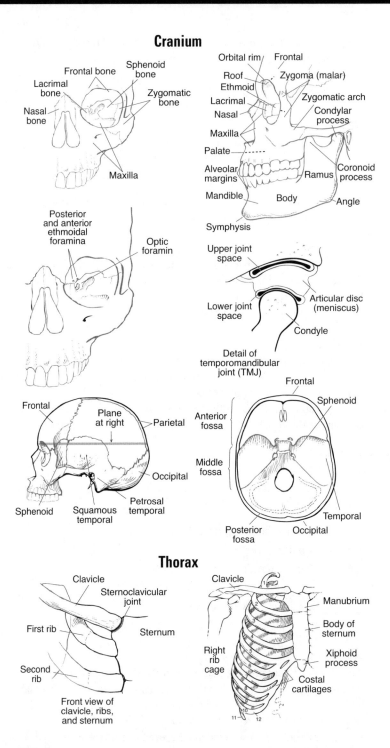

Cranium

Thorax

Neck and Thorax

The neck is comprised of the seven cervical bones of the vertebral column. The first cervical vertebra, the atlas, is named for the support of the head. The second cervical vertebra, the axis, contains a peglike process called the dens that project up through the ring of the atlas and makes a pivot on which the atlas and head rotate. The seventh cervical vertebra, called the vertebra prominens, is marked by a spinous process that can be seen and felt at the base of the neck.

The thorax refers to the chest and lies between the neck and abdomen. The sternum (breastbone) and ribs in front and the dorsal vertebrae in back form the skeletal frame

CODING AXIOM

The types of bones that make up the skeletal system may be classified either by shape (long, short, flat, and irregular bones), or by location instead of shape (sutural and sesamoid bones).

of the thorax. This thoracic frame encloses and protects the organs within, which include the heart, lungs, and esophagus. The chest and abdominal cavities are separated by a muscular structure, the diaphragm.

Spine

The spine is the common name applied to the structure of bone or cartilage surrounding and protecting the spinal cord. It is also called a vertebral column or backbone. The spine is the major part of the skeleton and attached to it are the skull, shoulder bones, ribs, and pelvis. The spinal column contains 33 vertebrae: seven cervical vertebra in the neck; 12 thoracic vertebra in the region of the thorax (chest), which provide attachments for 12 pairs of ribs; five lumbar vertebrae in the small of the back, and five fused sacral vertebra forming the sacrum. A variable number of vertebrae are fused together to form the bottom of the sacrum.

Disks are found between the vertebrae that allow the back to flex or bend. They are filled with a liquid in the nucleus.

Spine

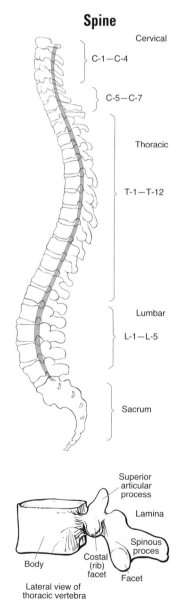

 DEFINITIONS

Bursa. A sac lined with synovial membrane that contains synovial fluid. Bursae are found between tendons and muscles at friction points.

Cartilage. A type of dense connective tissue (hyaline, elastic, and fibrocartilage) that is found in joints. Hyaline cartilage is at joints over the ends of long bones; fibrocartilage is found at other body sites, such as the pubic symphysis, intervertebral discs, menisci of the knee, and the point where the hip bones fuse anteriorly.

Cyst. An elevated encapsulated mass containing fluid, semisolid, or solid material with a membranous lining.

Ganglion. A fluid filled cyst within fibrous, muscle, or bone tissue attached to a tendon sheath; ganglions are frequently found in the hand, wrist, or foot and may connect to a underlying joint.

Hemarthrosis. The presence of blood in the joint cavity.

Shoulder/Upper Extremity

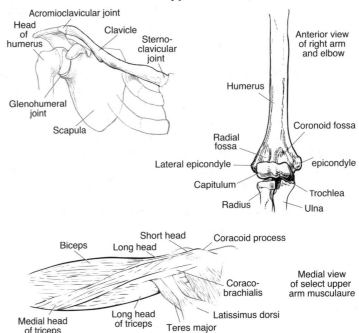

Shoulder Girdles

The pectoral or shoulder girdles attach the bones of the upper extremities to the axial skeleton; each of the two shoulder girdles consists of a clavicle and a scapula. The clavicles, or collarbones, are long bones and among the most frequently broken bones in the body due to falling on outstretched arms.

Separation of the shoulder refers to the dislocation of the acromioclavicular joint. The scapulae, or shoulder blades, are large, triangular, flat bones in the dorsal part of the chest (thorax) between the second and seventh ribs.

Upper Extremities

There are 60 bones in the upper extremities, which include the bones of the humerus in the arm, ulna and radius in the forearm, carpals (wristbones), metacarpals (palm bones), and phalanges in the fingers of the hand. The humerus is the longest and largest bone of the upper extremity and articulates with the scapula and at the elbow with both the ulna and radius. The olecranon is the bony prominence that extends from one end of the ulna. The ulna is the medial bone of the forearm, located at the side of the little finger. The radius is the lateral bone of the forearm, situated on the thumb side.

Wrist, Fingers, and Hand

The wrist bone consists of eight small bones, called the carpals, connected to each other by ligaments.

There are four bones in each of the two transverse rows of the wrist.

The scaphoid bone is on the thumb side of the wrist, close to the lower arm bones. The palm is made up of the five bones of the metacarpus. The heads of the metacarpals are commonly called the knuckles. There are 14 phalanges, or bones of the fingers, in each hand. The fingers each have three phalangeal bones; the thumb, or pollex, has no middle phalanx.

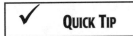

QUICK TIP

Carpal tunnel syndrome occurs when there is pressure on the median nerve as it passes between the bones of the wrist and the carpal ligament on the palmar side of the wrist.

Hand/Wrist

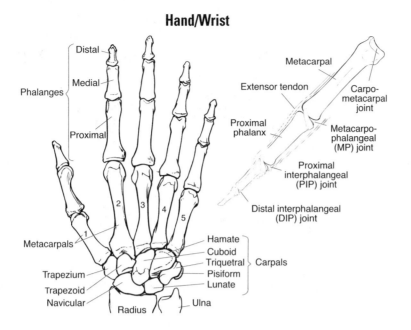

Pelvis and Hip

The pelvic (hip) girdle consists of the two coxal bones, commonly called the pelvic or hipbones, which connect anteriorly at the symphysis pubis and posteriorly at the sacrum. The pelvic girdle provides support for the lower extremities. The sacrum and the coccyx form the pelvis.

The hip is a ball-and-socket joint, which gives it stability and movement. The round head of the femur fits inside the acetabulum in the pelvis.

Lower Extremities

The lower extremities are composed of 60 bones, similar to the number of bones in the upper extremities. Each lower extremity includes the femur in the thigh, patella (kneecap), fibula and tibia in the leg, tarsals, metatarsals, and phalanges in the toes. The femur is the longest and heaviest bone of the body.

The knee has three joints:

- The medial joint (medial tibial plateau and medial femoral condyle)
- The lateral joint (lateral tibial plateau and lateral femoral condyle)
- The kneecap (patellofemoral) joint (patella and femoral trochlear notch); the patella, or kneecap, is a small, triangular bone anterior to the knee joint

Hip

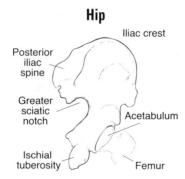

Lower Extremity

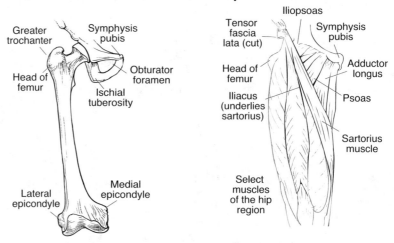

The anterior cruciate ligaments (ACL) are located inside the knee joints and attach the femur to the tibia.

Articular cartilage is a tough, elastic tissue that covers the ends of bones in joints.

Each lower extremity also includes the tarsals, metatarsals, and phalanges in the toes. The tibia, or shinbone, is the larger, medial bone of the leg and bears the major portion of the weight of the leg.

The top ankle joint is composed of three bones:

- The tibia
- The fibula
- The talus

The leg bones (tibia and fibula) form a pocket around the top of the anklebone (talus) which allows the foots up and down bending. The subtalar is where the talus connects to the calcaneus (heel bone) and provides the foot's ability to rock from side to side. Three sets of fibrous tissues connect the bones and provide stability to both joints. The bumps on either side of the ankle are the ends of the lower leg bones; the bump on the outside of the ankle (lateral malleolus) is part of the fibula; the smaller bump on the inside of the ankle (medial malleolus) is part of the tibia.

Foot and Toes

The talus and calcaneus are on the posterior part of the foot and the talus is the only bone of the foot that articulates with the fibula and tibia. The calcaneous, or heel bone, is the strongest tarsal bone and bears the weight of the leg transmitted from the talus during walking.

The metatarsus consists of five metatarsal bones and, like the metacarpals of the palm of the hand, each metatarsal consists of a base, shaft, and head. The phalanges of the foot resemble those of the hand; all but the big toe consists of a base, shaft, and head. The large toe, or hallux, has the proximal and distal phalanges.

📖 **DEFINITIONS**

Arthroscopy. Many joint procedures are performed using arthroscopy where an endoscope (a hollow tube with optically enhanced features, a light source, and a side port for introduction of surgical instruments) is used.

Bunion. A bony prominence on the inside of the foot near the great toe.

Foot and Ankle

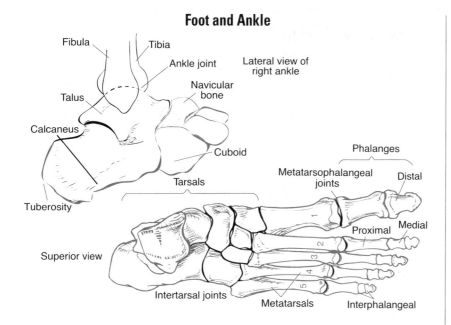

Fibula
Tibia
Ankle joint
Lateral view of right ankle
Talus
Navicular bone
Calcaneus
Cuboid
Tuberosity
Tarsals
Phalanges
Metatarsophalangeal joints
Distal
Proximal
Medial
Superior view
Intertarsal joints
Metatarsals
Interphalangeal

RESPIRATORY SYSTEM

The respiratory system functions as an air distributor and a gas exchanger, to supply oxygen and remove carbon monoxide from the body's cells. All parts of the respiratory system, except the microscopic alveoli of the lungs, function as air distributors. Only the alveoli sacks and ducts serve as gas exchangers. In addition to air distribution and gas exchange, the respiratory system and its structures provide for functions such as yawning, sneezing, coughing, hiccups, sound production (including speech), and the sense of smell (olfaction). The respiratory system also assists in homeostasis (regulation of pH in the body).

Anatomy of the Respiratory System

The upper respiratory tract is located outside the thorax (the chest cavity), and is composed of the nose, the pharynx (nasopharynx, oropharynx, and laryngopharynx), and the larynx. The first three subsections of this section contain codes related to the nose, the accessory (paranasal) sinuses, and the larynx. The lower respiratory tract, contained within the thorax, consists of the trachea, the bronchial tree and the lungs.

The respiratory system functions as follows. Air enters the body through the nose, where it is warmed, filtered, and humidified as it passes through the nasal cavity. The air passes the pharynx and from the pharynx into the trachea (the windpipe). The epiglottis, a muscle flap in the pharynx, prevents food from entering the trachea. The upper part of the trachea contains the three parts of the larynx and the vocal chords. At its base, the trachea divides into the left and right primary bronchi. Each bronchus divides into smaller branches known as segmental bronchi. These divide into tiny bronchioles that terminate in the microscopic ducts and alveoli sacs of the lungs where gas exchange takes place.

The lungs are large, paired organs in the thorax. The right lung has three lobes. The left lung cavity contains two lobes and encloses the heart. Thin sheets of epithelium (the pleura) separate the inside of the chest cavity from the outer surface of the lungs and the heart.

Nose

The external portion of the nose protrudes from the face and consists of bone and cartilage overlaid by skin which contains many sebaceous (oil producing) glands. The joining of the two nasal bones with the frontal bone of the skull forms the root of the nose. The nose is surrounded beneath and on both sides by the maxilla face bone. The cartilaginous structure that forms the outer side of each nostril (the anterior nares) is called the ala. The nostrils open into an area called the vestibule, lined with epithelium with many coarse hairs (vibrissae) and sebaceous and sweat glands.

External Nose

The external nose is made up of bone and cartilage covered with skin on the outside and mucous membrane on the inside.

The nose root is the area of the nose attached to the forehead. It is located in the surface area that exists between the eyes in the upper portion of that space. The bridge of the nose is located between the eyes in the mid to lower portion of that space. The tip of the nose is called the apex. The dorsum (dorsum nasi) of the nose is the outside area between the root (top) and the apex (bottom) of the nose. The nasal alae (ala) are the broad portions of the outside area of the nostrils. The external nares (nostrils) are the two openings in the nose that lead to the internal nose.

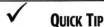

QUICK TIP

Children frequently aspirate foreign bodies in the right main brochus. Hypoxia might result from the objects restricting breath.

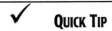

QUICK TIP

The cartilage in the nose is quite rigid, whereas the cartilage in the ear is "soft." This distinction may be used by physicians in documentation when describing cartilage in other parts of the body.

Respiratory System

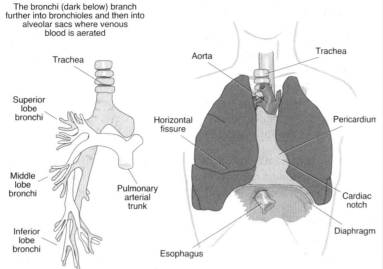

The bronchi (dark below) branch further into bronchioles and then into alveolar sacs where venous blood is aerated

Trachea

Superior lobe bronchi

Middle lobe bronchi

Inferior lobe bronchi

Pulmonary arterial trunk

The pulmonary arteries (white above) deliver venous blood to the lungs where it is oxygenated and converted into arterial blood

Aorta

Trachea

Horizontal fissure

Pericardiun

Cardiac notch

Diaphragm

Esophagus

The right lung is larger and heavier than its counterpart due to space lost to the bulge of the heart at the cardiac notch

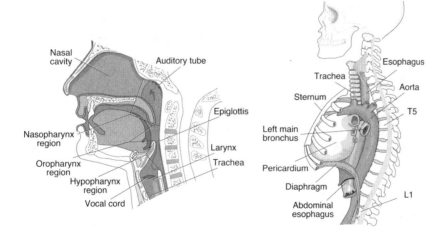

Nasal cavity

Auditory tube

Nasopharynx region

Epiglottis

Oropharynx region

Larynx

Hypopharynx region

Trachea

Vocal cord

Esophagus

Trachea

Aorta

Sternum

T5

Left main bronchus

Pericardium

Diaphragm

L1

Abdominal esophagus

Internal Nose

The internal nose is a large cavity that is made up of the tissues and bone. The paranasal sinuses (frontal, sphenoidal, maxillary, and ethmoidal) and nasolacrimal ducts open into the internal nose; some of the sinuses form the lateral walls of the internal nose. The soft palate and other bones, such as the palatine bones form the base.

The nasal cavity, the internal portion of the nose, lies over the roof of the mouth. The palatine bones form the floor of the nose, separating the nasal cavity from the mouth cavity. The roof of the nose is separated from the cranial cavity by part of the ethmoid bone, called the cribriform plate, which has multiple openings permitting branches of the olfactory nerve to enter the brain.

The nasal cavity is partitioned down the middle by the septum. This structure consists of the perpendicular plate of the ethmoid bone, the vomer bone, vomeronasal cartilage, and septal nasal cartilage. The septum has a rich blood supply.

The nasal cavity opens into the vestibule inside of the nostrils and continues to the respiratory area where there is bone in three shelves (formed by the nasal cavity) called the superior, middle, and inferior nasal turbinates (nasal conchae). The turbinates come close to the nasal septum, and subdivide the nasal cavity into passageways through nasal meatuses (superior, middle, and inferior). The air passes from the vestibule of the nose, into the respiratory portion of the nose, and into the next major segment of the upper respiratory tract—the pharynx.

The internal nose merges with the external nose on the outside through the external nares. It continues from the external nares and, in the back (posteriorly), connects with the nasopharynx (throat) through the internal nares (choanae).

Paranasal Sinuses

There are four pairs of paranasal sinuses named from the bones in which they are found: the frontal, maxillary, ethmoid and sphenoid. Each sinus is an air-containing space lined by respiratory mucosa and produces secretions that drain into the nasal cavity.

The right and left frontal sinuses are above the eye sockets, and the maxillary sinuses are on each side of the nose. The sphenoid sinuses lie deeper, at the midline, and are close to the pituitary gland and the optic nerve. The ethmoid sinuses are collections of small air cells that open independently into the upper nasal cavity. The sinuses serve both to lighten the bones of the skull and to provide resonating chambers for speech.

Larynx

The larynx is the organ of speech, and also functions to close the glottis during swallowing to prevent aspiration of food or drink into the respiratory tract. Folds of mucosa line the larynx. The upper folds are called the false cords; the lower folds are called the true vocal cords and vibrate to produce the necessary sounds for speech.

The larynx is between the hypopharynx and trachea and is anchored in position by the thyroid cartilage, cricoid cartilage, and arytenoid cartilage.

Trachea and Bronchi

The trachea and bronchi with their many branches resemble an inverted tree trunk and its branches and are commonly referred to as the bronchial tree.

CLINICAL NOTE

The hypopharynx (laryngopharynx) breaks into two parts—the esophagus and larynx. The larynx is the voice box and consists of three single and three pairs of cartilage.

Sinuses

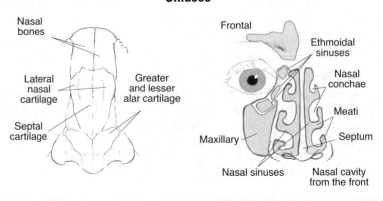

Larynx

Epiglottis

Hyoid bone

Thyroid cartilage

Vocal cord

Cricoid cartilage

Cervical trachea

Anterior ethmoidal artery

Posterior ethmoidal artery

Spheno-palatine artery

Hard and soft palate

Tongue

Palantine tonsile

Vocal cords

Arytenoids

Overhead view of vocal cords

The trachea, or windpipe, extends from the larynx in the neck to the branches of the primary bronchi in the thorax. It is usually about 11 centimeters long by 2.5 centimeters in diameter. It is a flexible, tubular structure formed by approximately 20 C-shaped rings of cartilage that are embedded in smooth muscle. The trachea is lined with specialized epithelium tissue that produces and moves mucus up and out of the respiratory tract, keeping the lungs and air passages free.

The trachea divides at its lower end into two primary bronchi. The right bronchus is slightly larger and more vertical than the left (accounting for aspirated objects lodging more frequently in the right bronchus). As each bronchus enters the lung, it divides into smaller branches called secondary bronchi; these continue to further branch into tertiary bronchi and small bronchioles. The structure of the primary bronchi is similar to the trachea; however, the cartilaginous rings become complete, versus C-shaped, as the bronchi enter the lungs. The bronchi are lined with ciliated mucosa, similarly to the trachea.

The trachea and the bronchi distribute air to the lungs' interiors, and, similar to the other anatomical components of the respiratory tract, they cleanse, warm, and humidify inspired air.

Lungs and Pleura

The lungs are pyramidal or cone-shaped organs that extend from the diaphragm (the base of the lung) to above the clavicles (the apex) and lie within and against the rib cage (the costal surface). Each lung is divided into lobes by fissures. The left lung is partially divided into two lobes (superior and inferior) and the right lung into three (superior, middle, and inferior). The lobes of the lung are further subdivided into functional units, called bronchopulmonary segments; each served by a tertiary bronchus. There are 10 segments in the right lung and eight in the left.

The primary bronchi, the pulmonary blood vessels, and folds of pleural tissue are bound together and to the mediastinum by connective tissues. They form the root of

	DEFINITIONS

Hypercapnia. Excess carbon dioxide in the blood.

Hypoxemia. Not enough oxygen in the blood.

the lung, and enter each lung through a slit, called the hilum. Upon entering the substance of the lung, the bronchus, the pulmonary veins, and arteries divide and subdivide, ultimately forming a dense network of capillaries and alveoli, or air cells. The capillaries and alveoli provide an enormous surface area (estimated at 85 square meters) for gas exchange referred to as the respiratory membrane. The outer surface of the lungs is covered by closely adherent visceral pleura.

The lungs perform two functions: the distribution of air and exchange of gases. The tubes of the bronchial tree perform delivery of air into the alveoli. Gas exchange between air and blood is the joint function of the alveoli and the network of capillaries that surround them.

The pleura are the sac-like membranes of serous epithelium that divide the thoracic cavity into three divisions. The lungs occupy two pleural divisions. The mediastinum is the central division occupied by the esophagus, the trachea, the large blood vessels of the thorax, and the heart. The layer of membrane that lies against the organs is called the visceral pleura and the outer lining of the cavity is the parietal pleura. The space formed between these two layers is called the pleural space. The pleura provide protection and lubrication to allow for movement, expansion, and contraction of the visceral organs and the thoracic cavity.

Respiratory System

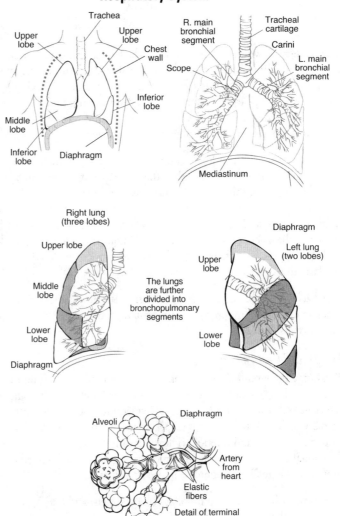

CARDIOVASCULAR SYSTEM

The cardiovascular system includes the heart, pericardium, and blood vessels. It distributes the gases provided by the respiratory system while bringing waste products back for cleansing via blood.

Anatomy of the Cardiovascular System

The heart pumps blood through a series of blood vessels (located throughout body) to the body tissues. The blood is pumped back to the heart through a separate series of vessels.

The inside of the heart is divided into four chambers: two atria (right and left) and two ventricles (right and left). Valves between the heart chambers, the pulmonary trunk, and the aorta prevent the back-flow of blood into the chambers. The valves consist of flaps called cusps. The ends of the cusps, between the atria and ventricles, extend into the ventricles and connect to the papillary muscles that are held in place by the fibrous chordae tendineae.

Venous blood enters the heart through the superior and inferior vena cava where it is directed into the coronary sinus and into the right atrium. The right atrium contracts, pumping blood through the atrioventricular (tricuspid valve) and into the right ventricle. The right ventricle pumps the blood through the pulmonary semilunar valve and into the pulmonary trunk. A right and a left pulmonary artery carries the blood into the lungs where the carbon dioxide saturated venous blood is pumped through small blood cells for an exchange of oxygen from the alveoli.

The oxygen-rich blood from the lungs is returned to the heart through four pulmonary veins and into the left atrium. The blood passes from the left atrium to the left ventricle, through the atrioventricular (bicuspid) valve. The ventricle contracts, pumping the oxygenated blood through the aortic (semilunar) valve and into the aorta (the largest artery of the body). The blood is directed to the heart (myocardium) through the coronary arteries and to the rest of the body through the vascular system.

In the inside of the heart, the chambers are separated by the interatrial and interventricular septum into right and left sides.

In addition to innervation by the autonomic nervous system, the heart has an internal conduction system in the myocardium that is composed of specialized muscle tissues that direct the contraction of cardiac muscle cells. The sinoatrial (SA) node (pacemaker) is a mass of cells on the right atrium. The SA node triggers the cardiac cycle. Action potentials send out impulses that pace the contractions of the atria. The impulses spread and hit the atrioventricular (AV) node located at the inferior portion of the interatrial septum. Action potentials from the AV node are sent via conduction fibers (bundle of His) to the top of the interventricular septum. The conduction fibers run down the sides of the heart septum to specific areas of the ventricles. It is here that special (Purkinje) fibers tell the ventricles to contract.

The heart has three layers and is kept in place by the pericardium the outer most layer of the heart. The hearts three layers are:

- The pericardium comprises an inner layer of parietal and visceral tissue called the serous pericardium. The pericardial cavity (space) between the parietal and visceral tissue contains pericardial fluid.
- The middle (muscle) layer of the heart is called the myocardium.
- The innermost layer is called the endocardium, lines the myocardium and covers the valves of the heart (and their tendons).

 CLINICAL NOTE

There are four phases to every heartbeat:
1. The atria relax and fill with blood from main veins.
2. Blood moves from the atria, through the tricuspid and mitral valves, and into the ventricles.
3. Ventricles contract, forcing blood through the aortic and pulmonary valves into the main arteries.
4. Ventricles relax and the cycle begins again.

Each cycle circulates about 70 ml of blood and takes less than a second to complete.

 KEY POINT

Knowledge of cardiac and neck vessels is essential in assigning the correct codes for cardiac and vascular catheterizations.

Circulatory System: Arterial

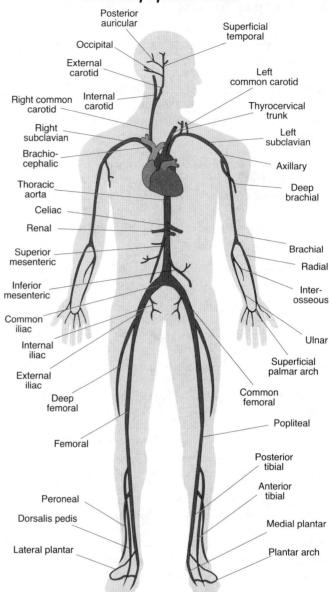

Posterior auricular
Superficial temporal
Occipital
External carotid
Left common carotid
Internal carotid
Right common carotid
Thyrocervical trunk
Right subclavian
Left subclavian
Brachio-cephalic
Axillary
Thoracic aorta
Deep brachial
Celiac
Renal
Brachial
Superior mesenteric
Radial
Inferior mesenteric
Inter-osseous
Common iliac
Ulnar
Internal iliac
Superficial palmar arch
External iliac
Common femoral
Deep femoral
Popliteal
Femoral
Posterior tibial
Anterior tibial
Peroneal
Dorsalis pedis
Medial plantar
Lateral plantar
Plantar arch

Circulatory System: Venous

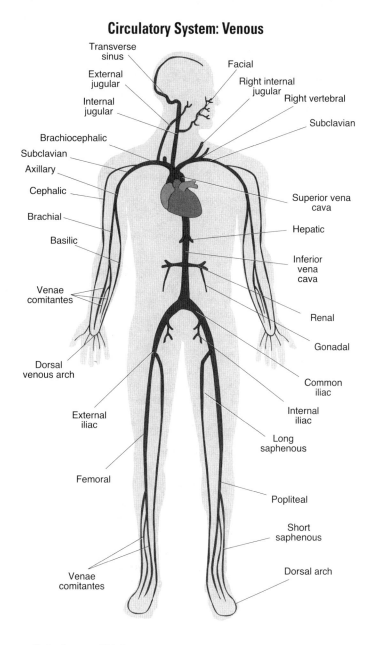

Coronary Arteries and Veins

The coronary arteries supply blood to the myocardium of the heart. They are separated into the left and right coronary artery. Both the right and the left coronary artery are divided into branches, such as:

- Left coronary artery branches:
  — Anterior interventricular branch
  — Circumflex branch
- Right coronary artery branches:
  — Posterior interventricular branch
  — Marginal branch

The hepatic portal vein delivers unoxygenated blood from the gastrointestinal tract, spleen, pancreas, and gallbladder to the liver.

Heart

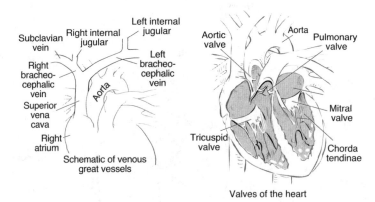

Schematic of venous great vessels

Valves of the heart

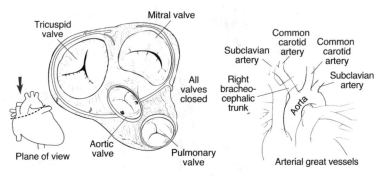

Plane of view

All valves closed

Arterial great vessels

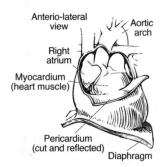

Vessels

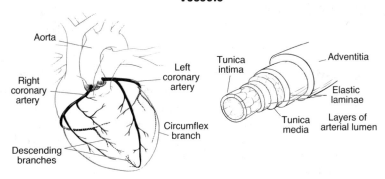

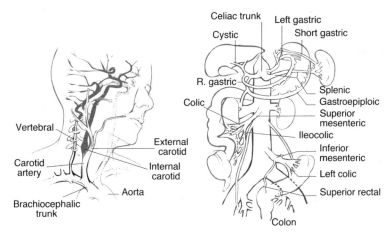

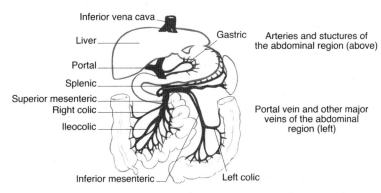

Arteries and stuctures of the abdominal region (above)

Portal vein and other major veins of the abdominal region (left)

LYMPHATIC SYSTEM

The lymphatic system includes the lymph nodes, spleen, thymus gland, and bone marrow and serves to protect and bathe our cells.

Anatomy of the Lymphatic System

The lymphatic system is the common name for the circulatory vessels that collect the fluid that bathes the tissue cells and carry the fluid to the bloodstream proper. The lymphatic system has primary importance in transporting digested fat from the intestine to the bloodstream, removing and destroying toxic substances, and helping the body resist the spread of disease. The portions of the lymphatic system that collect the tissue fluids are known as lymphatic capillaries, which allow the passage of large-molecule proteins, produced as a result of tissue breakdown, into the lymphatics for transport away from the tissues.

Spleen

The spleen is a flattened, oblong organ that removes disease-producing organisms and worn-out red blood cells from the bloodstream. The spleen is situated in the upper left abdominal cavity, in contact with the pancreas, the diaphragm, and the left kidney. It is supported by bands of fibers that are attached to the peritoneum. The spleen has several important functions. For example:

- Stores and releases blood in cases of emergency (e.g., hemorrhage)
- Produces B cells
- Rids the body of bacteria, worn-out (damaged) red blood cells, and platelets by a process called phagocytosis

If the spleen is removed, other organs such as the liver and bone marrow compensate.

Bone Marrow

Bone marrow is a highly vascular connective tissue found in the long bones and certain flat bones that is the origin of blood cells. Stem cells can develop into many other types of cells, such as blood stem cells in the bone marrow. Blood stem cells can mature and change into all types of blood cells such as white blood cells, red blood cells or platelets.

Lymph Nodes

Lymph nodes, more commonly called the lymph glands, are bean-shaped organs containing large numbers of leukocytes, embedded in connective tissue. Lymph refers to the clear, sometimes yellow fluid that flows through the tissues in the body, through the lymphatic system and then into the bloodstream. All the lymph being returned along the lymphatics to the bloodstream must pass through several of these nodes, which filter and destroy infectious and toxic material. During any infection, the nodes become enlarged because of the large number of phagocytes produced.

Thymus Gland

The thymus gland consists of lymphatic tissue and contains a few small areas of epithelial tissue known as Hassall's corpuscles. The thymus gland grows through puberty, then shrinks gradually and the lymphatic tissue is replaced by fat. The gland plays a role in the early development of the immune response system.

Mediastinum and Diaphragm

The mediastinum is the mass of tissue between the pleurae of the lungs and extends from the sternum to the vertebral column. The mediastinum has superior, anterior, middle, and posterior sections and includes all of the contents of the thoracic cavity, except the lungs proper. The thymus lies within the anterior and superior sections; the thoracic aorta within the posterior; the heart and the great vessels in the middle; and the esophagus and trachea in the superior section.

The diaphragm is a wide muscular partition separating the thoracic cavity from the abdominal cavity and is attached to the lumbar vertebrae, the lower ribs, and the sternum or breastbone. The esophagus, aorta, veins, nerves, and the lymphatic and thoracic ducts pass through the three openings of the diaphragm.

Lymphatic System

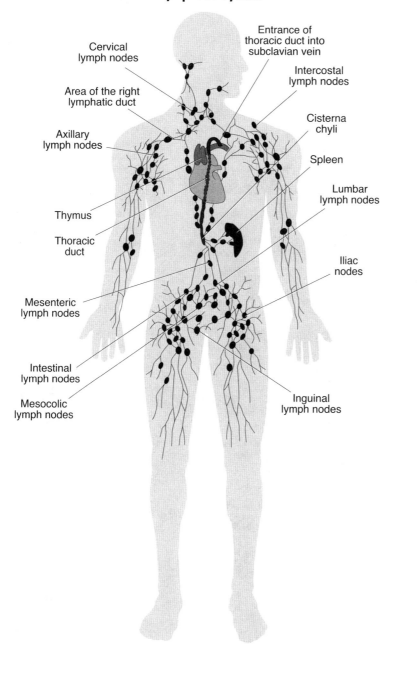

Lymph

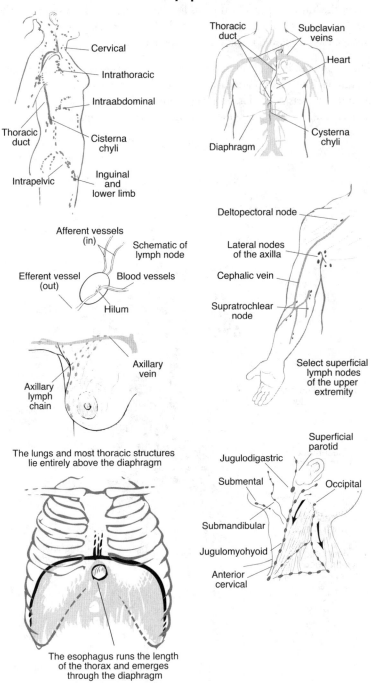

The lungs and most thoracic structures lie entirely above the diaphragm

The esophagus runs the length of the thorax and emerges through the diaphragm

DIGESTIVE TRACT

The digestive system is a group of organs forming a continuous tube beginning where foods and liquids enter the body at the mouth and ending where the waste products are finally excreted through the anus. There are other organs and tissues that support digestion but are outside this continuous tube; these include the salivary glands, the gall bladder, the pancreas, and the liver that provide secretions containing chemicals critical for the digestion and the utilization of nutrients by the body.

Digestive Tract

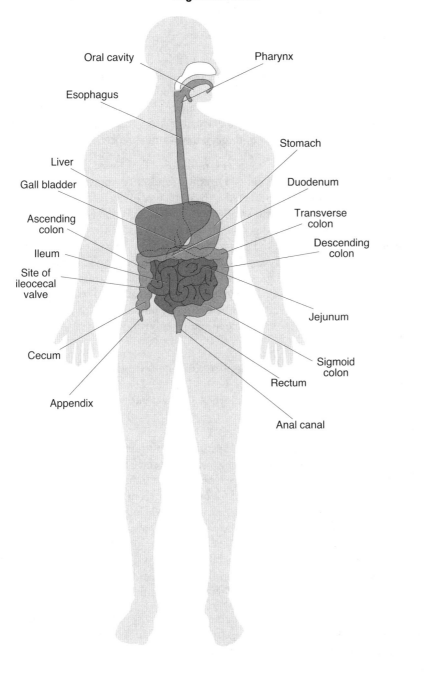

DEFINITIONS

ANUG. Acute necrotizing ulcerative gingivitis, also known as trench mouth, Vincent's angina, or fusospirochetosis.

Anatomy of the Digestive Tract

The anatomical digestive system begins at the mouth, continues in the pharynx and esophagus, to the stomach, the small and large intestines, and finally, the rectum and anus. Digestion involves both mechanical and chemical processes that break down and change food chemically so that it can be absorbed as simple, soluble substances into the blood, the lymph systems, and body tissues. Mechanical actions include chewing in the mouth, churning action in the stomach, and intestinal peristaltic action. These mechanical forces move the food through the digestive tract and mix it with secretions containing enzymes that accomplish three chemical reactions: the conversion of carbohydrates to simple sugars, the breaking down of proteins into amino acids, and the conversion of fats into fatty acids and glycerol.

Digestive Process

The process of digestion begins in the mouth. Food is ground by the teeth into small particles and mixed with saliva to form a soft mass. The tongue traps and forces clumps of this mixture into the pharynx and esophagus where it is squeezed by peristolic action into the stomach. The stomach churns and mixes the food with hydrochloric acid and enzymes and gradually releases the materials into the upper small intestine (the duodenum) through the pyloric sphincter.

The wall of the gastrointestinal tract is made up of four layers: the mucosa, submucosa, muscularis and serosa. Digestive glands may empty their products into the lumen (inner tube of the digestive tracts) by way of ducts. The majority of the digestive process occurs in the small intestine where most foods are hydrolysed and absorbed. The products of digestion are actively or passively transported through the wall of the small intestine and assimilated into the body. The stomach and the large intestine (colon) can, however, also absorb water, alcohol, certain salts and crystalloids, and some drugs. Water-soluble digestive products (such as minerals, amino acids, and carbohydrates) are transferred into the blood system and transported to the liver. Fats, resynthesized in the intestinal wall, are picked up by the lymphatic system, and enter the blood stream through the vena caval system, bypassing the liver.

Remaining undigested matter, together with cellular debris from the digestive tract, is passed into the colon where water is extracted. This comparatively solid mass (the stool) is propelled into the rectum, where it is held until excreted through the anus.

Mouth

The lips (labia) are highly mobile structures that surround the mouth opening. They contain skeletal muscles, primary of which is the orbicularis oris, the sphincter muscle that encircles the mouth and lies between the outer skin (integument), and the mucous membranes of the interior (or buccal) aspect of the lips. The labial glands, which are similar to salivary glands, are between the muscle and mucous membrane tissues. The lips also have many sensory nerves and abundant capillary vessels that produce the normal reddish color. The external margin of the lips (the vermilion border) marks the boundary between the skin of the face and the mucous membrane that lines the alimentary canal of the digestive system. The commissure of the lip is the angle or corner of the mouth at the junction of the upper and lower lips.

The vestibule of the mouth is the part of the oral cavity inside the cheeks and lips and outside the dentoalveolar structures (the teeth and gums of the jaw). It includes the mucosal and submucosal tissue of the lips and cheeks, and the labial and buccal frenulum, or frenum. These are the soft, connecting folds of membrane, which support and restrain the lips and cheeks. Secretions from the salivary glands lubricate the vestibule.

Mouth

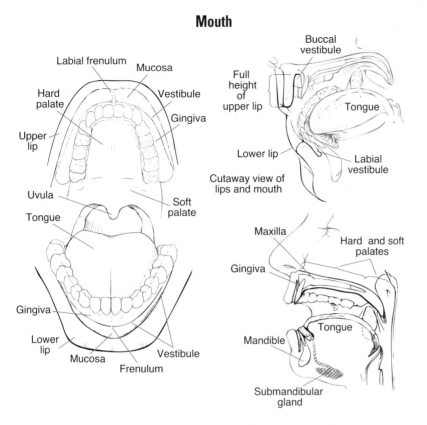

Upper Digestive Tract

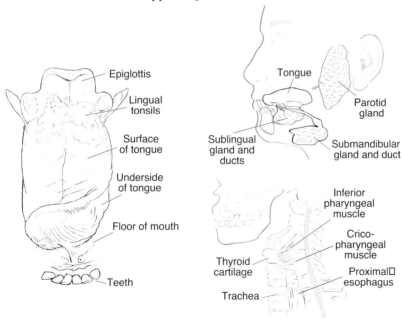

Tongue

The tongue is a strong muscle attached to the floor of the mouth within the curve of the mandible jawbone. It is anchored to muscles at the rear of the mouth, which attach to the base of the skull and to the hyoid bone (a small, U-shaped bone, at the back of the tongue). The muscle fibers of the tongue are heavily supplied with nerves, which provide for manipulation and safe placement of food in the mouth and between the teeth for chewing. The underside of the tongue is attached to the floor of the mouth by membranes that form a distinct vertical fold in the centerline, called the frenulum linguae.

The tongue contains mucous, serous, and lymph glands. The lymph glands at the back of the tongue form the lingual tonsils.

The surface of the tongue is covered with the lingual membrane, a specialized tissue with a variety of papillae protruding from it. These papillae nodules produce the characteristic rough surface of the tongue. Between the papillae are the taste buds, the sensory nerve organs that provide the sensations of flavor. The tongue also aids in swallowing and in the formation of sounds of speech.

Dentoalveolar

These are processes of the maxillary (upper) and mandible (lower) jawbones, and include the dental arches, which contain the sockets for the teeth. The root of each tooth is seated in a bony socket of alveolar bone that is lined with periodontal membrane. The tooth is attached within its socket by periodontal ligaments, and cushioned, as it emerges from the socket, by the gingiva (gums).

Palate and Uvula

The palate is the bony and muscular partition that divides the oral and nasal cavities. The bony, hard palate at the front of the mouth is formed by parts of the maxillary and palatine bones. These are covered above by the mucous membrane of the floor of the nasal cavity and underneath by the mucoperiosteum of the roof of the mouth. This tissue contains the palatine blood vessels, nerves and mucous glands. The muscular, soft palate lies behind the bony palate and forms an arch (called the fauces) partly dividing the mouth from the oropharynx, and the oropharynx from the nasopharynx. At the middle rear of this arch is a small cone-shaped process composed of connective, glandular, and muscle tissue, called the uvula.

Salivary Glands and Ducts

The salivary glands are typical of the digestive system's accessory glands. They are located outside the alimentary canal, and their secretions are conveyed or emptied into the lumen of the digestive tract via ducts.

There are three pairs of compound tubuloalveolar salivary glands: the parotids, submandibulars, and sublinguals. These three pairs of glands are responsible for secretion of about one liter of saliva each day.

The parotids are the largest paired salivary glands. They are pyramid-shaped and lie between the skin and the masseter muscle in front of and below the ear. The parotid (or Stenson) ducts are about five centimeters long and open into the mouth opposite the second upper molars, and secrete watery, serous saliva containing digestive enzymes.

The submandibular are mixed glands that produce both serous (enzyme) saliva and mucous. These are walnut-sized irregular shaped glands below the mandibular angle of the jawbone, under the back part of the floor of the mouth. The submandibular (Wharton) ducts open into the mouth on either side of the lingual frenulum.

The sublingual glands are the smallest salivary glands, located in front of the submandibulars and under the mucous membrane on the floor of the mouth. They drain only mucous saliva onto the floor of the mouth through eight to 20 (Rivinus) ducts.

The other, small salivary (buccal) glands, which are found in the mucosa lining of the cheeks and mouth, contribute only five percent of the total saliva, but are important to the comfort and hygiene of the mouth tissues.

Pharynx, Adenoids, and Tonsils

The pharynx, or throat, is a muscular, tubular structure lined with mucous membrane and extends about 12.5 centimeters from the base of the skull down to the esophagus, in front of the cervical vertebrae. Three anatomical divisions make up the pharynx:

- Nasopharynx, which lies behind the nose down to the soft palate
- Oropharynx, located behind the mouth from the soft palate down to the hyoid bone at the back of the tongue
- Laryngopharynx, which extends from the hyoid bone to the esophagus

The openings in the pharynx are the eustachian tubes, the posterior nares, the fauces (the opening from the mouth), the slit-like opening into the larynx, and the final opening into the esophagus.

Opposite the posterior nares in the nasopharynx are the pharyngeal tonsils. When enlarged, these are called adenoids (hence adenoidectomy is the term for their removal). The palatine tonsils, located behind and below the arch of the fauces, are tissues of the oropharynx. The palatine tonsils are commonly removed by a tonsillectomy. The lingual tonsils are at the base of the tongue and rarely removed.

The pharynx serves as a pathway for the digestive and respiratory tracts to the esophagus and trachea, respectively, and provides definition in speech production (phonation) (i.e., vowel sounds are formed by changes in shape of the pharynx).

Esophagus

The esophagus is the first segment of the digestive tube, or alimentary canal, proper. It is a collapsible tube about 25 centimeters long that extends from the end of the pharynx, travelling behind the trachea (windpipe) and the heart. Leaving the thoracic cavity through the diaphragm, the esophagus enters the abdominal cavity below. Circular muscle fibers, called the cardiac or lower esophageal sphincter, guard the entry of the esophagus into the stomach.

Stomach

The stomach is the pouchlike structure at the end of the esophagus. Two sphincter muscles divide it from neighboring portions of the alimentary canal: the cardiac or lower esophageal sphincter at its entrance, and the pyloric sphincter at its exit into the duodenum/small intestine.

The stomach lies in the upper abdominal cavity, below the diaphragm and liver, mostly to the left of the median line. Its size and position are variable because an adult stomach is able to distend from a collapsed state to accommodate a volume of up to one liter or one and one-half liters; it can be pushed up and down with inspiration and expiration.

DEFINITIONS

Gastroesophageal reflux dystrophy (GERD). A weakening of the lower esophageal sphincter allowing reflux of the stomach contents into the esophagus. One form of GERD is commonly defined as "heartburn."

Lymphatic drainage of the head, neck, and face

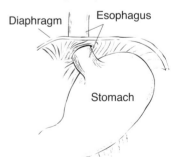

There are three divisions of the stomach: the fundus, the body, and the pylorus. The fundus is the enlarged portion to the left above the cardiac sphincter. The body is the central part, and the pylorus is the lower narrowing portion.

Similar to other parts of the digestive tract, the stomach lining is four-layered. Two of the layers have special modifications. The epithelial lining, the gastric mucosa, has folds and depressions (rugae and gastric pits) with numerous gastric glands that produce essential digestive juice including mucus, enzymes, hydrochloric acid, and intrinsic factor. The thick muscle of the stomach wall, the muscularis, has a three-layered criss-cross of muscle fibers that enable an efficient mixing action for the stomach contents.

The stomach has several critical functions. Among the primary functions is the stomach's storage capacity for partially digested foods that is churned, mixed, and moved into the duodenum. In addition, the stomach is a secretory organ that secretes gastric juices and an intrinsic factor to protect B12 prior to the vitamin's absorption. The stomach also absorbs some drugs, water, alcohol, and lactic fatty acids, produces gastrin hormone for digestive regulation, and helps destroy swallowed pathogenic bacteria.

Intestines (Except Rectum)

The small and large intestines are somewhat different in form and function. The small intestine is a six-meter long tube coiled into a loop in the abdominal cavity. Its three parts are: the duodenum (uppermost), the jejunum (middle), and the ileum (end). The duodenum leads from the pyloric sphincter of the stomach and is a C-shaped tube only about 12 centimeters long; it becomes the jejunum where the tube turns forward and downward abruptly. The jejunum is usually about 2.5 meters long and there is no clear demarcation as it changes to the ileum.

The wall of the small intestine, similar to the entire gastrointestinal tract, consists of five layers of tissue: the serosa (outer-most), the circular and longitudinal muscle layers responsible for peristalsis, the submucosa, and the mucosa. Its folds (plicae) and villi distinguish the mucosa of the small intestine. The villi are tiny, closely packed projections about one millimeter in length. Each villus has a covering, called brush border cells or microvilli, which produce digestive enzymes. This specialized lining significantly increases the surface are of the small intestine. Goblet cells on the villi and in the intestinal crypts in the lining produce mucus. The crypts in the intestinal lining also serve as a site of rapid mitotic cell division, providing for continual renewal of the lining. Specialized secretory cells in the base of the crypts produce enzymes that inhibit bacterial growth in the small intestine. The mucosa also contains clusters of lymph nodules (Peyer's patches) and numerous single lymph nodes called solitary nodes.

The small intestine is the major organ of digestion and absorption, which it achieves through chemical and mechanical processes. The mechanical process of intestinal motility involves segmentation and peristalsis. Segmentation is a forward and backward movement of the gastric contents within segments of the intestine, which mixes foods with the digestive juices and brings the digested food into contact with the specialized mucosa lining to facilitate absorption. The peristaltic action propels the intestinal contents along the alimentary canal. Chemical digestion is performed with the addition, in the small intestine, of pancreatic juice, bile from the liver and concentrated by the gall bladder, and the intestinal juice produced directly by the mucosa.

 DEFINITIONS

EGD. Common abbreviation for esophagogastroduodenoscopy.

GE. Gastroesophageal.

GI. Gastrointestinal.

UGI. Upper gastrointestinal.

The large intestine is an organ also divided into three different sections: the cecum, the colon, and the rectum, which together form the lower part of the alimentary canal. The name "large intestine" refers to its diameter (averaging six centimeters), which is noticeably greater than the small intestine. It is, however, considerably shorter—only about 1.5 meters to 1.8 meters.

The cecum forms the first five centimeters to eight centimeters of the large intestine and is a blind pouch in the lower right quadrant of the abdomen, accessed from the ileum by the ileocecal valve. The lumen is below the ileocecal valve, or entrance, to the vermiform appendix.

The colon, which consists of the ascending, transverse, descending, and sigmoid portions, leads from the cecum. The ascending portion extends from the cecum along the front of the right abdominal wall beneath the liver, and bends sharply at a right angle to the left in a curve called the hepatic flexure. From there, the colon crosses the abdominal cavity as the transverse colon over to the left abdominal wall. At the splenic flexure (below the stomach and the spleen), begins the descending colon that traverses along the left rear abdominal wall to the pelvic region. The colon forms an angle from the pelvis to form an S-shaped curve called the sigmoid colon, which ends at the superior rectal valve.

The walls of the large intestine are distinguished by having the outer longitudinal muscle layer condensed to form three tapelike strips (taenia coli). Inside this the circular muscle layer forms small sacs, called haustra, that give the rest of the wall its puckered appearance. In older adults, who eat low-fiber foods, diverticula may form in the intestinal wall, which are abnormal, saclike outpouchings that may become inflamed—a condition called diverticulitis. The presence of mucosa is also a notable modification of the large intestine. The glandular goblet cells produce the lubricating mucous, which coats the feces as they are formed.

Water and ion reabsorption and the formation and temporary storing of feces are the major functions of the colon.

Meckel's Diverticulum and the Mesentery

Meckel's diverticulum is the remains of the yolk stalk of the embryo. The mesentery is a part of the peritoneum. The peritoneum is the large, continuous sheet of serous membrane that lines the walls of the abdominal cavity and binds the abdominal organs together. The mesentery is a fan-shaped projection of the peritoneum. At its attachment, in the lumbar region of the back of the abdominal wall, the mesentery is only 15 centimeters to 20 centimeters long; however, the loose outer edge, which encloses the jejunum and the ileum, is six meters long. The construction allows free movement of each coil of the intestine, and helps prevent constriction or strangulation of the intestinal tube.

Appendix

The vermiform appendix is a blind, wormlike tubular organ, averaging eight centimeters to 10 centimeters in length usually found behind the cecum or over the pelvic rim in the right lower quadrant of the abdomen. The entrance to the appendix is in the blind end of the cecum, below the ileocecal valve.

Rectum

The last 16 centimeters to 20 centimeters of the intestinal tube are called the rectum. The terminal portion of the rectum is referred to as the anal canal and its mucosa forms vertical folds called anal columns. Each of these contains blood vessels, which

DEFINITIONS

Helicobacter pylori. A type of bacterium found in the digestive tract that causes gastritis and is associated with peptic ulcer disease. Commonly called *H. pylori.*

CLINICAL NOTE

Often thought to be a vestigial organ in humans, the appendix' function remain uncertain. Some biologists believe that the appendix serves to assist in production of intestinal bacteria, or flora, which normally inhabit the colon and are thought to both help prevent disease and aid in the digestion or absorption of essential nutrients.

in cases where they become distended are called hemorrhoids. The columnar folds are effaced when the rectum is distended.

There are also usually three permanent transverse folds in the rectum, known as Houston's valves. Occasionally, two or as many as four valves are present. These rectal valves support the weight of fecal matter after the colon performs the mass peristalsis of fecal matter into the sigmoid colon and rectum. Without the support of these valves, urgent sensation to defecate occurs.

The anus is the opening of the rectum to the exterior and controlled by two sphincter muscles. The internal sphincter is formed by smooth muscle, while the external sphincter (superior and subcutaneous) is striated muscle to enable, in combination, voluntary control of defecation.

Liver

The liver has two major lobes and two minor lobes. To the front, the large right lobe is separated from the smaller left lobe by the falciform ligament, which is a fold of the peritoneum. The caudate lobe, which is near the inferior vena cava, and the quadrate lobe, which is next to the gallbladder, are underneath. The falciform ligament attaches the liver to the front abdominal wall and the coronary ligament holds it to the diaphragm. The porta of the liver (a transverse fissure in the organ) is where the hepatic artery, portal vein lymphatics, and nerves enter the liver and where the hepatic ducts exit.

Each lobe of the liver is divided into numerous lobules by small blood vessels and fibrous strands. These strands form the supporting framework for the liver, called the Capsule of Glisson, which is an extension of the heavy connective tissue capsule that envelops the entire liver. Despite this protection, the liver is easily lacerated because of its soft and highly vascular composition. Although the liver is the largest internal organ of the body, it is only one cell to two cells thick (liver cells, hepatocytes, are one cell to two cells thick and separated from each other by large capillary spaces called sinusoids). The hepatic plates are arranged into hexagonal or pentagonal functional units called liver lobules. In the middle of each lobule is a central vein and at the periphery of each lobule are branches of the hepatic portal vein and hepatic artery, opening into spaces between hepatic plates.

Arterial blood and portal venous blood, containing nutrient molecules absorbed in the gastrointestinal tract, mix as the blood flows from the periphery of the lobule to the central vein. The central veins of the lobules converge to form two hepatic veins that carry blood from the liver to the inferior vena cava. Bile is produced in the liver by the hepatocytes and secreted into thin channels, called bile canaliculi, within each hepatic plate. The canaliculi are drained peripherally by bile ducts, which drain into hepatic ducts that carry bile away from the liver. As a result, blood travels in the sinusoids and bile travels in the opposite direction to prevent the mixing of blood and bile in the lobules of the liver.

The sinusoids in the liver are lined with specialized cells that remove bacteria, old red blood cells, and other particles from the blood. This detoxification process is one of the many functions of the liver. It also produces bile for the digestive process in the gastrointestinal tract and metabolizes absorbed food nutrients (carbohydrates, proteins and fats). In addition, the liver acts as a storehouse for several substances, including minerals and vitamins.

📁 CLINICAL NOTE

The liver is the largest gland in the body, usually weighing about 1.5 kilograms. It is roughly wedge-shaped and located under the diaphragm in the right upper part of the abdominal cavity.

Biliary Tract

The biliary system is the bile-producing system that consists of the liver, gallbladder, and their associated ducts. From the liver, the right and left hepatic ducts join to form the common hepatic duct, which delivers bile to the junction of the cystic duct of the gall bladder and the common bile duct. The gallbladder lies on the undersurface of the liver, attached by areolar connective tissue, and is a pear-shaped sac, 7 centimeters to 10 centimeters long and 3 centimeters wide; it can store from 30 mls to 50 mls of bile. The walls of the gallbladder have serous, muscular, and mucous layers, which fold in rugae, mimicking the structure (function) of the stomach to expand and contract as it fills, concentrates, and empties.

Bile enters the gallbladder from the hepatic and cystic ducts for storage. During storage, the bile is concentrated five- to tenfold. When bile is needed for digestion, the gallbladder contracts and ejects the concentrated bile. The bile flows down the common bile duct, which connects to the pancreatic duct, and a short tube formed by the union of the two ducts dilates into an ampulla, called the ampulla of Vater. Sphincter muscles control the flow as the bile is ejected into the duodenum at a structure called the major duodenal papilla.

Pancreas

The pancreas is a fish-shaped gland that and extends horizontally behind the stomach from the curve of the duodenum to the spleen. The pancreas has two different types of glandular tissue: the exocrine, which secretes digestive enzymes, and the endocrine, which produces hormones.

The main pancreatic duct extends horizontally through the pancreas from its tail at the spleen to where it joins the common bile duct in the ampulla of Vater. Pancreatic digestive juices are ejected into the duodenum at the major duodenal ampulla. The endocrine glandular tissue, which represents only about two percent of the mass of the pancreas, is embedded in the exocrine tissue in small clusters called pancreatic islets

The pancreas produces digestive juices to assist in the breakdown of food for absorption and hormones that regulate how products of absorption are metabolized.

Abdomen, Peritoneum, Omentum

The umbilicus (navel), the most frequently used "landmark" of the abdominal surface, is ordinarily at the level of the fourth lumbar vertebra.

The wall of the abdomen provides a strong girdle of muscles to support and protect the abdominal cavity and its internal organs. The muscles are arranged in three layers. The external oblique is the outermost muscle. The middle layer is the internal oblique, and the innermost layer is the transversus abdominis. In addition to the three sheets of muscles, the rectus abdominus muscle runs down the midline of the abdomen, from the thorax to the pubis. The rectus abdominus protects the abdomen and flexes the spinal column.

The parietal layer is inside the muscular layers of the abdominal layer. The parietal layer is a serous membrane, part of the peritoneum, which covers most of the organs and holds them in place; the mesentery, a fan-shaped projection enveloping the loops of the small intestine, is the longest of the peritoneum. A similar fold, called the transverse mesocolon, attaches the transverse colon to the back of the abdominal wall. The omentum, another projection of the peritoneum, is a double-fold of fatty membrane that hangs down in front of the intestines; it contains blood vessels, nerves, lymph vessels, and lymph nodes and stores fat. The fat forms in spotty

 DEFINITIONS

BS. Bowel sounds.
IBS. Irritable bowel syndrome.
UC. Ulcerative colitis.

 DEFINITIONS

Pancreatitis. Inflammation of the pancreas.

 CLINICAL NOTE

Munro's point, which is midway between the umbilicus and the left hip or pelvic bone, is another important landmark and a common point for abdominal punctures for inserting instruments used in diagnostic procedures.

deposits that give the omentum the appearance of a lace apron hanging down over the front of the intestines.

There are two parts to the omentum: the greater omentum, which descends from the greater curvature of the stomach and the first section of the duodenum, and the lesser omentum, which attaches from the liver to the stomach and duodenum.

CLINICAL NOTE

As well as providing physical protection and enabling movement of the organs, the omentum limits the spread of infection in the abdominal cavity by compartmentalizing infected areas away from the rest of the abdomen.

Digestive Tract

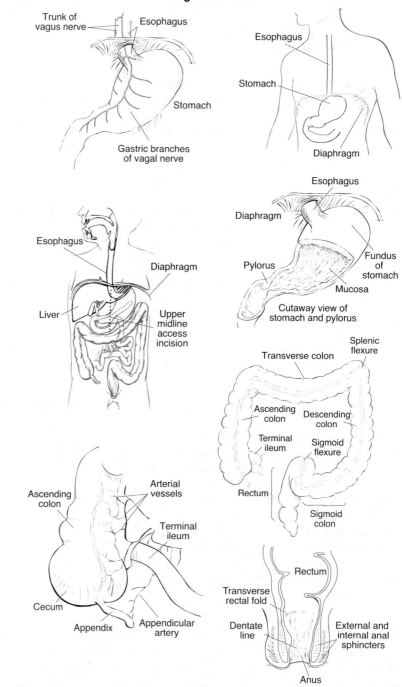

URINARY SYSTEM

The urinary system produces and excretes urine, a transparent yellow fluid containing unwanted wastes, mostly excess water, salts, and nitrogen compounds.

Anatomy of the Urinary System

The major organs of the urinary system are the kidneys (two), ureters (two), bladder (one), and the urethra (one). The kidneys are paired organs between the parietal peritoneum and the posterior abdominal wall (retroperitoneal), from the last thoracic vertebrae to the third lumbar vertebrae.

Kidney

The kidneys may be considered the body's blood filter and serve several functions. For example, they:

- Maintain water balance, ensuring that the amount of water in body tissues remains at a constant level
- Regulate the composition of blood by controlling blood volume
- Control calcium levels in the blood to maintain healthy bones
- Eliminate the waste the body cells deposit in the blood while retaining elements (e.g., potassium) necessary for the proper functions of the bodies cells and tissues
- Filter blood pumped from the blood and send the filtered blood through the renal veins for a return trip to the heart
- Stimulate the body to make red blood cells

Ureter

Renal calyces are cup-like projections in each kidney that drain urine into a large cavity called the renal pelvis. Two ureters (tubes)—one from each of the kidneys—arise in the renal pelvis and drain and transport the urine in a process called peristalsis. There are three layers within the ureters: the inner layer, or mucous coat, is continuous with the linings of the renal tubules and the urinary bladder; the middle layer, or muscular coat, is composed of smooth muscle fibers; the outer layer, or fibrous coat, is connective tissue.

The ureters deposit the urine into the bladder where it is stored until released from the body. A valve at the entrance to the bladder restricts urine backflow into the ureters or the renal pelvis.

Bladder

The bladder lies in front (anterior) of the rectum in men, and in front (anterior) of the vagina in women. Pelvic floor muscles support the bladder. The wall of the urinary bladder consists of four layers, as follows:

- The inner layer, or mucous coat, is layered with epithelial cells.
- The second layer, or submucous layer, is made up of connective tissue and elastic fibers.
- The third layer, or muscular coat, is interlaced to form the detrusor muscle, a portion of which forms an internal urethral sphincter that controls excretion of urine.
- The outer layer, or serous coat, is made of the parietal peritoneum on the upper surface of the urinary bladder and the outer coat is composed of fibrous connective tissue.

 CLINICAL NOTE

Each kidney contains about one million microscopic coiled channels, called nephrons, which filter the blood and produce urine in the process. Waste materials pass from the nephrons into the renal pelvis. From the renal pelvis, waste trickles out of the kidney into the ureter, which empties into the urinary bladder, which expands and contracts according to the volume of urine it contains. A sphincter muscle surrounds the bladder's outlet and prevents spontaneous emptying.

 CLINICAL NOTE

Nerve endings in the bladder are stretched during the filling phase and send information to the cortex that is perceived as fullness, discomfort, or pain. The normal adult bladder can store up to about one pint of urine, which is voided through the urethra to the outside of the body. An internal and external urinary muscle sphincter controls the urine flow and prevents continual release.

45

Urogenital Tract

Medullary ray
Minor calyx
Major calyx
Renal pelvis
Papilla
Ureter

Cutaway detail of right kidney

Capillaries
Bowman's capsule
Collecting tubule
Vein
Artery
Glomerulus

Schematic of nephron, the tiny filtering mechanism of the kidney

Kidney
Adrenal gland
Bladder
Upper ureter
Urethra
Prostate (male)

Posterior view of male bladder and prostate

Vas deferens
Bladder
Ureters
Seminal vesicle
Prostate

Ovary
Uterus
Colon
Recto-vaginal septum
Kidney
Ureter
Pubic bone
Bladder
Urethra
Anus
Vagina

Sideview schematic of female urogenital system

Posterior view showing location of kidneys and ureters

Spleen
Liver
Left kidney
12th rib
Ureters
Right kidney
Sacrum
Iliac crest

Urethra

The urethra is a tube that directs urine from the bladder to outside of the body. Mucous glands, called urethral glands, are dispersed throughout the urethra and secrete mucous into the urethral canal. The urethra and urethral sphincters are striated muscle. These muscles contract to hold the urethra and bladder neck closed during filling. They relax just prior to urination. The combined action of the contraction of the bladder's smooth muscles and the relaxation of these striated muscles causes the bladder neck to raise and open, and the bladder to empty.

Renal System

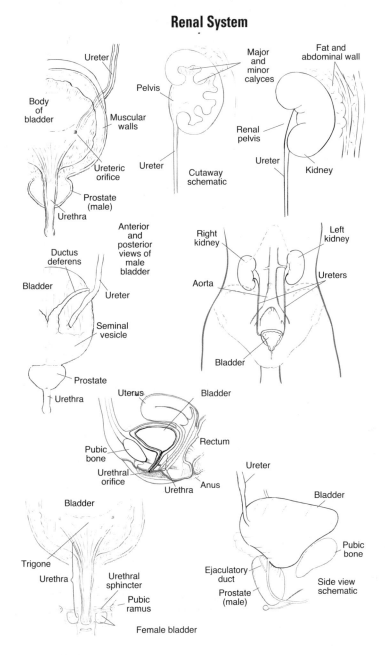

Male Genital System

Males have two perineal openings, one for passing urine and semen through the tip of the penis, and the anus located behind the scrotum.

Penis

The penis consists of two parts, the shaft and the glans. The shaft is made up of three cylinders that swell with blood when the penis is sexually stimulated causing it to enlarge and harden. The fold of skin (frenulum) that passes from under the glans of the penis to the skin covering the penis shaft is called the frenulum preputii. The urethra is a tube that goes from the bladder to the tip of the penis. In men, the urethra has two functions: urination and ejaculation. A muscle prevents urine from mixing with the semen during ejaculation.

Male Genitalia

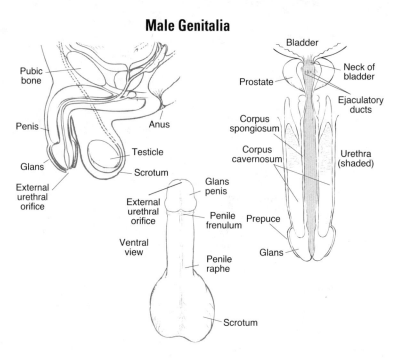

Testis

The testicles are two oval-shaped glands that produce male hormones and sperm. It is normal for one testicle to hang lower in the scrotum than the other.

Epididymis

Sperm is continuously produced in the seminiferous tubules, which are inside each of the two testicles. When sperm leave a testicle they enter one of the epididymides. Inside each epididymis is a thin, tightly coiled tube where, as the sperm move through, they undergo a maturation process that gives them the ability to move forward.

Vas Deferens/Spermatic Cord

Sperm enter one of the vas deferens, a tube that sperm travel through prior to ejaculation. The spermatic cord consists of the vas deferens, testicular artery, nerves, and veins that drain the testes. The spermatic cord is about 45 centimeters long and passes from the testicle, through the inguinal canal, over the bladder and forms an ampulla before the ejaculatory duct. Sperm collects in the ampulla prior to being expelled out through the urethra at ejaculation.

Seminal Vesicles

The seminal vesicles are glans next to the ampulla. They secrete liquids important for the survival of sperm. On each side of the urethra at the ejaculatory duct, each vas deferens joins with the opening of a seminal vesicle, and the seminal vesicles connect to the urethra. These seminal vesicles produce an alkaline fluid that contains fructose (a nutrient for sperm). Surrounding the urethra is the prostate gland. Fluid from the seminal vesicles and fluid from the prostate gland mix together as semen and enter the urethra.

Prostate

The prostate is a gland that surrounds the urethra at the neck of the bladder. The prostate supplies fluid that goes into semen.

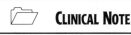 **CLINICAL NOTE**

The total volume of semen in each ejaculate is around one teaspoon and contains 120 million to 600 million sperm.

Female Genital System

The female genital system can be divided into external and internal organs. The entire area of the external female genital anatomy is called the vulva. The internal organs are within the pelvis.

Vulva

Females have three perineal openings: the urinary opening or urethra, the opening into the vagina, and the anus. The mons pubis is a collection of fatty tissue that protects the pubic bone and is covered by skin and pubic hair. The labia majora extend from the mons pubis to the anus. They cover the urinary and vaginal openings and are in turn covered by pubic hair. The labia minora, or inner lips, are folds of moist skin that lie inside the outer lips and extend from just above the clitoris to below the vaginal opening.

The clitoris is a sensitive organ that lies just under the mons. It is covered by the inner lips that can be pushed back to reveal the tip (the head or glans). The urinary opening is just under the clitoris. It is the outer part of the urethra, the tube from the bladder.

The vaginal opening is behind the urinary opening. The vagina lies between the urethra and the rectum.

Vagina

The vaginal opening is behind the urinary opening. The vagina lies between the urethra and the rectum. A muscular canal, it extends from the vulva to the cervix of the uterus. The vagina is approximately 6 to 10 centimeters long.

Female Genitalia

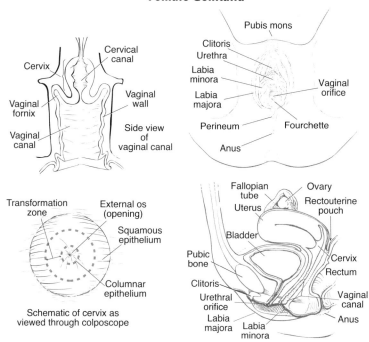

Uterus

The uterus has two main parts: the cervix and corpus. The cervix is the neck of the uterus and is approximately the lower third of the organ. More tubular in shape, it extends downward to the vagina. The cervical orifice is the opening between the vagina and cervix and the area where Pap smear samples are taken.

The corpus, or main portion of the uterus, is a muscular organ. The uterus is approximately 7.5 centimeters in the nonpregnant woman. The uterus is in front of the bowel and behind the bladder and usually tilts anteriorly. The top of the uterus is the fundus, where a horn on either side connects to a fallopian tube. The uterus will stretch to accommodate a growing fetus.

Fallopian Tubes

A fallopian tube extends from each horn of the uterus to the ovary and is approximately 8 centimeters in length. The larger end is divided into feathery, finger-like projections known as fimbria. The fimbria help to move the egg from the ovary into the fallopian tube. Fertilization of the egg occurs in the fallopian tube where secretions encourage fertilization. The fertilized egg then moves into the uterus to attach to the uterine wall for the duration of the pregnancy.

Ovaries

The ovaries are small, oval glands about 4 centimeters long positioned adjacent to the fallopian tube fimbria. Each ovary produces eggs and the hormones estrogen, progesterone, and relaxin. The ovum, or unfertilized egg, matures within the ovary and at a specified point of development approaches the surface of the ovary and bursts free. Women, at birth, have about 60,000 eggs of which approximately 400 will mature over her lifetime.

ENDOCRINE SYSTEM

The endocrine system is a made up of glands that includes the thyroid, parathyroid, pancreas, ovaries, testes, adrenal, pituitary and hypothalamus. The endocrine glands produce and secrete hormones that regulate metabolism, reproduction, growth, and development.

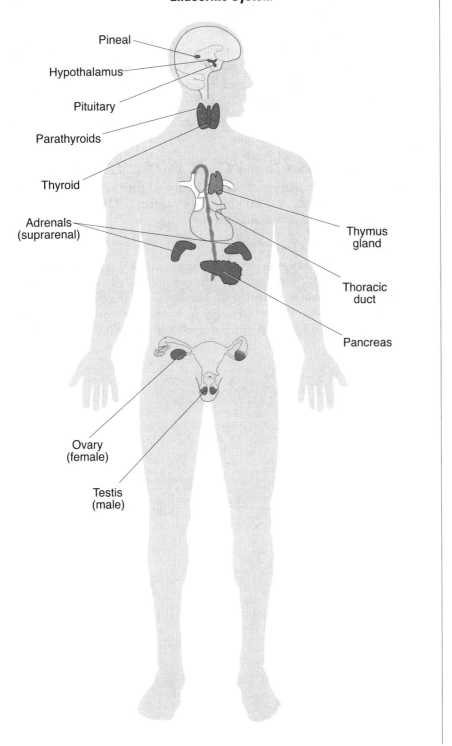

Endocrine System

Anatomy of the Endocrine System

The endocrine glands include:

- Pituitary gland (hypophysis): one, located in the sella turcica of the sphenoid bone
- Thyroid glands (right and left lateral lobes): two, located immediately below the larynx
- Parathyroid glands (superior and inferior): two pairs, embedded in the back (posterior) portion of the thyroid glands
- Adrenal glands: two, one located above (superior) each kidney
- Pancreas (the pancreas is an exocrine and endocrine gland): one, located to the back (posterior) and slightly below (inferior) the stomach
- Ovaries: two, located in the pelvic cavity
- Testes: two, located in the scrotum
- Thymus: one, located in the superior mediastinum, to the back (posterior) of the sternum between the lungs

Parathyroid, Thymus, Adrenal Glands, and Carotid Body Parathyroid

The parathyroids are four glands behind the thyroid gland at the front of the neck that produce the hormone called parathyroid hormone (PTH). This hormone maintains the level of calcium in blood and bones.

Thymus and Thymus Carotid Body

The thymus gland consists of lymphatic tissue and areas of epithelial tissue, called Hassall's corpuscles. The thymus grows through puberty, after which the gland shrinks, and the tissue is replaced by fat. The thymus gland is thought to play a role in the immune response. The carotid bodies are oval nodules located at the fork of the carotid arteries that monitor the oxygen content of the blood and help regulate respiration.

 DEFINITIONS

Goiter. Abnormal enlargement of the thyroid gland not affecting hormone production.

Hyperthyroidism. Overproduction of thyroid hormone.

Hypothyroidism. Underproduction of thyroid hormone.

Endocrine System

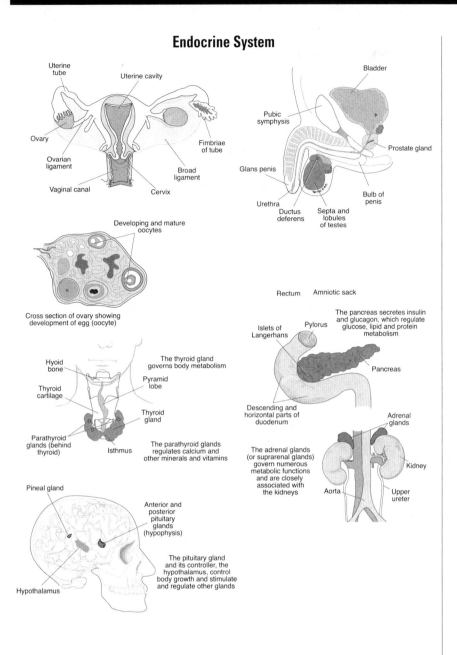

Uterine tube

Uterine cavity

Ovary

Ovarian ligament

Vaginal canal

Cervix

Fimbriae of tube

Broad ligament

Bladder

Pubic symphysis

Glans penis

Urethra

Ductus deferens

Septa and lobules of testes

Bulb of penis

Prostate gland

Developing and mature oocytes

Cross section of ovary showing development of egg (oocyte)

Rectum

Amniotic sack

Hyoid bone

Thyroid cartilage

Parathyroid glands (behind thyroid)

Isthmus

The thyroid gland governs body metabolism

Pyramid lobe

Thyroid gland

The parathyroid glands regulates calcium and other minerals and vitamins

Islets of Langerhans

Pylorus

The pancreas secretes insulin and glucagon, which regulate glucose, lipid and protein metabolism

Pancreas

Descending and horizontal parts of duodenum

The adrenal glands (or suprarenal glands) govern numerous metabolic functions and are closely associated with the kidneys

Adrenal glands

Kidney

Aorta

Upper ureter

Pineal gland

Anterior and posterior pituitary glands (hypophysis)

Hypothalamus

The pituitary gland and its controller, the hypothalamus, control body growth and stimulate and regulate other glands

NERVOUS SYSTEM

The nervous system controls the reception of stimuli, the transmission of nerve impulses, and the activation of muscle. There are two divisions in the nervous system: the central part (spine and skull) and the peripheral part that extends throughout the remainder of the body.

Anatomy of the Nervous System

The nervous system controls the reception of stimuli, the transmission of nerve impulses, and the activation of muscle. The two divisions in the nervous system are the central part (spine and skull) and the peripheral part that extends throughout the remainder of the body.

Twelve pairs of cranial nerves connect to the brain by passing through openings in the skull, or cranium, and 31 pairs of spinal nerves pass through openings in the vertebral column, developing major branches and associated complexes known as peripheral nerves. Both cranial and spinal nerves convey impulses to the central nervous system (afferent impulses, also referred to as sensory) and also carry messages outward (efferent, also referred to as either somatic or visceral motor impulses).

Neurons are the conducting cells of the nervous system and transmit nerve impulses from one part of the body to another. The cell body of a neuron conducts sense impressions and others conduct muscle responses, called reflexes, such as those caused by pain.

Spine and Spinal Cord

The meninges, tough membranous protectors of the central nervous system, cover the brain and spinal cord. The meninges are arranged in three layers, the thickest and toughest being the outside membrane, the dura.

Extracranial Nerves, Peripheral Nerves, and Autonomic Nervous System

The various types of nerves include the following:

Facial nerve. Sole source of motor supply to the muscles of facial expression.

Greater occipital nerve. General sensory and motor nerve of the skin and scalp of the back of the head.

Infraorbital nerve. Maxillary branch of the trigeminal nerve; sensory in nature. It transverses the infraorbital groove and emerges on the face where it supplies the internal and external nasal areas as well as the upper lip and lower eyelid.

Inferior alveolar nerve. Enters the mandible via the mandibular foramen and passes along the mandibular canal until it exits through the mental foramen. While in the canal, it innervates the teeth of the mandible.

Lingual nerve. Lies anterior to the inferior alveolar nerve and is the sensory nerve to the anterior tongue, the floor of the mouth, and to the gingivae. It lies in mucosa medial to the third molar.

Mental nerve. Branch of the inferior alveolar nerve and passes to the face through the mental foramen. It provides sensation to the lower lip, chin, and the mucous membranes, gingiva, and teeth of the front mandible.

Phrenic nerves. The two phrenic nerves arise mainly from the fourth cervical nerve. Each is a motor nerve to a side of the diaphragm and serves in the breathing function. The right nerve also plays a role in liver function.

✓ QUICK TIP

The level of spinal injury can often be determined by symptoms or area the associated nerve endings enervate.

 DEFINITIONS

Encephal. Pertaining to the brain.
Intra. Within.
Mening. Pertaining to the lining of the brain and spinal cord.
Sub. Below.
Supra. Above.

Pudendal nerve. Serves most of the perineum and the external anal sphincter; also the sensory nerve of the external genitalia in males and females.

Sciatic nerve. Enters the buttock through the greater sciatic foramen. It lies under the gluteus maximus and enters the thigh where it descends to the middle back of the leg.

Supraorbital nerve. The ophthalmic branch of the trigeminal nerve and sensory in nature. It enervates the lateral part of the forehead and the front part of the scalp.

Sural nerve. A distal branch of the sciatic nerve under the skin and fascia of the back of the lower leg where it enervates the outer ankle muscles and skin.

The autonomic nervous system is one of the two main divisions of the nervous system, and controls the action of the glands; the functions of the respiratory, circulatory, digestive, and urogenital systems; and the involuntary muscles in these systems and in the skin. The sympathetic branch of the autonomic nervous system stimulates the heart, dilates the bronchi, contracts the arteries, and inhibits the digestive system in preparation for physical activity. The parasympathetic branch, or craniosacral division, of the autonomic nervous system prepares the body for feeding, digestion, and rest.

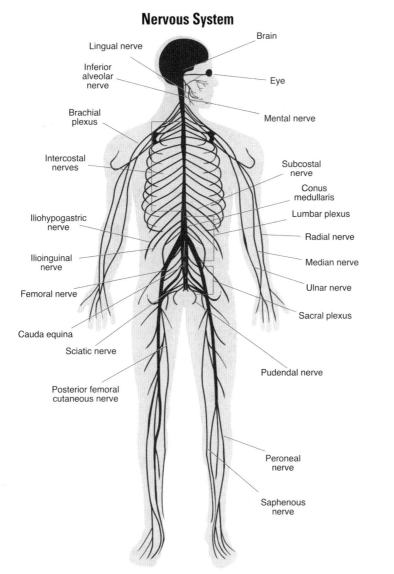

Nervous System

Brain and Nervous System

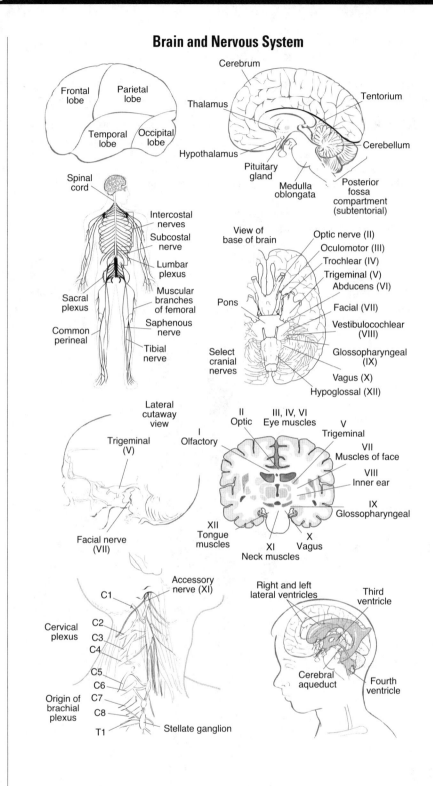

EYE—OCULAR—AUDITORY

These organs are primary to our senses, providing us with the ability see and hear.

Eye

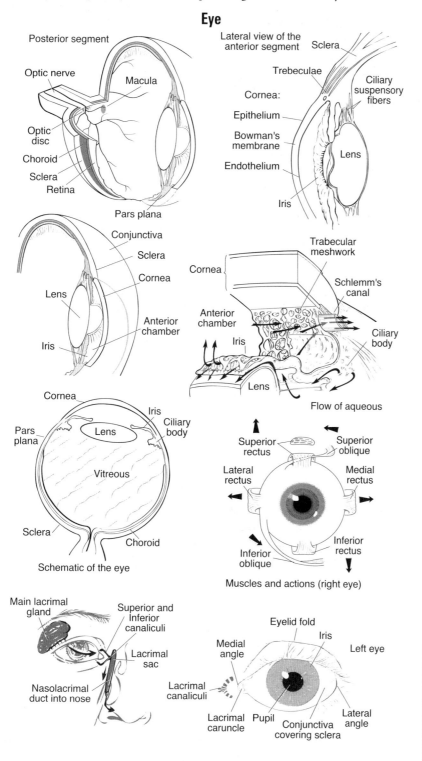

Posterior segment
Optic nerve
Macula
Optic disc
Choroid
Sclera
Retina
Pars plana

Lateral view of the anterior segment
Sclera
Trebeculae
Cornea:
Epithelium
Bowman's membrane
Endothelium
Iris
Ciliary suspensory fibers
Lens

Conjunctiva
Sclera
Cornea
Lens
Iris
Anterior chamber

Cornea
Trabecular meshwork
Schlemm's canal
Anterior chamber
Iris
Ciliary body
Lens
Flow of aqueous

Cornea
Iris
Ciliary body
Pars plana
Lens
Vitreous
Sclera
Choroid

Schematic of the eye

Superior rectus
Superior oblique
Lateral rectus
Medial rectus
Inferior oblique
Inferior rectus

Muscles and actions (right eye)

Main lacrimal gland
Superior and Inferior canaliculi
Lacrimal sac
Nasolacrimal duct into nose

Eyelid fold
Iris
Left eye
Medial angle
Lacrimal canaliculi
Lacrimal caruncle
Pupil
Conjunctiva covering sclera
Lateral angle

Anatomy of the Eye

The front parts of the eye (the cornea, pupil, and lens) are clear and allow light to pass through to the vitreous cavity, which is filled with vitreous gel. The light is focused on a thin layer of tissue called the retina, which covers the back inside wall of the eye. When the focused light hits the retina, a picture is taken. Messages are sent to the brain through the optic nerve so we can "see" the image.

Cornea

The cornea is the clear, protective window at the front of the eye that lies directly over the iris.

Iris, Ciliary Body

The uvea includes the iris, the ciliary body, and the choroid. The iris opens and closes to change the amount of light entering the eye. The ciliary body changes the shape of the lens inside the eye so it can focus. The choroid layer is next to the retina.

Posterior Segment

The gel-like vitreous is attached to the retina, optic nerve, macula and the large retinal blood vessels.

Retina or Choroid

The retina, in the posterior segment of the eye, has two parts: the peripheral retina and the macula. The macula is the small center, while the peripheral retina that surrounds the macula makes up 95 percent of the retina. The macula allows us to see details. The peripheral retina gives us peripheral vision.

Anatomy of the Ear

The three parts of the ear are the outer (external), middle, and inner ear. The definition of each follows:

- The outer, or external, ear is the visible ear, the ear canal, and the outside of the eardrum, a tough, flexible membrane also called the tympanic membrane. Sound waves travel through the outer ear to the eardrum to get to the middle ear. The tympanic membrane (eardrum) separates the outer ear from the middle ear. The membrane vibrates when sound waves strike it, beginning the process that converts the sound wave into a nerve impulse that travels to the brain. The auricle, or pinna, is another term for the external ear.

- The middle ear, just behind the eardrum, is a hollow chamber that contains the three smallest bones of the body, the incus, malleus, and stapes, which carry sound to the inner ear. The eustachian tube leads from the back of the throat to the middle ear and keeps the middle ear cavity filled with air.

- The inner ear is housed in the bony labyrinth of the skull and contains the cochlea, the organ of hearing; the three semicircular canals and two other structures, called the utricle and the saccule, which contain the balance sense organs. Soft tissue of the inner ear is made of sensory cells, supporting cells, and nerve fibers arranged in a pattern on a thin, elastic membrane. Channels filled with fluid surround the soft tissue of the inner ear.

Sound Conduction

Sound is transported in the following ways:

Air conduction. Transportation of sound from the air, through the external auditory canal to the tympanic membrane and ossicular chain, ending at, but not including,

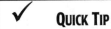
QUICK TIP

The bones of the ossicular chain, the incus, malleus, and stapes, are more commonly known as the anvil, hammer, and stirrup.

the cochlea. Testing air conduction establishes the patency or nonpatency of these mechanisms.

Bone conduction. Transportation of sound through bone where the source of sound is placed on the skull or teeth and the vibration stimulates the cochlea, bypassing normal air conduction routes. Bone conduction requires operational sensorineural hearing mechanisms.

Sensorineural conduction. Transportation of sound from the cochlea to the acoustic nerve and central auditory pathway to the brain.

Ear

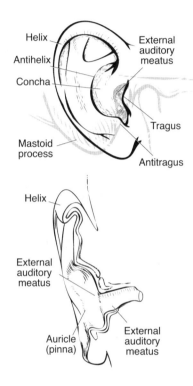

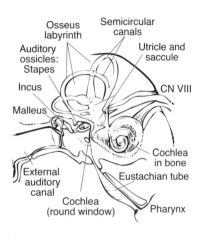

Auditory System

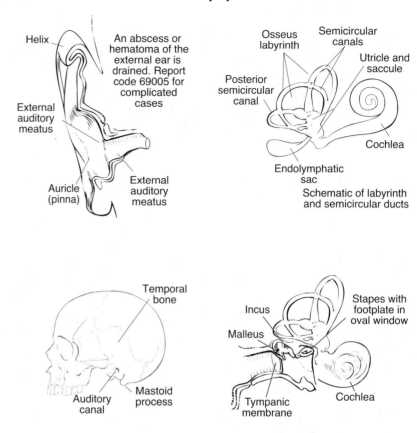

Helix

An abscess or hematoma of the external ear is drained. Report code 69005 for complicated cases

External auditory meatus

Auricle (pinna)

External auditory meatus

Osseus labyrinth

Semicircular canals

Utricle and saccule

Posterior semicircular canal

Cochlea

Endolymphatic sac

Schematic of labyrinth and semicircular ducts

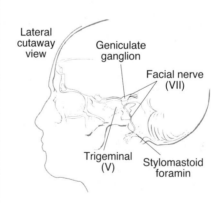

Temporal bone

Auditory canal

Mastoid process

Incus

Malleus

Stapes with footplate in oval window

Tympanic membrane

Cochlea

Lateral cutaway view

Geniculate ganglion

Facial nerve (VII)

Trigeminal (V)

Stylomastoid foramin

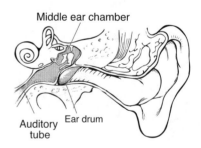

Middle ear chamber

Auditory tube

Ear drum

PLANES

References are made to imaginary planes that pass through the body. The median plane runs vertically through the center of the body, dividing it exactly into the right side and the left side. Any number of sagittal planes run parallel to the median plane. Coronal planes run at right angle to the median plane. Horizontal planes run at right angle to both the median plane and the coronal planes.

Terms Denoting Relationship

A number of terms are used to describe a body part relative to the anatomical position. The following terms and definitions are essential to accurate description for all manner of medical references.

Anterior. To the front of, or nearer to the front. The nose is on the anterior surface of the head. The anterior surface of the hand is the palm. (Also, ventral.)

Posterior. To the back of, or nearer to the back. The heel occupies the posterior part of the foot. (Also, dorsal.)

Superior. Toward the top of the body, or toward the head. The esophagus is superior to the stomach, to which it is attached. (Also, cranial, cephalic.)

Inferior. Toward the lower part of the body, or toward the feet. Immediately inferior to the diaphragm lies the abdominal cavity. (Also, caudal.)

Medial. Toward the middle or toward the medial plane. The external auditory canal extends medially to the tympanic membrane, or ear drum.

Lateral. Farther away from the middle or away from the medial plane. The heart lies in the left lateral compartment of the mediastinum.

Terms That Compare Positions

The following is a list of words used to compare the positions of various anatomical structures. These are common terms and precise usage is important.

Proximal. Nearest to the point of origin, or nearest to the trunk. The thoracic portion of the aorta is proximal to its passage through the diaphragm.

Distal. Farthest from the point of origin, or farthest from the trunk. The patella, or kneecap, partially overlies the most distal portion of the femur.

Superficial. Closest to the surface. The epidermal layer is superficial to the dermis.

Interior. Nearer the center. Two chambers divided by a septum occupy the interior of the heart.

Exterior. Farther from the center. The muscular exterior of the esophagus works to facilitate swallowing.

Positional Terms

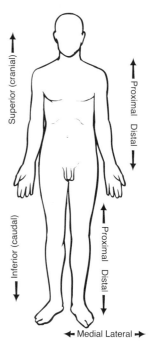

Movement Terms

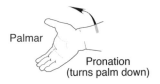

Palmar

Pronation
(turns palm down)

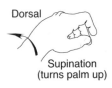

Dorsal

Supination
(turns palm up)

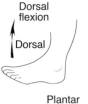

Dorsal
flexion

Dorsal

Plantar
flexion

Plantar

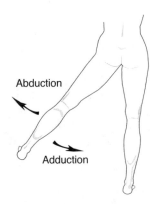

Abduction

Adduction

Terms that Denote Movement

The following select terms define movements, usually of the limbs, but also of other parts of the body. A knowledge of these terms is particularly useful for medical coders in the interpretation of operative reports.

Flexion. The movement causing decreased angle of a joint.

Extension. The movement causing increased angle, or straightening, of a joint.

Abduction. The movement away from the median plane.

Adduction. The movement toward the median plane.

Eversion. The movement, usually of the foot at the ankle, away from the medial plane.

Inversion. The movement, usually of the foot at the ankle, toward the medial plane.

Afferent. Conveying toward a center. For example, afferent nerves carry impulses to the central nervous system.

Efferent. Conveying away from the center. For example, efferent nerves carry information away form the central nervous system to muscles and glands.

Supination. The movement of the lower arm that rotates the palm and forearm anteriorly (as in the anatomical position).

Pronation. The movement of the lower arm that rotates the palm and forearm posteriorly (opposite position of supination).

Approaches to Medical Terminology

The language of human anatomy comprises more than 4,500 words. Most of these terms can be broken down into the following components/elements:

Word root. The foundation of the medical term and the source of its meaning.

Prefix. If present, is found at the beginning of the word. A hyphen may follow a prefix (e.g., sub-)

Suffix. Found at the end of the word. All medical terms have a suffix.

Combining vowels. Usually "o" joins the root to a suffix or to another root.

When words are divided into their component parts even complex words can be understood.

Word Root

Word roots contain the fundamental meaning of a term. Word roots are usually terms that can stand alone as the main portion of a medical term. The root is the foundation of the word and the source of its meaning. All medical words have one or more roots. A prefix, suffix, or combining vowel may accompany it. Most medical words are formed by combining a root word with a suffix. As the name implies, the word root is the central part of the word and the key to its meaning. Variations are found in how clearly the root presents within the word. The root *mamm* is derived from the Latin *mamma,* for breast. The root is clear in terms such as submammary or mammotropic. Others can be more obscure.

In the medical term arthr/itis, *Arthr-* (which means *joint*) is the word root.

In the medical term hepat/itis, *Hepat-* (which means *liver*) is the word root.

Because the word root contains the fundamental meaning of the word, each medical term contains one or more word roots.

Suffix

The suffix is a word part attached to the end of the word root to modify and give specific meaning to the word root. The suffix often describes a condition of, or action to, a body part.

Examples:

In the medical term hemangioma, *-oma* (which means *mass or tumor*) is the suffix.

In the medical term hepat/ic, *ic* (which means *pertaining to*) is the suffix.

Hepat is the word root for *liver*; therefore, *hepatic* means *pertaining to the liver*.

In the medical term hepat/itis, *itis* (which means *inflammation*) is the suffix. The term *hepatitis* means *inflammation of the liver*.

The suffix appears at the end of a medical term. It is used to modify the meaning of a word; therefore, not all medical terms have a suffix. Suffixes can also be used alone as separate terms. In medical terms, suffixes often indicate the procedure, condition, disorder, or disease.

Examples:

Lysis (lytic) means destruction, breakdown, separation.

A surgeon performs lysis of adhesions of the ovary. The surgeon separates and removes adhesions from the ovary.

Hemolysis is the separation, breakdown, and/or destruction of red blood cells.

Emesis (emetic) means vomiting.

Hematoemesis is vomiting blood.

The emetic is given to a patient to cause vomiting when a poison is swallowed.

Prefix

The prefix is a word part attached to the beginning of a word root to modify its meaning and to make the meaning of that term more specific. Not all medical words contain a prefix. Prefixes are often used to indicate location, time, or number.

Examples:

In the medical term sub/hepat/ic, *sub* (which means *under*) is the prefix.

*Hepa*t is the word root for *liver*, and *ic* is the suffix for *pertaining to*. The medical term *subhepatic* means *pertaining to under the liver*.

In the medical term intra/ven/ous, *intra-* (which means *within*) is the prefix.

ven- (which means *vein*) is the word root, and *-ous* (which means *pertaining to*) is the suffix.

The word *intravenous* means *pertaining to within the vein*.

Combining Vowel

The combining vowel is usually an o, (i, or u are also used frequently), and is used between two word roots or between a word root and a suffix to ease pronunciation.

Examples:

In the word therm/o/meter, *o* is the combining vowel used between two word parts.

QUICK TIP

If a term has more than one root, there are no rules as to which goes first. *Oste/o/arthropathy* could very well be *arthr/o/oste/o/pathy*.

KEY POINT

When connecting a word root with a suffix, a combining vowel is usually not used if the suffix begins with a vowel. When connecting two word roots, a combing vowel is usually used even if the vowels are present at the junction. The combining vowel is used to ease pronunciation; therefore, not all medical terms will have combining vowels.

In the medical term arthr/o/pathy, *o* is the combining vowel used between the word root *arthr* and the suffix *-pathy* (which means disease).

See CD-ROM for additional word parts.

SUMMARY

This chapter begins by covering the basics of medical language. It gives a history of the evolution of medical nomenclature from Greek and Latin words. One of the objectives is to analyze words by dividing them into component parts. The next step is to relate the medical terms to the structures and functions of the human body. The student learns to relate body systems to corresponding medical fields and specialties.

DISCUSSION QUESTIONS

The following discussion questions and issues are for your consideration upon completion of this chapter. A full series of test questions on this chapter are found on the accompanying CD-ROM, and in the instructor's manual.

Terminology

- What do you think is the rationale behind a systematized structure of medical terminology? Is Greek and Latin terminology obsolete in our Americanized culture?
- What are eponyms and why are they sometimes problematic to clear communication? Think of areas that might hinder clear communication of medical details. What might be the implications of unclear or confusing communication of medical information?
- Think about the broader nature of word roots. Try to identify Greek and Latin word roots in commonly used English words. Do the same for prefixes and suffixes.
- What are some of the better references for medical terms? Are you a confident speller? Can you easily find hard-to-spell words in your preferred references?

Anatomy

- Think about organizational approaches to human anatomy. Where do you think early anatomists made their biggest errors?
- Think about the ethical considerations of dissection and study of the human body.
- Are you comfortable approaching human anatomy through its major systems? Choose a major system and name as many component subsystems as you can. Try the exercise on other systems.
- Practice using correct terminology for movements and directions. Describe a random person within view, or in a photo, using terms for movement and directions. What aspect is the head facing? Describe the position of all extremities.

Chapter 2: Insurance Basics

INTRODUCTION

As you prepare to enter the field of medical coding, it is important to keep in mind that medical codes act as a kind of language. The language serves a variety of purposes and is interpreted by man and machine alike. Health statistics and utilization patterns are compiled and analyzed through the codes. But a major purpose of medical codes is to communicate services to health insurers.

The numeric and alphanumeric codes are the language that health insurance computers understand. And for better or worse, insurance reimbursement in all its forms drives the financial end of the health care industry today.

HISTORY

Insurance as a concept dates to the cradle of civilization, with laws pertaining to commercial insurance in the codes of Hammarabi. The practice of pooling risk to cover losses was developed largely by the commercial shipping industry in the 17th and 18th centuries. Venture capitalists of the time began the practice of signing their names under the amount they were willing to guarantee against risk, which gave rise to the term underwriter. But insurance against personal health failure is much more recent.

The first sickness insurance policy written in this country is thought to have been sold during the 1840s in Boston. Railroad and mining companies began early employer sponsored insurance in the late 19th century. But coverage was usually limited to occasional fitness checks by the company physician. Montgomery Ward stores offered a more comprehensive plan to its employees as early as 1910. And the earliest Blue Cross insurance plan was launched in association with Baylor University in Texas in the late 1920s. Formed as a not-for-profit organization with chapters in several states, the Blue Cross Commission was established in 1937.

The post-World War II era saw the meteoric growth in health insurance that influences so many sectors of the health services industry today. Squeezed by wartime wage and price restraints and a limited labor force, many manufacturers turned to nonwage benefits to attract qualified workers. Health insurance proved an effective incentive and the movement enjoyed the added support of powerful trade unions. A negotiated tradition of sharing the cost between workers and employers was established. To boost the trend, health insurance benefits were not considered taxable to either the employee or employer. Employer-sponsored health plans boomed in the 1950s and 1960s.

MEDICARE AND MEDICAID

The mid-1960s also saw the introduction of the federal Medicare program. Enacted in 1965, Medicare offered hospital and physician services coverage to people aged 65 and older. As enacted, Medicare covered hospital services for up to 90 days with up to 100 days of extended aftercare and home health services. The inpatient deductible was originally set at $40. Patient coinsurance began after 60 days of hospitalization

OBJECTIVES

In this chapter, you will learn:

- Insurance terminology
- About care options and payers
- The difference between Medicare Part A intermediaries and Part B carriers
- How to distinguish between participating and nonparticipating providers
- About the Medicare physician fee schedule (MPFS) and RBRVS
- The basics of insurance fraud and abuse

DEFINITIONS

Provider. An all-inclusive, generic term for people or institutions that provide health care. The provider may be a physician, hospital, pharmacy, other facility, or other health care provider.

Self-funded plan. A plan where the risk is assumed by the employer rather than the insurer Also called a self-insured plan. The employer generally pays claims directly from a general fund account. An insurer is usually hired to manage the plan.

and was set at 25 percent of cost. Physician services at that time carried a $50 per calendar year deductible and 20 percent coinsurance.

The Medicaid program followed soon after, and was structured to address essential health care needs of individuals meeting poverty-level guidelines. Unlike Medicare, the Medicaid program is administered and partially funded by the states. But enabling legislation was at the federal level and each state must meet minimum guidelines in order to receive supplemental federal funding.

The Medicare program has evolved significantly since 1965. Coverage has been extended to disabled individuals under age 65. And patients with end-stage renal failure are also covered. Coverage and patient costs have also changed over the years, but perhaps the most significant difference from 1965 is the government's method of reimbursement for services.

During the early years of the program, reimbursement for all medical services was based on reasonable charges. As cost containment strategies came into place in the late 1980s, however, reimbursement moved toward a schedule of set fees for physician services. Hospitals came to be reimbursed according to a complex formula based on the diagnostic severity of the patient caseload. Medicare's role in setting trends in health care reimbursement is detailed later in this chapter.

HEALTH INSURANCE TODAY

The 21st century promises to be an exciting era in American health care. Every day we read about advancements in the treatment and prevention of health threats. But the cost of today's health care remains a concern. Public programs such as Medicaid and Medicare must balance the need to provide high-quality health care against the need to keep tax burdens reasonable. Today, more than 18 percent, or 43.1 million, of Americans under the age of 65 lack health care coverage. A large percentage of the uninsured are members of working families. Yet low incomes and unavailability of employer-sponsored plans make health insurance beyond the reach of many Americans.

Health insurance is a means to guard against unexpected economic loss due to accidental or other catastrophic medical conditions. Health plans may sell individual coverage, group coverage, or both. Individual coverage is insurance that is purchased directly by an individual and may also cover family members. Group insurance is through an employer or other sponsor, such as a union or professional association. The group arranges for health coverage for its employees or members, often on a bid basis. The group sponsor generally determines the benefits offered to employees or members.. The choice of benefits may be limited or extensive.

PAYER COMPARISONS

The following section lists some of the larger private insurers, organization types, and government payers.

Blue Cross and Blue Shield Plans

Blue Cross was founded as a not-for-profit health organization to provide hospital insurance benefits. In most states, this plan has merged with its counterpart, Blue Shield, which offers physician services benefits. The Blue Cross/Blue Shield Association (BCBSA) is the oldest and largest group of health insurance companies in the country. The group has 47 independent, locally operated member companies in the 50 states, the District of Columbia, and Puerto Rico. Some have formed regional

 DEFINITIONS

Participating provider. A provider who has contracted with the health plan to deliver medical services to covered persons. The provider may be a physician, hospital, pharmacy, other facility, or other health care provider who has contractually accepted the terms and conditions set forth by the health plan. Also known as network or in-network provider.

groups. According to BCBSA, 25 percent of the U.S. population is covered by an association member.

Blue Cross/Blue Shield plans range from self-funded to fully insured. Self-funded plans are used by large corporations and other entities that have sufficient funds to underwrite their own health care needs. These companies hire a locally operated BCBS organization to manage the plan, process the claims, and negotiate physician contracts. Self-funded plans offer many advantages, including shields from many state regulations.

Fully insured plans involve the purchase of insurance from BCBS in addition to the plan management services previously mentioned. Employers choose from the variety of benefit options available from the local BCBS plan. Premium payments are adjusted accordingly, and include the financial responsibility of payment for covered claims.

Each BCBS plan differs in its corporate structure and policies. Some offer managed care through preferred provider organization (PPO) plans, health maintenance organization (HMO) plans, point of service (POS) plans, and traditional indemnity plans. Each company is an independent franchise of the association and a variety of insurance products are sold, including Medicare supplement, small business plans, and plans tailored to individuals. Some BCBS plans act as regional carriers—the contractors that manage and process Medicare Part B claims. And some serve as fiscal intermediaries—the contractors that manage and process Medicare Part A claims.

Health Maintenance Organizations

Managed care is a health care system that assumes both the financial risks and the delivery risks associated with providing comprehensive medical services to a voluntary enrolled population in a particular geographic area, usually in return for a fixed prepaid fee. The most common form of managed care is the health maintenance organizations (HMO) model. Generally speaking, HMOs may embrace many coverage issues and in varying degrees to manage the provision of health care to subscribers. A hallmark of this type of insurance model is a level of administrative control over patient access to specialty services. HMOs must follow pertinent requirements of the Public Health Service Act as well as other federal and state regulations.

Health Maintenance Organization Medicare

This structure is a type of Medicare managed care plan where a group of doctors, hospitals, and other health care providers agree to offer services to Medicare beneficiaries for a set amount of money every month. As in any HMO, all care is from providers of the plan.

Point of Service (POS) Plan

A point-of-service health plan allows the covered person to choose to receive a service from a participating or nonparticipating provider, with different benefit levels associated with the use of participating providers. Under a POS plan, a non-participating provider may bill the subscriber the deductible and a percentage of the remaining costs, up to a set limit. When the costs exceed the limit, the HMO assumes the remaining expenses.

Preferred Provider Organization (PPO)

A preferred provider organization (PPO) typically contracts on behalf of employer groups or other plans with hospital and physician providers at reduced rates. PPO providers have agreed to accept a specific negotiated amount as payment in full for

 KEY POINT

Three major categories for managed care:
- Health maintenance organizations (HMO)
- Preferred provider organizations (PPO)
- Point of service (POS) plans

 DEFINITIONS

Fee-for-service. A traditional type of reimbursement system that provides physicians and other health care providers with a payment that does not exceed the billed charge for each unit of service provided.

services provided to the patient. They generally bill the insurance plan directly and the plan pays them directly. The hospitals and physicians participating in the preferred provider network generally are called either preferred or participating providers. Usually, there is an incentive to the patient to use a preferred provider. A patient who visits a physician who is not a preferred provider likely will have to pay a higher co-payment or deductible for covered services. Providers offer discounts to PPOs in anticipation of achieving additional patient volumes or to minimize the chances that their patient volume will go to another provider. A PPO arrangement can be insured or self-funded.

Exclusive Provider Organizations (EPOs)

An exclusive provider organization (EPO) is a variation of a PPO. EPOs contract with providers on a discounted basis, but enrollees must receive care within the network (receive services only from network providers). EPOs, like PPOs, provide no penalties to providers if the patient opts to obtain care outside the network. Instead, the enrollee assumes responsibility for out-of-network costs.

Third-Party Administrator (TPA) and Administrative Services Organization (ASO)

TPAs and ASOs are neither health plans nor insurers, but organizations that provide claims paying functions for the clients they service. Many self-insured groups, such as employers and union trusts use third-party administrators (TPA) or administrative services organizations (ASO) to manage and pay their claims. In lieu of paying premiums to health insurers who would charge group premiums, these self-insured groups generally assume the risk of the provision of such services on their own, usually with some "stop loss" insurance. The self-insured group may contract directly with providers, and it may use the services of a PPO.

Fee-for-Service (FFS), Also Called 'Indemnity Plans'

This is a payment system in which the insurer either reimburses the group member or pays the provider directly for each covered medical expense after the expense has been incurred. Although many of these kinds of payers survive, they are not viewed as managed care organizations. Usually, the patient has assigned his or her benefits to the indemnity carrier, who in turn pays the provider directly. Many of the indemnity carriers have attempted to include PPO-like characteristics to reduce costs.

Medicare

The laws of the Medicare program are found in Title XVIII of the Social Security Act. The Centers for Medicare and Medicaid Services (CMS), established by the Department of Health and Human Services (HHS), is responsible for the implementation of all rules, regulations, and health related policies governing the Medicare program. Medicare is the largest public payer for health care.

The Medicare program consists of three parts. Part A (hospital insurance) covers inpatient care in hospitals, critical access hospital care, and skilled nursing facility care. It also covers hospice care, some home health care, and certain blood services. Part B (medical insurance) covers physician care, outpatient hospital care, and other related health services that Part A does not cover, such as some of the services of physical and occupational therapists, and some home health. Part B helps pay for covered services and supplies as deemed medically necessary. Part B is a voluntary program for which the beneficiary pays a monthly premium. Some persons reaching age 65 choose not to enroll in Medicare Part B. A third type of Medicare coverage, MedicareAdvantage (formerly Medicare +Choice) is a Medicare HMO.

 DEFINITIONS

Medically necessary. Services or supplies that:

- Are warranted for the diagnosis or treatment of a medical condition
- Are used for the diagnosis, direct care, and treatment of a medical condition
- Meet the standards of good medical practice in the local community
- Are not solely for the convenience of the patient or the doctor

Medicare coding varies for outpatient and inpatient services. Outpatient coding is based on ICD-9-CM diagnosis codes and the Healthcare Common Procedure Coding System (HCPCS), which includes the CPT coding system. Coding for inpatient Medicare services is based on ICD-9-CM diagnosis and procedures codes that combine to make up more than 500 diagnosis-related groups (DRG), which is Medicare's basis for payment of inpatient claims.

The Medicare program is addressed constantly throughout this book, since it is a major force in health care. In general, the program serves retired people over age 65, some people with disabilities under age 65, and patients with end-stage renal disease (permanent kidney failure requiring dialysis or transplant). Starting July 1, 2002, people younger than age 65 who have Lou Gehrig's disease (amyotrophic lateral sclerosis, or ALS) are eligible to receive Medicare benefits the first month that they receive disability form Social Security or the Railroad Retirement.

Medicare is mandated to pay for services deemed medically necessary and reasonable for the diagnosis and treatment of illness and injury. Medicare is not required to pay for noncovered and undocumented services.

Determining Medicare as Secondary Payer

Medicare is in many instances not the primary insurer of beneficiaries. Some beneficiaries who are 65 years or older have spouses whose employment coverage extends to a Medicare beneficiary. Certain automobile coverage can be the primary as well.

Medicare beneficiaries who receive Veterans Administration benefits will see the VA coverage as the primary payer. Workers' compensation coverage is also ordinarily primary over Medicare. Other situations may arise as well, and office personnel should review primary and secondary coverage issues.

Medigap coverage, discussed later in this chapter, is secondary to Medicare and pays after Medicare has paid its portion of the claim.

Medicaid

The federal and state governments jointly administer the Medicaid programs, which may also go by names such as Welfare, Title XIX, or Medi-Cal. Medicaid payers share certain characteristics: all are subject to the same federal guidelines; all have unique, individual guidelines for claims submissions; and each publishes a handbook that outlines and updates the Medicaid rules for that state. Medicaid helps pay medical costs for some people with limited incomes and resources. People with Medicaid may get coverage for nursing home care and outpatient prescription drugs that are not covered by Medicare. The Medicaid and Medicare programs are major sources of payment to nursing facilities.

Long-Term Care

Long-term care insurance is sold by private insurance companies and usually covers medical care and non-medical care to help with personal care needs, such as bathing, dressing, using the bathroom and eating. Generally, Medicare does not pay for long-term care. Medicare covers skilled nursing facility (SNF) care following a related three-day hospital stay. The benefit is usually limited to 100 days per benefit period. Medicaid pays for nursing homes for people who qualify for the program with limited income and resources.

Medigap (Medicare Supplement Insurance Policies)

Many Medicare beneficiaries purchase private supplemental insurance, commonly known as Medigap, to cover Medicare deductibles, coinsurance amounts, or

 FOR MORE INFO

For free booklets about Medicare and related topics: Call 1-800-MEDICARE (1-800-633-4227) 24 hours a day, including weekends.

Visit the website, www.cms.hhs.gov

 FOR MORE INFO

For more information about Medigap policies, call 1-800-Medicare (1-800-633-4227).

noncovered services of the program. A Medigap policy is a health insurance policy sold by a private insurance company to fill gaps in original Medicare plan coverage. Medigap policies must follow federal and state laws.

Medigap policies may be purchased individually from national organizations such as the American Association of Retired Persons (AARP), or from the last employer before retirement if offered.

TRICARE and TRICARE for Life

TRICARE, formerly known as CHAMPUS, provides health insurance benefits to military personnel (active and retired) and their dependents. TRICARE for life (TFL) includes expanded medical coverage for Medicare eligible retired members of the National Guard and Reserves. Medicare-eligible family members and widow/ widowers are also eligible, as are certain former spouses. TRICARE patients can seek medical care from nonmilitary providers.

Workers' Compensation

All states require workers' compensation benefits to provide medical and disability coverage for employees who are injured, contract an illness or disease, or become disabled as a result of their employment. In most states, employers voluntarily provide these benefits, but the criteria vary for mandatory coverage. Some states require employers to carry workers' compensation coverage only if they hire a certain number of people. A workers' compensation payer may contract with employers to offer a PPO type of contract for initial care of an injury or illness.

Employee or Union Health Coverage

Many large corporations, unions, or public employer groups have their own health coverage for employers (self-insured). A third party administrator might manage the program using the employer's funds.

Veterans Administration Benefits

The Veterans Health Administration (VHA) provides medical, surgical, and rehabilitative care to veterans. When veterans have commercial insurance, the VA can bill the private insurance carrier for services related to nonrated illnesses or injuries. A rated illness or injury is one determined to be a service-connected disability.

 FOR MORE INFO

U.S. Department of Veterans Affairs can be reached at 1-800-827-1000 for information about Veterans benefits and services. For more information visit the website www.va.gov

THE REIMBURSEMENT PROCESS

The above material offers just a thumbnail sketch of the major types of insurance plans circulating in the health care system. As you enter the field of medical coding, a familiarity develops with the policies and protocols of the major payers serving your physicians' patients. Some general rules apply to nearly all payers, however.

COVERAGE ISSUES

Insurers reimburse physicians only for covered services, and then only to the extent delineated by contract. Contractual language typically requires services to be medically necessary, established and effective, safe, and consistent with accepted medical standards. Furthermore, a service must be fully documented in the patient's medical record. The treating physician provides the documentation, which should contain evidence to support medical necessity of the service or procedure. A popular adage in medical reimbursement circles is that "if it isn't documented it didn't happen." Insurers simply won't pay for undocumented claim submissions.

PAYMENT METHODOLOGIES

Many years ago insurance companies simply paid patients or physicians for the billed cost of medical services. Payment, or fee-for-service as it is known, was based on an amount deemed "usual, customary, and reasonable" for a given service. Known as the UCR system, health providers were paid the lowest of:

- The provider's actual charge for the service
- The provider's customary charge during a defined time period
- The prevailing charge in the area

Medicare's payment system was similar and was referred to as "customary, prevailing, and reasonable." Essentially, under both Medicare and the private insurance systems physician services were reimbursed based on the physician's actual fees. Neither system made any attempt to reimburse physician services based on the work requirements and practice expense or cost of providing the medical care.

FEE SCHEDULES AND RELATIVE VALUES

However, as health care costs skyrocketed in the 1970s and 1980s, both government and private sector payers began evaluating alternative reimbursement methodologies. The UCR system was successfully challenged over time by a system of fee schedules. A fee schedule in its simplest form is a price list for medical services. Whether imposed by payers or negotiated between physician groups and payers, fee schedules have largely replaced the UCR system.

A concept closely linked to fee schedules is that of a relative value scale (RVS). Relative values of services are defined in terms of units, with more complex, more time-consuming services having higher unit values than less complex, less time-consuming services. Each individual medical service is assigned a particular number of relative value units (RVU) that indicates its value compared with a reference service. Furthermore, each service is compared with all other physician services so that each service is given a value that reflects its cost or value when compared with all other physician services.

By way of simplified example, a common medical service such as the treatment of strep throat is deemed the reference service and given the value 1. A group of medical experts will then evaluate another medical service, say heart bypass surgery, as being one hundred times more difficult than treatment of a sore throat. That surgery, then, is assigned a relative value of 100. A single layer laceration repair of the finger might have a value of 5, while an open reduction and internal fixation of a wrist fracture might have a value of 15. These values are directly related to the differing levels of complexity and the amount of time required to perform the procedures. In reality, considerations such as malpractice insurance and other overhead costs also go into the assignment of RVUs. This type of relative value system is known as "resource-based."

A monetary value is then assigned per relative value. In our simplified example, the assigned value is $36. Reimbursement for the sore throat visit then is $36 (1 x 36 = 36) and the finger laceration repair is $180 (5 x 36 = 180). Once again, in reality much more is involved in determining the relative value. But these are the basic mechanics of establishing a relative value fee schedule.

The most comprehensive effort devoted to the development of a resource-based relative value scale (RBRVS) was performed under federal contract by Harvard University. The result of the Harvard study is the Medicare physician fee schedule

 DEFINITIONS

Relative value scale (RVS). Ranking of all physician services based on the intensity of the procedure or service being performed. A relative value unit (RVU) is a specific value assigned to a procedure that is multiplied by a dollar conversion factor to determine a monetary value for the procedure.

DEFINITIONS

Health care services. Processes that contribute to the health and well-being of a patient. Services may be provided in a variety of health care settings including nursing, medical, surgical, or other health related services.

Inpatient. A patient who receives health care services and who is provided room, board, and continuous nursing service in a unit or area of the hospital.

Outpatient. A patient who receives care without being admitted for inpatient or resident care.

Patient. A patient is an individual who is receiving or who has received health care services. This could include a person who is deceased.

KEY POINT

Medicare Part A coverage includes inpatient hospital, skilled nursing facilities, hospice and home health. Most people do not have to pay for Part A.

Medicare Part B coverage provides payment for physician services provided in a variety of settings, including, but not limited to the physician office, an inpatient and outpatient hospital setting, and ambulatory surgery center.

FOR MORE INFO

For information about electronic claims, see http://www.cms.hhs.gov/hipaa/hipaa2/TCS Form Instructions.asp.

DEFINITIONS

Electronic data interchange (EDI). The transference of claims, certifications, quality assurance reviews, and utilization data via computer.

---

that has been in use since the early 1990s. Following the lead of Medicare, many private payers began using RVS fee schedules to reimburse physicians for their services.

CAPITATION

Another payment method is known as capitation. This system is designed for health care spending. Capitation contracts are often negotiated between certain payers and their high volume practices—oftentimes primary care practices. Generally, one primary care provider is designated the gatekeeper for a patient's overall management. Payment is based on a dollar amount per enrolled insurance subscriber. The amount does not vary according to the actual number of patients in the member population seen by the provider. Subsequently, health care in a capitated system depends on shared risk, or the ability to successfully manage a practice or a specialty clinic according to fees paid on this "per capita" basis.

As you can see, the system varies significantly from fee-for-service health plans. Under capitation, incentive depends upon providing quality care in the most appropriate and lowest cost setting, whereas incentives in a fee-for-service system depend on volume and number of procedures actually performed. More than 30 percent of HMOs reimburse physicians under capitation formulas.

INPATIENT AND AMBULATORY SYSTEMS

In this introduction to insurance we have noted that payers make a distinction between hospital insurance and coverage for physician services and procedures. Medicare services are divided into Part A for hospital coverage and Part B for physician services. The BCBSA originally was divided in much the same way.

Payment methodologies are also divided somewhat along these lines. Hospitals and certain other acute care settings, or inpatient facilities as they are known, are reimbursed according to a system known as DRGs. Developed by the federal government for Medicare purposes, the system assigns reimbursement to diagnoses that are grouped according to severity and similarity. Inpatient coding and DRGs are addressed in greater depth in chapters 6 and 7.

Along somewhat similar lines, the federal government has recently introduced a reimbursement system for a wide range of hospital facility services performed on an outpatient basis. This system reports services performed in specialty clinics operated by hospitals. Known as ambulatory payment classifications (APC), this aspect of medical coding is addressed in chapter 8, but readers should be clear on the distinction between various payment methodologies.

CLAIM SUBMISSION

As you will learn in the following chapters, medical codes are the communication link between health care providers and payers. Diseases and injuries, examinations and procedures, and medical equipment and supplies are all communicated by these codes.

Today, of course, much of this communication takes place digitally over computer links. Many claims are already submitted electronically.

In 1996, the Health Insurance Portability and Accountability Act (HIPAA) became law. It requires, among other things, that the HHS establish national standards for electronic health care transactions and code sets. October 16, 2002 was the original

---

deadline for covered entities to comply with these new national standards. However, the deadline for compliance with HIPAA electronic health care transactions and code sets standards was extended for most covered entities one year to October 16, 2003. The electronic formats currently used are 837i for institutional claims such as inpatient hospital services, and the 837p for professional claims such as physician services. Both formats incorporate elements that were previously contained in the paper versions of the billing formats.

It is increasingly difficult to submit paper claims to private insurance companies. The medical codes are transferred by means of a form. Known throughout the industry as the CMS-1500 (formerly HCFA-1500), this two-sided claim form was universal—it was used everywhere medical claims are submitted for reimbursement. The CMS-1500 was primarily used for Part B billing. The UB-92 was used for billing Part A services. In the future, the paper CMS form will be replaced with electronic submission of claims.

COMMON INSURANCE TERMINOLOGY

Accidental injury. An injury caused by an external force or element such as a blow or fall that requires immediate medical attention.

Admission. A registered inpatient, admitted for at least 24 hours, to a hospital, skilled nursing facility or other health care facility. The period of entry as an inpatient into a facility until discharge. In counting days of inpatient care, the date of entry and the date of discharge count as the same day.

Allowable costs. A predetermined amount allowed or paid for services rendered or supplies furnished, by any health care provider, which qualify as covered expenses.

Assignment. If the contracted provider accepts assignment, the provider agrees to accept the amount approved by the carrier as payment in full.

Calendar year. The inclusive period of time from January 1 of any year through December 31 of the same year.

Carrier. An entity that may underwrite, administer, or sell a range of health benefits programs. May also refer to an insurer or a managed health plan.

Coinsurance. The portion of covered health care costs the covered person is financially responsible for, usually according to a fixed percentage after a deductible requirement is met.

Copayment. A cost sharing arrangement in which a covered person pays a specific charge for a specified service, such as $10 for an office visit. The covered person usually is responsible for payment at the time the health care is rendered. Typical copayments are fixed or variable flat amounts for physician office visits, prescriptions, or hospital services.

Deductible. The amount of eligible expense a covered person must pay each year out of pocket before the plan will make payment for eligible services.

Group health coverage. Health care coverage that you are eligible for based on your employment, or your membership in or connection with a particular organization or group, that provides payment for medical services or supplies.

Lifetime maximum. The maximum amount insurance will pay on your behalf for covered services you received while you are enrolled.

QUICK TIP

A basic premise of medical coding is knowing the "par" or "non-par" status of the physicians you bill for. This pertains to Medicare as well as other major private payers. A par or participating provider in Medicare agrees to accept assignment: that is acceptance of the Medicare allowable as payment in full. Non-par or nonparticipating providers can bill the beneficiary for a balance over and above the Medicare amount. However, the provider must bill the beneficiary and accept the Medicare payment through the beneficiary, rather than directly through Medicare. The participation contracts are made on a yearly basis.

FRAUD AND ABUSE ISSUES

According to the insurance industry, the most common type of health insurance fraud involve false claim schemes. Billing false claims to obtain undeserved payment for services, procedures, and/or supplies that were not provided is a common tactic. Misrepresentation of provided services is another. Misrepresentation of diagnoses, and of patient identity are also used.

It is illegal to charge for a service that was not performed or to double bill for a service. Double billing is charging more than once for the same service. Resubmittal of charges with a different billing date is a common tactic.

Some provider offices intentionally "upcode," which means to charge a more complex service than was actually performed. In most instances this is considered an abusive practice. Upcoding also sometimes occurs inadvertently. Insurance investigators look closely for billing patterns that indicate a conscious effort to gain unearned reimbursement.

The National Health Care Anti-Fraud Association works in cooperation with several large insurance companies to develop computer systems that detect suspicious billing patterns. And federal legislation gives the U.S. Office of Inspector General (OIG) jurisdiction over private insurance plans as well as public ones.

Additional information pertaining to Medicare fraud and abuse is found in chapter 6.

SUMMARY

Whether you plan to work for a clinic-based health care provider, an insurance office, or a major inpatient facility, it is important to understand various types of health insurance plans. Insurance and reimbursement have become an important element in today's health care. A knowledge of its basic elements is essential to a successful medical coding career.

The following discussion questions and issues are for your consideration upon completion of this chapter. A full series of test questions on this chapter are found on the accompanying CD-ROM and in the instructor's manual.

DISCUSSION QUESTIONS

- Think about the nature of health insurance. How has it changed from your parent's time? Or your grandparent's time?
- Can you determine if a Medicare claim should be billed to a Medicare Part A Intermediary or Part B carrier? Can you determine when Medicare is the secondary insurer? Do you understand the difference between a participating and nonparticipating provider?
- Review in your mind the basic elements of a resource based relative value scale? Can you explain the key elements to a lay audience?
- Do you understand how poor coding practices can place a health care provider in legal jeopardy?

📖 DEFINITIONS

Miscoding. Using a code number that does not apply to the procedure.

Unbundling. (1) Breaking a single service into its multiple components to increase total billing charges. (2) Providers billing separately for health care services that should be combined according to industry standards or commonly accepted coding practices.

Upcoding. Provider billing for a procedure that reimburses more than the procedure actually performed.

Chapter 3: Coding Physician Services and Procedures

INTRODUCTION

As touched on in the previous chapter, insurance billing and reimbursement are key factors in health care and, for this reason, so is procedure coding. Procedure codes tell third-party payers what was provided during an encounter and let payers know what should be reimbursed. Known informally as CPT codes or procedure codes, this reporting system communicates the services of health care providers to the payers. Like the CMS-1500 or UB-92 claim form on which they are reported, the codes are common to practices and clinics all over the country.

CPT HISTORY

The *Physicians' Current Procedural Terminology* (CPT) coding system is a standardized system of five-digit codes with descriptive terms used to report the medical services and surgical procedures performed by physicians and other health care providers (e.g., nurse practitioners, physical therapists, and chiropractors). These services are known as professional services. In addition, CPT codes are used to report the technical or facility component of most outpatient services including laboratory, radiology, and same day surgery. The CPT coding system was developed and is updated annually and published in January by the American Medical Association (AMA) and includes procedures that are consistent with contemporary medical practice and reflective of new technology used by physicians in many locations. The CPT coding system codes communicate to other providers, patients, and mostly to payers, the procedures performed during a medical encounter.

For this reason, accurate coding is essential for proper reimbursement from third party payers (insurance companies, Medicare, Medicaid) and for compliance with government regulations.

Prior to 1966, no uniform coding system existed to report physician services performed in the outpatient setting. Insurance companies developed their own coding systems for tracking physician services and procedures. The first edition of the CPT code book was published by the AMA in 1966 as a companion piece to *Current Medical Terminology (CMT)*, a manual of preferred medical nomenclature, then in its third edition, to establish a uniform reporting method for physician services and procedures. The pocket-sized first edition of the CPT book (5 x 7 inches, 163 pages) contained a listing of four-digit codes and brief descriptions to report a full range of medical procedures and services. Each code was cross-referenced to then-available diagnosis codes, which were the *Standard Nomenclature of Diseases and Operations (SNDO)* and the *International Classification of Diseases, Adapted (ICDA)*. Editors of the first edition cited a variety of sources in developing the work, including the Social Security Administration, the Blue Shield Manual of Statistical Requirements, and the Relative Value Studies of the California Medical Society. The four-digit codes did not approximate those of today's CPT book.

 OBJECTIVES

In this chapter, you will learn:
- About the coding sets and practices used in the physician offices
- The basics of coding
- About the physician billing operation

 KEY POINT

The "technical" component reflects the resources such as the cost of equipment, technician salaries, treatment rooms, supplies and the utilities in support of professional services.

CODING AXIOM

Guidelines are used throughout the CPT book to provide definitions and direction for appropriate use of the codes for each section.

Modifiers are used to report that a procedure or service has been altered in some way, but not enough to change the basic code definition.

KEY POINT

CPT codes are also known as HCPCS Level I codes.

QUICK TIP

HCPCS Level III codes, assigned by local carriers, were eliminated December 31, 2003, as part of the Health Insurance Portability and Accountability Act (HIPAA) of 1996.

KEY POINT

Category III codes were included in the 2002 edition of the CPT code book as temporary codes to report emerging technologies.

The 1970 second edition of the CPT book marked the genesis of the coding manual familiar to today's medical office workers. Many of the five-digit codes and expanded descriptions in this work remain unchanged to this day. The number of codes far exceeded those available to users of the first edition. The second edition was developed with assistance from a handful of members of medical professional societies, a practice that would evolve into today's 100-member CPT Advisory Committee.

The third edition of the CPT book was first published in 1973 and offered new features such as alphabetic modifiers and starred procedures marked with an asterisk. Deleted codes (but not new codes) could be found in an appendix. This edition also saw the medical codes moved to the front of the code listings, a benchmark that would stand for almost 20 years until the introduction of the Evaluation and Management codes in 1992.

The fourth edition of the CPT book, published in 1977, began the custom of significant yearly revisions, usually concentrated within a small number of sections. Since then, medical office coders across the country have made an annual ritual of analyzing the code changes and their related effects on coding and billing for their practices.

Before 1983 only private insurance groups used the CPT coding system to report physician services and procedures. Medicare also determined a need for a procedural coding system, one which would also feature a coding system for supplies and non-physician services. The federal agency in charge of Medicare, the Department of Health and Human Services, developed HCPCS, or Healthcare Common Procedure Coding System in that year. Medicare's system adopted the already established CPT coding system to assign codes for physician services and procedures. The CPT coding system then became the first level (Level I) of this new HCPCS coding system.

The second level of HCPCS (Level II) is a national coding system to describe supplies, certain drugs, ambulance and nonphysician services not usually contained in the CPT code book. These codes are developed by Centers for Medicare and Medicaid Services (CMS) and take precedence over Level I or CPT codes for Medicare and Medicaid billing. Although created by CMS, the codes are widely accepted by other third party payers.

The HCPCS system and volume 3 of the *International Classification of Diseases, Ninth Revision, Clinical Modification (ICD-9-CM)* (see chapter 7) are the only medical procedure coding sets used throughout the United States. Volume 3 of ICD-9-CM is used by hospitals for coding inpatient services and HCPCS is used for coding health care practitioner procedures and services in all settings.

The fourth edition of the CPT code book is the current tool to report physician services and procedures. The AMA recently developed a fifth edition and its implementation is currently underway. A new level of CPT codes were introduced with the 2002 edition of the CPT code book. Those codes, known as category III codes, were included as temporary codes for use with emerging technologies, services, and procedures.

WHO USES CPT CODES?

CPT codes are mandated by federal standards as a national code set. In fact, Medicare and state Medicaid carriers are required by law to use these codes for the payment of health insurance claims. And almost all commercial insurance payers process claims using CPT codes.

Although required by most insurance companies, the mere existence of a CPT procedure code does not imply coverage under any given insurance plan. In other words, just because there is a CPT code for a medical procedure or service does not mean that a payer is obligated to reimburse physicians for the service.

DOCUMENTATION AND THE CPT CODE BOOK: REVIEWING THE SOURCE DOCUMENT

Documentation and communication are two vital links in the CPT coding system. The coder must rely on the physician, nursing staff, medical assistants, and/or the office manager to provide complete and legible facts. If the information is unclear or illegible, the coder should verify services or procedures performed with the appropriate staff member before attempting to select codes. Questionable information can result in inaccurate claim submission as well as denied or delayed payment to the practice.

The coder first reviews the source document to identify all physician and nonphysician services and to determine the need for modifiers due to services differing from standard practices or special circumstances. Many types of source documents (e.g., medical records, encounter forms, superbills, operative reports, etc.) are used to identify a patient's diagnosis and the services provided. The operative report shown on the next page is an example of a document for coding. The source document furnishes information such as the diagnosis and the procedural statement. The procedural statement is the first step toward assignment of a CPT code.

The difficulty in coding a procedure exists when the terminology contained in the medical record does not match the descriptions in the CPT book, or when the procedure cannot be found.

Understanding the definitions of medical terms and the intricacies of the coding system allows any procedure or service to be coded. If you cannot locate the procedure in the CPT book, do not assume that a code does not exist. It may be just a matter of tracking down the clues.

For example, the physician documents the procedure as "core decompression, right hip." The index does not list core decompression or decompression of the hip. An understanding of the procedure helps in coding. Core decompression of the hip involves drilling a hole into the femoral head to allow drainage of fluid from the bone, usually due to infection. To locate the appropriate code, look under the main term "hip," subterms "bone" and "drainage." Turn to the musculoskeletal subsection to review the code. The appropriate code is 26992 Incision, bone cortex, pelvis and/or hip joint (e.g., osteomyelitis or bone abscess).

Consult a physician, nurse, or published medical resource to determine the meaning of unfamiliar terms. To ignore terms that you do not understand could reduce coding accuracy.

A sample operative report is included here to demonstrate the link between documentation and the assignment of the correct code. Read the following operative report and note all the key words that have been underlined.

 KEY POINT

Consult a physician, nurse, or published medical resource to determine the meaning of unfamiliar terms.

Example:

Operative Report

Preoperative Diagnosis: <u>Occluded thrombosed arteriovenous</u> (AV) fistula, left forearm, and chronic renal failure.

Postoperative Diagnosis: Same

Operation(s): <u>Fogarty thrombectomy of Gor-Tex fistula</u>, left forearm, and <u>revision of the venous end</u>.

Description of Operation: With the patient on the operating table in the supine position after adequate axillary block anesthesia had been administered, his left forearm and upper arm were sterilely prepared and draped in the usual fashion.

An incision was made through the old incision just distal to the antecubital fossa and carried through skin and subcutaneous tissue. Hemostasis was obtained with electrocautery. The venous and arterial ends of the graft were exposed. The venous end appeared to be occluded from thrombosed vein. There was another excellent basilic vein medial to it and quite large. This was a branch going off laterally.

The venous end of the graft was transected and no bleeding was seen from the venous end, and the vein was totally thrombosed. The entire portion of the <u>graft</u> connected to this vein <u>was removed</u> and the <u>veins ligated</u> with stick ties of 4-0 Prolene suture. The <u>graft was thrombectomized</u> with the 4 Fogarty catheter and the <u>arterial line thrombectomized</u> with excellent inbleeding into the graft. The graft was injected with heparinized saline solution and the vascular clamp applied. The basilic vein was dissected proximally towards the distal end of the forearm and surgeon was able to get plenty of vein <u>to anastomose it end-to-end to the existing graft</u>. The <u>vein was ligated</u> with 2-0 silk suture distally and transected; there was a valve right at this area. The valve was removed under direct vision and the vein spatulated to fit to the 6 mm. <u>Gor-Tex graft</u> and it was anastomosed to it with a running suture of 6-0 Gor-Tex. The clamp was removed with an excellent thrill palpable and excellent flow through the graft. No leaks were seen.

The wound was irrigated with antibiotic solution and subcutaneous tissue closed with running suture of 3-0 Vicryl and the skin with a running subcuticular suture of 4-0 Dexon. Steri strips were applied and sterile dressing applied. The patient went to the recovery room in stable condition. He tolerated the procedure well. He was given Phenaphen #3 one to two every four to six hours as needed for pain and to return in two weeks for follow-up evaluation.

The description of the procedure performed is thrombectomy of a Gor-Tex fistula with a revision of the venous end. The key terms are anastomosis, thrombectomy, fistula, and revision. Locate the term anastomosis in the index. Arteriovenous fistula is the first subterm under anastomosis and the coder is directed to codes 36819, 36820, 36821, 36825–36830, and 36832–36833. Review the codes and narratives in the in the tabular listing of the CPT book.

Code 36822 is used for insertion of cannula for prolonged extracorporeal circulation. The medical record does not support the use of this code. The next code selection might be 36825–36830. These codes are used for creation of the arteriovenous fistula. Since the record indicates revision of an AV fistula, these codes are not the appropriate choice.

Now review codes 36832 and 36833. The narratives of these codes indicate a revision of the arteriovenous fistula, with or without thrombectomy, autogenous graft or nonautogenous graft. The narrative of code 36833 contains all the key words pulled directly from the medical record. Documentation supports this code choice.

CPT CONVENTIONS

Understanding the complex procedure coding process begins with a careful study of the CPT manual introduction. Understanding the format of the text and its support tools ensures accurate coding, which in turn streamlines claims processing. Essential

---

📖 DEFINITIONS

Specialist in medicine. Generally a physician who has had advanced training (residency years, fellowships, etc.) in one or more clinical areas of practice (e.g., cardiology, or the study of the cardiovascular system).

A cardiologist (usually an internist with specialized advanced training) is a physician who practices cardiology.

information found in the CPT code book introduction includes formatting and guidelines.

The listing of a service or procedure and its code number in a specific section of the CPT book does not restrict its use to a specific specialty group. For example, a cardiologist may use codes from the medicine section and not just those codes from the cardiology section. Any service or procedure code may be used to designate the services rendered by any qualified physician or other healthcare provider.

Organization of the CPT code book is arranged in eight major sections as follows:

- Evaluation and management (99201–99499)
- Anesthesiology (00100–01999, 99100–99140)
- Surgery (10021–69990)
- Radiology (including nuclear medicine, radiation oncology, and diagnostic ultrasound) (70010–79999)
- Pathology and laboratory (80048–89399)
- Medicine, except anesthesiology (90281–99199, 99500–99600)
- Category II Codes (0001F–0011F)
- Category III Codes (0001T–0044T)

The sections are organized in numeric order. The E/M section is located at the beginning of the CPT book. Other than this section, the book is in numeric order. The first six major sections of the CPT book are further arranged in subsections. Subsections pertaining to a section are listed within the section guidelines. For example, the radiology subsections are:

- Diagnostic imaging
- Diagnostic ultrasound
- Radiation oncology
- Nuclear medicine

Following the medicine section of the CPT book are the new sections "Category II Codes and Category III Codes." These codes are easily identified as four numbers and the letter F or T, keeping with the five-digit format of CPT codes. Six appendixes follow the Category III codes:

- Appendix A—Modifiers
- Appendix B—Summary of Additions, Deletions, and Revisions
- Appendix C—Clinical Examples
- Appendix D—Summary of CPT Add-on Codes
- Appendix E—Summary of CPT Codes Exempt from Modifier 51

The CPT book's printed format has been designed to save space because many of the codes within a given section have a common procedure description with only a partial difference in the code definition. For example, as seen below, 50610 and 50620 share the common description of "Ureterolithotomy." The difference between the codes is that 50610 reports the "upper one-third of ureter," while 50620 is for the "middle one-third of ureter."

The key to interpret these codes correctly is the semicolon (;) in 50610. The semicolon separates the common portion of the description from the portion unique to that code. Whenever a code is indented, you must always refer to the preceding nonindented code for the common portion of the description. Thus, the indented

KEY POINT

The key to interpreting CPT code descriptions is the semicolon (;), which separates the common portion of the description from the portion unique to that procedure. Always refer to the preceding nonindented code for the common portion of the description when reporting an indented CPT code.

code 50620 does not repeat the common portion (that part immediately before the semicolon), but instead supplies its own unique information. Use caution when locating the common portion for the set of indented codes you are referencing. Some of the indentations pass from page to page but are always indented below the code for which there is a common portion.

50610   Ureterolithotomy; upper one-third of ureter
50620   middle one-third of ureter

The complete description of 50620 is: *Ureterolithotomy; middle one-third of ureter.*

✓ **QUICK TIP**

Each guideline must be reviewed to obtain a complete understanding of the proper use of the codes listed in the section.

GUIDELINES

Guidelines appear at the beginning of each of the eight major sections of the CPT book. The information contained in the guidelines provides definitions, explanations of terms, and section specific instructions. Each guideline must be reviewed to obtain a complete understanding of the proper use of the codes listed in the section. Generally, information listed in the guidelines is not repeated within the section, subsection, or within the code range. For example, the anesthesia section guidelines provide information about time reporting for anesthesia services.

Example:
   "Anesthesia time begins when the anesthesiologist begins to prepare the patient for the induction of anesthesia in the operating room or in an equivalent area and ends when the anesthesiologist is no longer in personal attendance, that is, when the patient may be safely placed under postoperative supervision."

Guidelines also appear at the beginning of subsections located within the major sections of the CPT code book and provide information unique to a particular range of codes. Guidelines are also found within the code ranges in a subsection. Information specific to a given code may be included as a parenthetical phrase following the code. Revised text in guidelines, notes, and parenthetical phrases is enclosed by "▶◀" symbols. For example, below code 76831 is a parenthetical phrase:

(For radiologic supervision and interpretation for transcatheter placement of extracranial ▶vertebral or intrathoracic carotid◀ artery stent(s), ▶use◀ Category III codes ▶0075T, 0076T◀)

When a code has been deleted, information specific to that code or range of codes may be included as a parenthetical phrase in code number order. The parenthetical phrase may also contain directions on where to go to find the correct code. For example:

▶(91032 and 91033 have been deleted. To report, see 91034, 91035)◀

●91034   Esophagus, gastroesophageal reflux test; with nasal catheter pH electrode(s) placement, recording, analysis and interpretation

The CPT book has many features to add ease to code selection. The top of each page contains a reference in the far left or far right corner for the codes listed on that particular page as well as the heading for the section and subsection.

The bottom portion of the page contains a reference for the commonly used symbols in the CPT code book such as the "▶◀" symbols for new or revised text.

CODE CHANGES

In order to stay current with the advances in medicine, the AMA's CPT Editorial Panel reviews the coding system and makes periodic changes to codes and their descriptions. These changes are posted on the AMA's website with the date these code changes are effective. Most code changes by the AMA occur annually and are effective January 1 of each year. The panel accepts information and feedback from providers about new codes and revisions to existing codes that could better reflect the service or procedure being provided. Appendix B consists of a summary of additions, deletions, and revisions to the current edition. Of these three types of changes, only summary descriptions of new codes appear in appendix B, making it necessary to refer to the main body of the CPT book for the full narrative description. Since code narrative changes (changes to the text) state only that the terminology has been revised, you must compare the new edition to the previous one to identify how the code descriptions have been changed. In most instances where only placement of the semicolon or other punctuation has changed, the description will read "grammatical change" only.

New codes are identified by a solid circle.

● 43644   Laparoscopy, surgical, gastric restrictive procedure; with gastric bypass and Roux-en-Y gastroenterostomy (roux limb 150 cm or less)

Revised codes are identified by a solid triangle.

▲ 19160   Mastectomy, partial (eg, lumpectomy, tylectomy, quadrantectomy, segmentectomy);

Deleted codes, when noted, are enclosed within parentheses.

(89350 has been deleted. To report, use 89220)

Codes with minor grammatical changes are not identified in the CPT code book with a symbol, but are identified in appendix B.

MODIFIERS

Modifiers, introduced in the third edition of the CPT book, allow coders to indicate that a service was altered in some way from the stated CPT code description, without actually changing the basic definition of the service. This 1973 addition to the CPT book provided an easy-to-use variable to coding.

The definitions as well as changes to modifiers can be found in appendix A. In addition, those modifiers related to the multiple procedures can be found in the surgery guidelines. Appendix A is divided into two sections. Modifiers for physician services are listed first and titled simply "Modifiers." Modifiers approved for ambulatory surgery center (ASC) hospital outpatient use are listed second and are divided into two subsections: CPT Level I modifiers and Level II (HCPCS/national) modifiers.

Modifiers can be reported in one way only. They must be appended to a CPT code, as in 15000-22.

The following is a sample from the CMS-1500 paper claims submission form.

QUICK TIP

CPT, ICD-9-CM, and HCPCS Level II codes are updated on a yearly basis. It is important to use only the most current version for accurate coding.

CODING AXIOM

Modifiers should be used to indicate that a service or procedure performed differs somewhat from the basic definition of the service.

21. DIAGNOSIS OR NATURE OF ILLNESS OR INJURY (RELATE ITEMS 1, 2, 3 OR 4 TO ITEM 24E BY LINE)

1 | 574.20   3 |___ ___

2 | 278.01   4 |___ ___

24.		A						B	C	D		E
		DATE(S) OF SERVICE						Place of Service	Type of Service	PROCEDURES, SERVICES, OR SUPPLIES (Explain Unusual Circumstances)		DIAGNOSIS CODE
	From			To						CPT / HCPCS	MODIFIER	
MM	DD	YY	MM	DD	YY							
03	02	2003	03	02	2003			21		47605	22 LT	1,2

25. FEDERAL TAX I.D. NUMBER   SSN   EIN   26. PATIENT'S ACCOUNT NO.   27. ACCEPT ASSIGNMENT? (For govt. claims, see back)   YES   NO

FOR MORE INFO

Consult *Ingenix Coding Lab: Understanding Modifiers*. This product explains modifiers in more detail and includes decision trees for their usage.

MODIFIER IMPACT ON REIMBURSEMENT

As mentioned earlier, modifiers communicate information to the payer about the procedure or service performed. For this reason, proper use of modifiers may affect reimbursement. Modifiers can indicate the following:

- A service or procedure represents only a professional component
- A service or procedure was performed by more than one physician
- Only part of a service was performed
- An adjunctive service was performed
- A bilateral procedure was performed
- A service or procedure was provided more than once
- Unusual events occurred
- A procedure or service was altered in some way

Always stay current on the latest guidelines for modifiers; and, it is equally important to be familiar with federal and commercial payer guidelines.

Some modifiers affect how a third-party will look at your claim for reimbursement, allowing, in most instances, additional reimbursement for properly placed modifiers. It is also possible to use multiple modifiers to provide information on one procedure. Modifiers that affect reimbursement should always be sequenced before other modifiers that are informational in nature when applied to the same CPT code. For instance, the use of modifier 22 Unusual procedural services, prompts additional reimbursement, whereas modifier LT Left side, used to indicate procedures performed on the left side of the body, is informational and does not affect reimbursement. Therefore, modifier 22 is placed in front of modifier LT on the claim form (block 24D of the claim form above).

Modifiers that usually affect reimbursement include the following:

21   Prolonged evaluation and management services

22   Unusual procedural services

26	Professional component
27	Multiple outpatient hospital E/M encounters on the same date
50	Bilateral procedure
51	Multiple procedures
52	Reduced services
53	Discontinued procedure
54	Surgical care only
55	Postoperative management only
56	Preoperative management only
57	Decision for surgery
58	Staged or related procedure or service by the same physician during the postoperative period
59	Distinct procedural service
62	Two surgeons
66	Surgical team
73	Discontinued outpatient hospital/ambulatory surgery center procedure prior to the administration of anesthesia
74	Discontinued outpatient hospital/ambulatory surgery center procedure after administration of anesthesia
78	Return to the operating room for a related procedure during the postoperative period
79	Return to the operating room for an unrelated procedure during the postoperative period
80	Assistant surgeon
81	Minimum assistant surgeon
82	Assistant surgeon (when qualified resident surgeon not available)
91	Repeat clinical diagnostic laboratory test

Appendix A in the CPT code book includes the list of modifiers that are approved for ASC hospital outpatient use. Modifiers were required on Medicare ASC hospital outpatient claims beginning July 1, 1998.

QUICK TIP

Modifiers can greatly affect reimbursement for a facility through coding policies that routinely use appropriate modifiers. Protocols that miss proper application of modifiers can cost a facility many thousands of dollars over the course of only several months.

ADD-ON AND MODIFIER 51 EXEMPT CODES

Icons preceding CPT codes in the CPT book specifically identify two types of services for which special coding rules apply. Add-on procedures are identified with a **+** prior to the five-digit procedure code. This **+** identifies services that are always performed with another service or procedure. In other words, add-on procedures are always secondary procedures and should never be reported alone. However, unlike other secondary procedures, add-on procedures are never appended with modifier 51. In addition to adding the icon, the CPT book has standardized the terminology related to add-on procedures. All add-on procedures include the parenthetical statement (list separately in addition to code for primary procedure) as part of the procedure description.

Modifier 51 exempt procedures are similar to add-on procedures and are designated with a ⊘. Modifier 51 exempt procedures may be reported alone, but are usually components of a larger service. Modifier 51 exempt procedures include secondary services that are directly related to the primary procedure.

CODING AXIOM

Add-on codes are exempt from the multiple procedure concept. No multiple procedure modifiers are necessary.

UNLISTED PROCEDURES

The first six sections of the CPT book (i.e., evaluation and management, anesthesiology, surgery, radiology, pathology and laboratory, and medicine) contain unlisted procedure codes. Use these codes when the procedure or service is not adequately described by an existing CPT code or a CPT procedure code with modifier. Select the unlisted procedure code from the appropriate section, subsection, or heading. For example, a procedure on the elbow that cannot be reported with an existing CPT code or combination of codes is reported with 24999 Unlisted procedure, humerus or elbow. Note that each section of the CPT code book contains multiple unlisted procedures codes. All unlisted codes may be found in the alphabetical index under "unlisted services and procedures."

With the implementation of Category II and III codes in the CPT manual, the use of unlisted codes has changed slightly. Coders must know the Category II and III codes and use a code from one of these sections if applicable instead of a Category I unlisted code. The unlisted codes do not offer specific information for data collection and the use of Category II or III codes include specifics for tracking, performance measurements, new emerging technology services and procedures.

THE CPT CODE BOOK INDEX

The alphabetic index is the starting point of all coding from the CPT book, but do not select codes solely based on information in the index—it is only a reference to the full listing of codes. Proper use of the CPT code book index is important to locate the appropriate code. Once the code is located, look it up in the appropriate section.

The CPT code book index provides a specific code, or range of codes, for procedures and services listed by main term alone, or a main term and up to three modifying terms. Main terms, or locators, are printed in boldface for easier and quicker access.

The index is set up to allow users to locate codes using various methods and to look up procedures or services using main terms. There are four basic methods to locate the codes:

- The main term that describes the procedure performed.
  Example: Appendectomy
- The body part or site where the procedure occurred.
  Example: Knee
- The condition that was treated.
  Example: Abscess
- Using synonyms, acronyms, or eponyms.
  Example: Bucca (*See* cheek), Barr Procedure (*See* Tendon, Transfer, Leg, Lower), BAER (*See* Evoked Potential, Auditory Brainstem)

The CPT book provides cross-references as instruction to the user to locate codes under a different main term. These cross references are of two types. The word "see" is used primarily for synonyms, eponyms, and abbreviations. The cross reference "see also" is used primarily to instruct the coder to locate a subterm under a different main term, if the term is not listed as a subterm under the current main term. An example is the main term "Collar Bone."

A review of the index is recommended in order to gain a familiarity with its setup. Once you have located the term, you will find a code, multiple codes, or range of codes. For example:

Bricker Procedure — 50820 (single code)

Frenotomy — 40806, 41010 (multiple codes)

Insemination — 58321–58322, 89268 (range of codes)

Once the code(s) are located, the next step is to look up the code in the appropriate section of the CPT code book. As we indicated, the codes are in numeric order, except for the E/M codes which are located in the front of the book for easy reference. Never assign a code from the index because there may be notes in the section or guidelines about appropriate use of the codes that are not available in the index.

Not all services included in some sections are listed in the index. If a procedure cannot be found in the index, turn to the appropriate section and review the subsections, headings, subheadings, and codes.

When locating the code take notice of any section guidelines or notes applicable to the code. Be careful to note that some of the guidelines and notes that pertain to a particular code are not always located directly above or below the code itself, but may be located above or below a section of codes. For example:

Notes pertaining to code 63081 are located below code 63091.

Instructional notes for diagnostic laparascopy (49320) are located above procedure code 43280.

THE 10 STEPS TO BASIC CPT CODING

When referencing the CPT code book, follow the 10 basic steps to ensure accurate and complete coding:

Step 1: Read the source document and code only from the information listed. Never assume any additional information. Review the chart note or operative report closely when selecting procedures to be coded.

Step 2: Using the information from the record, next analyze the procedure statement provided by the physician. Identify the main term and modifying terms (if applicable) for the procedure to be coded.

Step 3: Locate the main term in the CPT code book index. Main terms can be.

- The procedure performed
- The procedure's abbreviation
- The organ or anatomical site
- The condition or diagnosis
- A synonym for the main term
- An eponym

Step 4: Look for subterms indented below the main term.

Step 5: Jot down the tentative code or range of codes for each procedure. Entries in the CPT code book index provide a single code, two or more codes separated by a comma, or a range of codes to the right of the main term. Any code(s) identified should be considered tentative until checked in the appropriate section (e.g., medicine, surgery, etc.).

Step 6: Locate each tentative code in the appropriate section of the code book.

- When the tentative code is a single code, read its description carefully to make sure it accurately describes the service or procedure.
- When the tentative code is within a range of codes, read the descriptions for each code in the range, and then choose the one that most accurately describes the service or procedure.

Step 7: Read any instructional notes, and watch for diagnoses or specific procedures within code descriptions.

Step 8: Verify that the code matches the procedure statement provided in the record.

Step 9: Assign the code.

Step 10: If necessary, assign a modifier to the code.

This section provided instruction and general information needed to understand the basics of the CPT coding system. The following sections build on those basics and offer additional coding tips for each section of the CPT book.

EVALUATION AND MANAGEMENT SERVICES

The first section of the CPT code book is the evaluation and management (E/M) section. This section contains the codes applicable to all services commonly refered to as "visits," such as office or hospital level of service codes, hospital observation services, consultations, emergency department services, critical care services, neonatal intensive care, nursing facility services, custodial care services, home services, case management services, preventive medicine services, counseling, and/or risk factor reduction services, or newborn care.

The classification system for E/M services is first divided by place of service. Most main categories are further subdivided by type of patient and type of service.

Example:

    Hospital Inpatient Services
     Initial Hospital Care
     Subsequent Hospital Care
     Hospital Discharge Services

    Consultations
     Office or Other Outpatient Consultations
      New or Established Patient
     Initial Inpatient Consultation
      New or Established Patient
     Follow-up Inpatient Consultations

Because these codes represent the services most frequently performed by physicians (e.g., office, emergency department, inpatient visits), they have been placed, for convenience, at the beginning of the book.

Understanding how to correctly report E/M services is very important. Although E/M codes are not the most revenue intensive code set, they account for significant

KEY POINT

E/M codes were added in 1992 to provide definition to visits and to the different levels of service.

dollars for a practice because of the volume of these services (such as daily office visits).

E/M codes have been part of the CPT coding system since 1992, the year the codes were introduced to clarify documentation of these types of services. The codes were jointly developed by the AMA and the Centers for Medicare and Medicaid Services (CMS). The AMA holds copyright to the E/M codes and their descriptions, however.

The E/M codes are designed to standardize the way providers and medical coders report patient visits. The AMA and CMS have, over time, developed guidelines for the use of E/M codes. These guidelines supplement information already found in the CPT book and are summarized here.

E/M SERVICE GUIDELINES

Guidelines for E/M services are presented in the same arrangement as in other sections of the CPT code book. They are found at the beginning of the section and continue through many of the categories and subcategories. The guidelines are directions on how the codes within the section should be used and interpreted.

The E/M section is outlined below for ease of reference. Look at the sections in your CPT book to familiarize yourself with their location and applicable guidelines.

Office or Other Outpatient Services
New patient, 99201–99205

Established patient, 99211–99215

Hospital/Observation Services
Observation care discharge services, 99217

Initial observation care, 99218–99220

Hospital Inpatient Services
Initial hospital care—New or established patient, 99221–99223

Subsequent hospital care, 99231–99233

Observation or inpatient care services (including admission and discharge services), 99234–99236

Hospital discharge services, 99238–99239

Consultations
Office or other outpatient consultations, 99241–99245

Initial inpatient consultations—new or established patient, 99251–99255

Follow-up inpatient consultations—established patient, 99261–99263

Confirmatory consultations—new or established patient, 99271–99275

Emergency Department Services
New or established patient, 99281–99285

Other emergency services, 99288

KEY POINT

The E/M codes were jointly developed by the AMA and the CMS.

Pediatric Critical Care Patient Transport, 99289–99290

Critical Care Services, 99291–99292

Inpatient Neonatal and Pediatric Critical Care Services
Inpatient pediatric critical care, 99293–99294

Inpatient neonatal critical care, 99295–99296

Intensive (non-critical) low birth weight services, 99298–99299

Nursing Facility Services
Comprehensive nursing facility assessments—new or established patient, 99301–99303

Subsequent nursing facility care—new or established patient, 99311–99313

Nursing facility discharge services, 99315–99316

Domiciliary, rest home (e.g., boarding home) or custodial care services

New patient, 99321–99323

Established patient, 99331–99333

Home Services
New patient, 99341–99345

Established patient, 99347–99350

Prolonged Services
With direct patient contact, 99354–99357

Without direct patient contact, 99358–99359

Standby services, 99360

Case Management Services
Team conferences, 99361–99362

Telephone calls, 99371–99373

Care Plan Oversight Services, 99374–99380

Preventive Medicine Services
New patient, 99381–99387

Established patient, 99391–99397

Preventive medicine, individual counseling, 99401–99404

Preventive medicine, group counseling, 99411–99412

Preventive medicine, other, 99420–99429

Newborn care, 99431–99440

Special E/M Services
Basic life and/or disability evaluation services, 99450

Work related or medical disability evaluation services, 99455–99456

Other E/M services, 99499 (unlisted)

EVALUATION AND MANAGEMENT SERVICE LEVELS

E/M services within subcategories are arranged in levels, each with the same basic format:

- Place and/or type of service (hospital or newborn care, for example)
- A unique code with its definition
- Service content required by the code (what the physician has to do to use the code)
- A discussion about what constitutes counseling or coordination of care
- The severity (nature) of the presenting problem.
- Time (this is the typical time a visit of this level might take)

SELECTING A VISIT CODE

The key components in determining the correct level of E/M codes are 1) the history, which is the patient's account of the present illness or injury, the patient's past medical, social, and family history, as well as a review of the patient's body systems; 2) the examination, which includes a personal examination by the physician, as well as review of other data, such as x-rays or lab information, that provide the physician with an assessment of the patient's physical condition; and 3) the medical decision making, which is the assessment based on the history and examination as well as the plan for how to care for the patient's illness or injury, or even a plan for further assessment before determining the patient's status.

The E/M services are based on the intensity or complexity of the key components provided to the patient during an encounter. The CPT manual also includes the typical (average) time for some of the levels of service code descriptors. The indication of time should only be used as a supplementary factor to assist physicians and their staff in assigning the appropriate level of service. It is important to remember that time is not a key factor in determining code assignment, unless counseling or coordination of care accounts for more than 50 percent of face to face time spent with the patient and/or family.

To select the appropriate level of service, the coder must take the appropriate steps. First, determine the type of service provided (i.e., office, inpatient hospital, emergency department visit) and select the appropriate category, or subcategory, from the CPT manual. Second, read the guidelines found at the beginning of the subcategory to determine what special guidelines, if any, apply to that subcategory of E/M codes. Then determine the complexity of the medical decision making the service requires, the extent of the history obtained and the examination performed. The section guidelines contain information to help select the appropriate level. Review the code narratives in the appropriate category and subcategory. Each narrative includes the specific criteria that must be met or exceeded if the code is to be assigned. Finally, using the instructions in the code narratives, select the code that matches the levels of history, examination, and medical decision making involved.

NEW AND ESTABLISHED PATIENT SERVICES

Several code subcategories in the E/M section are based on the patient's status as either new or established. CPT code book guidelines clarify this distinction by providing the following time references:

CODING AXIOM

The level of E/M codes are determined according to the extent of the service provided for each key component, the history, examination, and medical decision making.

DEFINITIONS

CPT code:
99202   Office or other outpatient visit for the evaluation and management of a new patient, which requires these three key components:
An expanded problem-focused history;
An expanded problem-focused examination; and
straightforward medical decision making

DEFINITIONS

Group practice. Consists of a group of physicians of the same or varying specialties who have come together, usually as a professional corporation, to provide a variety of services to their patients.

A new patient is one who has not received any professional services from the physician, or another physician of the same specialty who belongs to the same group practice, within the past three years.

An established patient is one who has received professional services from the physician, or another physician of the same specialty who belongs to the same group practice, within the past three years.

The new versus established patient guidelines also clarify situations that occur when one physician is on call or covering for another physician. In this instance, you are instructed to classify the patient encounter the same as if it were for the physician who is unavailable.

SOAP NOTE

It is important to understand how physicians document their services for office visits, consultations, and hospital visits, as well as preventive care. Let us take a look at the familiar documentation approach known as the "SOAP" format.

The SOAP format is a nationally recognized and commonly accepted method of recording patient visits. The word is an acronym for Subjective, Objective, Assessment, and Plan.

A standard format like SOAP is a valuable way to record patient encounters in an organized and consistent manner. Without a systematic approach, patient information can turn into a lengthy, rambling, disorganized narrative that varies from physician to physician.

Another benefit of the SOAP format is that it mirrors the elements of the E/M levels of service as outlined in the CPT manual. By using the SOAP format, the individual components of an E/M service are easily recognized in the chart. Coding E/M services becomes faster and more straightforward.

Subjective
The subjective portion of the encounter includes all information the patient tells the physician. The physician makes sure that the patient's chief complaint, a history of the present illness, and a review of the affected systems are recorded. The subjective portion of the encounter correlates to the E/M history component.

Objective
The objective portion consists of observed, objective findings such as the patient's vital signs and the findings of the physical exam and any diagnostic tests. With the exception of the diagnostic tests, the objective information correlates to the E/M examination component.

Assessment
The assessment is basically a list of what the physician thinks is wrong with the patient and is typically documented by listing one by one the problems, diagnoses, and reasons that led the physician to those diagnoses.

Plan
The plan is the further workup or treatment planned for each problem in the assessment list. The plan is recorded in one of two ways. The physician may list all the problems together, then list separately the plans for the diagnoses. The other method involves listing each problem immediately followed by its plan. A plan details how the problem is to be treated and the final disposition.

CODING AXIOM

Professional services are those face-to-face services rendered by a physician and reported by a specific CPT code.

FOR MORE INFO

Consult *Ingenix Coding Lab: Understanding E/M Coding*. This product explains E/M coding in more detail and includes sample chart notes.

DEFINITIONS

SOAP. A common documentation format consisting of the following elements:

S—subjective
O—objective
A—assessment
P—plan

The components of history, examination, and medical decision making are keys to selecting the correct E/M codes. In most cases, all three components must be addressed in the documentation. However, in established, subsequent, and follow-up categories, only two of the three must be met or exceeded for a given code. Additional components—counseling, coordination of care, presenting problem, and time—are also a consideration for code selection.

History—First Key Component

The history has four distinct elements consisting of the chief complaint; history of present illness; past, family, and/or social history; and a review of systems. Each of the elements are defined as follows:

The chief complaint (CC) is part of the patient's history and is required for all levels of history. It is the patient's description of the problem, symptoms, conditions, diagnosis, or other factors that prompted the encounter.

The history component consists of:

- Chief complaint (CC)
- History of present illness (HPI)
- Review of systems (ROS)
- Past, family, and social history (PFSH)

The history of present illness (HPI) is a chronological description of the patient's present illness from the first sign or symptom to the present, or from the previous encounter to the present. It includes the following elements:

- Location (specific area where the problem presents)
- Quality (a description of the complaint such as a dull, aching pain)
- Severity (how bad is the problem?)
- Duration (how long has the problem been present?)
- Timing (when does the problem present itself? e.g., in the morning)
- Context (how did the problem begin?)
- Modifying factors (are there circumstances that alter the condition?)
- Associated signs/symptoms (a sign is a physical characteristic of an illness, a symptom; however, in this instance it is based on the patient's perception of illness)

The past, family and social history (PFSH) includes:

- Past history: prior major illnesses/injuries, prior operations, prior hospitalizations, current medications, allergies, immunization status, feeding/dietary status
- Family history: review of medical events in the family, including diseases which may be hereditary or place the patient at risk
- Social history: marital status/living arrangements, current employment, occupational history, use of drugs/alcohol/tobacco, education, sexual history

The review of systems (ROS) is an inventory of body systems obtained through a series of questions aimed at identifying additional signs/symptoms the patient may be experiencing. It includes: constitutional symptoms (fever, weight loss, etc.); eyes; ears/nose/mouth/throat; cardiovascular; respiratory; gastrointestinal; genitourinary; musculoskeletal; integumentary (skin, breast); neurological; psychiatric; endocrine; hematologic/lymphatic; allergic/immunologic.

CODING AXIOM

History is composed of four distinct elements:

- Chief complaint
- History of present illness
- Review of systems
- Past, family, and social history

DEFINITIONS

Presenting problem. A disease, condition, illness, injury, symptom, sign, finding, complaint, or other reason for the patient encounter.

The history component in E/M is categorized by four levels:

Problem focused. Chief complaint; brief history of present illness or problem.

Expanded problem focused. Chief complaint; brief history of present illness; problem-pertinent system review.

Detailed. Chief complaint; extended history of present illness; problem-pertinent system review (with limited additional systems); pertinent past, family, and/or social history directly related to the patient's problems.

Comprehensive. Chief complaint; extended history of present illness; review of systems related to present illness/problems (with review of all additional body systems); complete past, family, and social history.

Physical Exam—Second Key Component

The physical examination is the process of investigating or inspecting any symptomatic or involved body areas and/or organ systems using a variety of methods and techniques for the purpose of diagnosing the complaint, sign, symptom, or condition.

The physical exam component is similarly divided into four levels of complexity:

Problem focused. Limited exam of the affected body area or organ system.

Expanded problem focused. Limited examination of the affected body area or organ system and of other symptomatic or related organ systems.

Detailed. Extended examination of the affected body area(s) and other symptomatic or related organ system(s).

Comprehensive. Complete single organ system specialty examination or a general multisystem examination.

To correctly identify the body areas or organ systems for the second key component (physical examination), it is necessary to understand how the body areas and organ systems have been defined in the CPT book.

- **Body areas:**
  - Head, including the face
  - Genitalia, groin, buttocks
  - Neck
  - Back
  - Chest, including breasts and axilla
  - Abdomen
  - Each extremity
- **Organ systems:**
  - Eyes
  - Genitourinary
  - Ears, nose, mouth and throat
  - Musculoskeletal
  - Cardiovascular
  - Skin
  - Respiratory
  - Neurologic

☞ **KEY POINT**

A complete single organ exam is also considered a comprehensive level examination.

— Gastrointestinal

— Psychiatric

— Hematologic/lymphatic/immunologic

Medical Decision Making—Third Key Component

Medical decision making is the third key component and refers to the complexity of establishing a diagnosis and/or selecting a management option. This component is more complicated to determine than are the history and exam components.

The CPT book lists four types of medical decision making: straightforward, low complexity, moderate complexity, and high complexity. Any level of medical decision making requires that two of three elements are met or exceeded.

The following describes the four types of medical decision making:

Straightforward. Minimal risk of complications, and/or morbidity, or mortality; minimal complexity or no data; and a minimal number of diagnoses or management options.

Low complexity. Low risk, limited complexity of the reviewed data, and a limited number of diagnoses.

Moderate complexity. Moderate risk, moderate complexity of the reviewed data, and multiple diagnoses.

High complexity. High risk, extensive complexity of the reviewed data, and an extensive number of diagnoses.

Counseling

Counseling is defined in the CPT code book as a discussion with a patient and/or family concerning one or more of the following areas:

- Diagnostic results, impressions, and/or recommended diagnostic studies
- Prognosis
- Risks and benefits of management (treatment) options
- Instructions for management (treatment) and/or follow-up
- Importance of compliance with chosen management (treatment) options
- Risk factor reduction
- Patient and family education

An additional criteria for code selection revolves around counseling and coordination of care. Counseling, coordination of care, and the nature of the presenting problem are not major considerations in most encounters, so they generally provide contributory information to the code selection process. The exception arises when counseling or coordination of care dominates the encounter (more than 50 percent of the time spent). In these cases, time determines the proper code. Documentation of the exact amount of time spent will substantiate your selected code. For office encounters, count only the time spent face-to-face with the patient and/or family; for hospital or other inpatient encounters, count the time spent in the patient's unit or on the patient's floor, but be sure the time spent and counted is directed at caring only for that patient. The time assigned to each code is an average and varies by physician.

Along with the time, the medical record should indicate what was discussed during the encounter. If a physician coordinates care with an interdisciplinary team of

 DEFINITIONS

Medical decision making. This component of E/M comprises the intellectual aspect of a provider's services. The complexity of any medical decision bears on the value of the service.

 CODING AXIOM

When counseling or coordination of care dominate the patient encounter, then time becomes the dominant factor in code selection, with indifference to key components.

 DEFINITIONS

Interdisciplinary care. Involves two or more healthcare professions working in a collaborative manner for the benefit of the patient.

 DEFINITIONS

Documentation. The physician's written or transcribed notations about a patient encounter are known as documentation. Documentation may take the form of a detailed operative report, or just be a few written notes about a routine encounter. Source documentation must be the treating provider's own account of the encounter. These notes may be transcribed from dictation, dictated by the physician into voice recognition software, or be hand or type written. A signature or authentication accompanies each entry.

physicians or health professionals/agencies without a patient encounter, report it as a case management service (codes 99361 and 99362).

Next, match your assessment of key components against the requirements.

Once you've measured the extensiveness or complexity of each component as supported in the medical record, compare your results with the requirements of each code in the appropriate category or subcategory. Remember, these are minimal qualifications required for the code.

Evaluation and management guidelines note that the key components must meet or exceed the indicated level before the code can be reported for the service.

Nature of Presenting Problem

The CPT book identifies that the nature of the presenting problem is a nonkey issue although it can be considered contributory. As such, it is not appropriate to select the level of service solely on the presenting problem. The levels of presenting problem are defined as:

Minimal. Problem may not require physician presence, but a service is provided under the physician's supervision.

Self-limited or minor. Problem runs a definite and defined course, transient in nature and will not permanently change patient's health status or should resolve with management and patient compliance

Low severity. Problem with little risk of morbidity or mortality without treatment and expected recovery without impairment

Moderate severity. Problem with moderate risk of morbidity or mortality without treatment, uncertain prognosis or increased possibility of impairment

High severity. Problem with high or extreme risk of morbidity or mortality without treatment and high possibility of impairment

Although the nature of the presenting problem may indicate the severity of the problem, it is incorrect to use this as a final code selection tool. Oftentimes a condition that initially appears life threatening may not be as severe as first presented.

Time

According to CPT guidelines, evaluation and management (E/M) time will help the coder in the selection of a code as an indicator of the levels that may be appropriate if the documentation supports the performance of the E/M service. However, E/M time may not be the controlling factor for all services.

Under specific circumstances, E/M time may be the controlling factor in selecting a final E/M code. Time will be used as the main factor when counseling and coordination of care as described above constitute the majority of the service. For time to drive the code selection more than 50 percent of the time must be spent counseling.

The counseling and coordination of care must be documented and the time spent counseling as well as the total visit time must be documented. Code selection is based on the total time and not just the counseling and coordination of care.

Not all E/M codes have a time value assigned. For those services the other key components and instructions will determine the code selection.

MAIN CATEGORIES OF THE EVALUATION AND MANAGEMENT SECTION

Office or Other Outpatient Medical Services

The code range includes office and outpatient or other ambulatory facility services. Codes are subcategorized by new or established patient. These services are provided to patients who have not been admitted to a health care facility (i.e., hospital, skilled nursing facility [SNF], or comprehensive nursing facility [NF]).

Hospital Observation Services

These codes are used to report E/M services provided to a patient who is designated/admitted as "observation status" in a hospital. The patient need not be located in an observation unit designated by the hospital. When a patient is admitted to observation status in a hospital in the course of an encounter at another site of service, (e.g., physician's office or NF), all E/M services provided shall be considered as part of the initial observation care if performed on the same date as the admission to observation status.

Initial observation care is found in code range 99218–99220. Discharge from observation is coded to 99217. These codes are used for new or established patients. These codes may not be used for postoperative recovery observation if the procedure is part of a global surgical service (0, 10, or 90 days). For patients admitted and discharged from observation or inpatient status on the same day, report services with the appropriate code from the range 99234–99236.

Hospital Inpatient Medical Services

The code range is used to report E/M services provided to hospital inpatients. Codes are grouped by initial and subsequent hospital care. In addition to the codes for initial and subsequent hospital services, the CPT code book lists a code for discharge day management. Discharge of a patient often requires a final examination, discussion of treatment protocol, patient prognosis, and/or preparation of discharge records.

Consultations

The code range is used to report the service provided by a physician whose opinion or advice on a specific problem is requested by another physician. Codes are grouped by office, initial inpatient, follow-up inpatient, and confirmatory consultations. Distinction is not made between new and established patients.

A consultation includes services rendered by a physician whose opinion or advice is requested by a physician or other appropriate source for the further evaluation and/or management of a specific problem. The consultant must document the recommended course of action to the attending physician and treatment being initiated. When the consulting physician assumes responsibility for the continuing care of the patient, any subsequent service rendered will cease to be a consultation.

Emergency Department Services

The code range does not distinguish new or established patients. These codes are reserved to identify services provided in an emergency setting. An emergency department is defined as an organized 24-hour hospital-based facility that provides unscheduled services to patients needing immediate medical attention. Urgent care centers and ambulatory surgery centers are NOT considered emergency departments. The emergency department E/M codes do not have a time value associated with them. The code selection cannot be based upon time or counseling and coordination of care.

 QUICK TIP

The use and documentation of E/M codes receives a great deal of scrutiny from Medicare and its intermediaries. Documentation guidelines change frequently. If billing Medicare, be certain you are aware of the latest guidelines.

 QUICK TIP

A physician is a provider who has graduated from a four-year medical school and holds accreditation as either a Doctor of Medicine (MD) or a Doctor of Osteopathy (DO). To practice medicine, a physician must attend at least one year of residency (internship), which generally confers the title general practitioner. Specialists attend additional years of residency and usually sit for board certification in a chosen specialty (e.g., American Academy of Family Practitioners [AAFP]).

Patient Transport

This range of codes is used to report the physician's physical attendance and face-to-face contact with the critically ill or injured patient during interfacility transport.

Critical Care

The code range represents critical care as an all-inclusive service for the procedures listed below when provided on the same day by the same physician. Those services include vascular access procedures, chest x-rays, blood gases, interpretation of cardiac output measurements, blood pressure, ECGs, ventilator management, gastric intubation, and temporary transcutaneous pacing.

Neonatal Intensive Care

The code range covers neonatal intensive care. Guidelines explain the types of care rendered to the patient. The site of care is not the deciding factor in code selection, as care may be rendered in other than neonatal intensive care units. These codes are for reporting initial and subsequent care, per day, for physicians directing the care of a neonate or infant. These codes are used once per date of service, regardless of the number of times seen per day. These codes may be billed with a major therapeutic surgical procedure. The care includes management, monitoring, and treatment, including nutritional, metabolic and hematological maintenance, parent counseling and personal direct supervision of the health care team.

Nursing Facility Services

The code range groups services by new and established patient as comprehensive assessments or subsequent nursing facility care. These codes may also be used to report services to patients in psychiatric residential treatment centers. Within each group the code identifies the patient's problems and the types of care rendered. Nursing facilities that provide convalescent, rehabilitation, and long-term care are required to provide comprehensive functional capacity evaluations.

Prolonged Services

The code range contains two groups of codes, one for prolonged services with direct face-to-face services and one for indirect prolonged services. Face-to-face prolonged services are broken down one step further to services performed in an office, or other outpatient setting, and services performed in the inpatient setting. Services for prolonged care without direct face-to-face contact are to be used for services before and/or after direct face-to-face patient care (e.g., review of extensive records and tests, communication with other professionals, and/or the patient/family). Prolonged services are coded as the first hour and an additional code for each 30-minute block of time. Less than 30 minutes of prolonged care is not coded separately.

Physician Standby Service

The code is acceptable for monitoring EEGs, and standby for frozen section. It is to be used for standby services that require prolonged physician attendance. If standby of a surgeon results in the performance of a procedure, only the procedure code is reportable. Standby services should not be reported with other procedure codes and, according to CPT guidelines, when a physician provides standby services (at the request of another physician) and the services end with a performance of a procedure, the global surgical package rule applies and the standby code is not reported and is considered bundled to the procedure.

Case Management Services

The code range is used to report the services of a physician in the process of coordinating and controlling access to other healthcare services needed by the patient.

DEFINITIONS

Nursing facility assessments may include the following instruments:

MDS. Minimum data set, criteria for clinical information pertaining to residents of skilled nursing facilities.

RAI. Resident assessment instrument, an evaluation form for residents of skilled nursing facilities.

RAP. Resident assessment protocol, an evaluation criteria for residents of skilled nursing facilities.

QUICK TIP

Telephone call codes are not a covered benefit by most payers. Reporting such codes for internal tracking purposes may help in managed care contracting or in determining overall physician productivity.

This section contains two groups of codes: one for interdisciplinary medical team conference and one for telephone calls. Medical conferences are broken out by the amount of time, approximately 30 or 60 minutes. Among the telephone codes, three levels are available: simple or brief, intermediate, and complex or lengthy. Codes include examples of each.

Care Plan Oversight Services

The code range includes care plan codes including physician supervision of patients under care of home health agencies, hospice, or nursing facilities requiring complex or multidisciplinary care modalities involving regular physician development and/or revision of care plans; review of subsequent reports of patient status; review of related laboratory and other studies; communication with other health care professionals involved in the patient's care; integration of new information into the medical treatment plan and/or adjustment of medical therapy, within a 30-day period. Only one physician may report services for a given period of time, to reflect that physician's sole, or predominant, supervisory role with a particular patient. Care plan oversight codes are broken out by the amount of time of 15 to 29 minutes or 30 minutes or more. Services must be documented in the patient's medical record.

Preventive Medicine Services

Preventive medicine deals with keeping the patient well, rather than treating an established illness, although both may occur at these types of visits. Counseling/risk factor reduction is included. Codes are distinguished as provided to new and established patients. Codes are also arranged in each category by the age of the patient. These codes are appropriately used to report E/M services provided to a patient who presents without complaints.

Newborn Care

These codes are used to report services to normal and high-risk newborns. Attendance at delivery when requested by the delivering physician is also reported with the codes in this section.

Special Evaluation and Management Services

This series of codes covers any evaluative service a physician provides when no active management of the patient's problem is undertaken at the time of the encounter. If other E/M services and procedures are performed on the same date, report them with the appropriate E/M code in addition to the special evaluation code.

QUICK TIP

Newborn resuscitation is the provision of positive pressure ventilation and/or chest compressions in the presence of acute inadequate ventilation and/or cardiac output.

ANESTHESIA

Anesthesia services are reported by using a CPT code from the anesthesia section (00100–01999) and (99100–99140). Procedure codes in the anesthesia section (00100–01999) are divided into the following three types:

- Body region (e.g., head, neck, thorax, intrathoracic, spine, abdomen, perineum, pelvis, leg, shoulder, arm)
- Radiological procedures (e.g., hysterosalpingography, ventriculography, pneumoencephalography, cardiac catheterization, angioplasty, noninvasive imaging)
- Other procedures (e.g., physiological support for harvesting organs, region IV administration of local anesthetic, daily management of epidural drug administration)

The greatest number of codes in the anesthesia section are for procedures associated with surgery. These are arranged first by the site of the surgery and, second, by the surgical procedure involved.

Anesthesia Section Guidelines

Anesthesia services reported must be those performed by or under the responsible medical direction and/or supervision of a physician. Anesthesia services include, but are not limited to, general or regional supplementation of local anesthesia as well as other supportive services considered necessary by the anesthesiologist. Anesthesia services include the usual pre- and postoperative visits, intubation, the care by the anesthesiologist during surgery, the administration of fluids and/or blood, the usual monitoring services, and extubation. Usual forms of monitoring that are included in the anesthesia service are ECC, temperature, blood pressure, oximetry, capnography, and mass spectrometry. Unusual forms of monitoring such as central venous, intra-arterial or Swan Ganz monitoring are not included. If the third-party payer does not accept the anesthesia codes, the appropriate surgical procedure code and the amount of time may be reported instead. Obtain operative reports when necessary.

Services Included in Anesthesia Care

The following services are included in the provision of anesthesia care:

- Preoperative and postoperative visits (evaluation and management codes 99201–99420)
- Intubation (emergency intubation code 31500 unless modifier 59 is appended to the code to indicate it as a distinct or independent service)
- Esophageal intubation (91000) and/or gastric intubation code (91055, 91105)
- The care by the anesthesiologist during surgery (ventilation assist and management code 94656)
- The administration of fluids and/or blood
- Vascular access, reported by the code for introduction of a needle or intracatheter, vein, (36000*), a venipuncture code (36400–36425), or an IV infusion code (90781, 90781) should not be billed with an anesthesia procedure code because these procedures are performed for the administration of fluids anesthetic agents, and/or medications, and are included in the usual anesthesia service. Arterial puncture code (36600*) should not be billed with an anesthesia code. Blood transfusion codes (36430, 36440*) should not be billed with an anesthesia code (00100–01996).

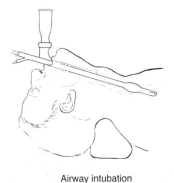

Airway intubation

Services Not Included in Usual Anesthesia Care

Usual monitoring services (e.g., ECG, temperature, blood pressure, oximetry, capnography, and mass spectrometry) are included in usual anesthesia care. Unusual forms of monitoring not included are:

- CVP catheter placement   36488*–36491*
- Arterial catheter placement   36620–36625
- Swan-Ganz catheter placement 93503

In addition, most third-party payers will not allow epidural, subarachnoid, subdural injections into the spine and spinal code (62310–62319) to be billed with anesthesia codes (00100–01996). The injection codes are being billed for the type of anesthesia provided and are considered to be included in the anesthesia code.

Qualifying Circumstances

The qualifying circumstances add-on codes are used to report some of the complex circumstances the anesthesiologist may encounter performing the administration of anesthesia. They may be used singly or in conjunction with each other (multiple add-on codes) for each anesthesia case. For example, a patient may be of extreme age and an emergency at the same operative session.

Use codes 99100–99140 to identify circumstances that affect the anesthesia service provided. When appropriate, more than one qualifying circumstance code may be used. The qualifying circumstance codes are:

+99100   Anesthesia for patient of extreme age, under one year and over 70 (List separately in addition to code for primary anesthesia procedure)

+99116   Anesthesia complicated by utilization of total body hypothermia (List separately in addition to code for primary anesthesia procedure)

+99135   Anesthesia complicated by utilization of controlled hypotension (List separately in addition to code for primary anesthesia procedure)

+99140   Anesthesia complicated by emergency conditions (specify) (List separately in addition to code for primary anesthesia procedure)

According to CPT guidelines, an emergency exists when delay in treatment of the patient would lead to a significant increase in the threat to life of a body part.

Remember, these codes are not reported alone, but are used as an additional description of circumstances that affect the anesthesia service provided. More than one code may be used.

Note that some payers consider these to be informational codes and do not assign a value or additional reimbursement. These codes are not paid for Medicare patients.

Conscious Sedation

When the same physician performing the surgery also provides conscious sedation for the patient's comfort, the conscious sedation codes from the medicine section in the CPT code book must be consulted. Conscious sedation is a state of sedation in which the patient remains conscious but is free of apprehension and fear through a depressed state of consciousness. The use of these codes requires the presence of an independent and trained observer to assist the physician in monitoring the patient's level of consciousness and physical status. To report conscious sedation, with or without analgesia, report CPT codes 99141 and 99142. While these codes are not add-on codes, they must be reported along with the primary surgical procedure code for the procedure performed by the surgeon providing the conscious sedation.

 KEY POINT

According to the CPT code book, an emergency exists when delay in treatment of the patient would lead to a significant increase in the threat to life of a body part.

 KEY POINT

Anesthesiologists do not report conscious sedation services with codes 99141 and 99142. The surgeon who performs the surgical procedure reports conscious sedation services.

CODING AXIOM

For anesthesia services encompassing multiple procedures, code only the most complex procedure.

DEFINITIONS

Bundled services. Items or services wrapped together for reporting and reimbursement purposes. The items or services may be related or unrelated, but all defined elements must be present to make a specific bundle.

Unbundling. Separately charging for health care services that are billed as part of a comprehensive surgical package.

QUICK TIP

The AMA has not developed a specific unbundling policy, but you can look in the following places for help to interpret how to apply the CPT codes:

- Format of the terminology listed in the introduction
- Listed surgical procedures
- Separate procedures
- Subsection information in the surgery guidelines
- Correct Coding Initiative (CCI)

Time

Because the billed units for anesthesia are largely based on time, it becomes a vital component of charge capture. For this reason, a clear definition of "anesthesia time" is provided by the CPT code book. Anesthesia time begins when the anesthesiologist starts preparing the patient for induction of anesthesia and ends when the patient is placed under postoperative supervision and care of the attending physician.

Multiple Surgical Procedures

When multiple surgical procedures are performed during the same surgical encounter (i.e., single anesthetic administration) report the anesthesia code for the most complex procedure only. The total time for all procedures is combined and reported.

SURGERY

Fragmentation and Unbundling

Before we begin a review of the surgery section of the CPT code book, it is important to understand a basic coding concept known as "bundling." Understanding unbundling and fragmentation can be accomplished by first defining the term, "bundle." A bundle is a defined set of items or services wrapped together in a group, bunch, or package. The items in the bundle can be related or unrelated, but all defined elements must be present to make a specific bundle. Consider a bundle that includes one dozen apples and oranges. Although at first it may seem that the apples and oranges are unrelated, they are both types of fruit and have been put together in a fruit bundle. Anyone purchasing this fruit bundle expects that all the apples and oranges are present (i.e., the buyer is purchasing the entire dozen). If, however, one of the apples is removed, and billed separately, in addition to paying the cost per dozen, the person buying the bundle is being charged twice for the apple.

Of course when it comes to coding, a bundle has nothing to do with apples and oranges. Instead, unbundling relates to CPT surgical codes and the global or package concept. Unbundling or fragmentation primarily occurs two ways.

First, unbundling occurs when minor integral services are reported separately or in addition to a major procedure. Unfortunately, since all minor components of a procedure may not be listed explicitly, it is sometimes difficult to determine which services are integral to a given procedure.

One way to approach this is to ask what services are normally performed with a given procedure. A simple example is an excision of a skin lesion. To excise the skin lesion, an incision must be made. An incision is always integral to an excision of a lesion and should not be billed separately. However, an incision is not described in the excision of skin lesion codes. It is implicit because it must be performed with every excision.

Second, unbundling occurs when a single procedure with two or more explicitly described components is broken into its component parts and reported with several CPT codes instead of the single CPT code for the combined service. A simple example of this type of unbundle is illustrated with the procedure for a combined abdominal hysterectomy with colpo-urethrocystopexy. Because the two components of this procedure are frequently performed together, a combined code 58152 has been assigned to describe this service. However, it is also possible to perform each of the components separately (abdominal hysterectomy, 58150 and colpo-urethrocystopexy, 51840 or 51845). When the combined procedure is performed during a single surgical session, it must be reported with the bundled CPT code 58152. If it is reported with code 58150 in conjunction with 51840 or 58145, it is considered unbundled or fragmented.

Unbundling is considered by payers a form of inappropriate billing. The rationale is simple. Unbundled services frequently net more reimbursement than reporting the single bundled CPT code.

The Centers for Medicare and Medicaid Services (CMS) adopted the Correct Coding Initiative (CCI) unbundling guidelines, an evolving list of codes that cannot be reported in combination with other codes for Medicare claims. As previously stated, the CPT book does not have a specific guideline for unbundling. Instead, payers and other interested parties have developed guidelines for bundled procedures from information that is listed in the CPT book. The four most common areas of the CPT book used for these interpretations are the format of the terminology listed in the introduction, listed surgical procedures, separate procedures, and subsection information in the surgery guidelines. Look at these four areas and how payers may interpret the guidelines. Keep in mind that while most payers will have many common rules and interpretations, they will have some rules specific to their company. Make an effort to understand these differences, requesting written documentation for rules that differ significantly from accepted health care practices.

Unbundle Prevention

You can take some easy steps to avoid problems with fragmentation or unbundling:

- Use a current CPT book as well as the current rules, regulations, and provider manuals for Medicare and for the private payers with whom you have a contractual arrangement. A current copy of CCI should be on hand.

- Educate yourself on the CPT book guidelines as well as the rules and regulations of your payers.

- When using a preprinted charge ticket or routing sheet, specify the exact CPT code and description. Always have an area on the charge ticket for the physician to indicate that a service should be coded by hand and code from the operative report or medical record. Many providers feel reimbursement is better by coding directly from the record or operative report.

- Update codes on your charge ticket annually.

- Create charge tickets or routing sheets to avoid fragmented billing. For example, the abbreviation "SP" might be used to indicate the code is a separate procedure, alerting the coder that this should not be reported when related, or integral, to a major procedure.

- Query the physician if documentation is not adequate to support the codes selected.

- Use the correct modifiers as appropriate to clarify or append circumstances that can arise within global package time periods.

As payers become increasingly proficient in interpreting CPT codes, coders must exercise caution when reporting integral procedures, even when benefits are allowed. Medicare and Medicaid closely monitor physicians' billing practices for possible abusive or fraudulent billing. Private payers also have mechanisms in place to scrutinize claims.

The Surgery Section

Each subsection is arranged by body system, then anatomical site, starting with the top of the body progressing downward, and then from the outside to the inside of the body and finally by type of procedure.

 KEY POINT

Unbundling, whether intentional, is considered by payers a form of inappropriate billing. The rationale is simple. Unbundled services frequently net more reimbursement than reporting the single bundled CPT code.

 FOR MORE INFO

The Correct Coding Initiative edits should be referenced before submitting a claim with multiple procedures.

For example, look under "Urinary System" in your CPT book. You will notice the following hierarchy:

Urinary System
    Kidney
    Ureter
    Bladder
    Urethra

Understanding the organization of the surgery section often helps locate the correct procedure code. You will notice that most of the surgical sections begin with "Incision," "Excision," "Introduction," "Repair," "Laparoscopy," "Endoscopy," etc.

For example, by examining your CPT book, you will see under "Kidney" the following procedures:

Incision
Excision
Renal Transplantation
Introduction

By becoming familiar with the organization of the CPT code book, as well as an understanding of the anatomy of the body, you will find it helpful when the physician's documentation does not readily point toward the main term in the index. For example, the appropriate code for the repair of a patient's lacerated knee is not found under the main term "repair" in the CPT code book index. "Laceration repair" is listed, but the index instructs the coder to "See Specific Site." "Knee" is listed, but without mention of "laceration repair." "Repair" is listed under "Knee," but refers to repairs of the "ligament, meniscus, or tendon," since the laceration occurs to the skin of the knee. The procedure, repair, would be performed on the skin, a part of the integumentary system of the body. One way to locate the code range in the index is to look under the main term "Skin" and find the modifying term "Wound Repair." Through familiarity with the CPT code book and the structure of the surgery section, however, the coder can turn to the integumentary system subsection and scan down the listing under "Skin, Subcutaneous and Accessory Structures" to find the subheading "repair." Checking further, the coder finds the range of codes that includes the site, "Knee," is 12001–12007.

Standard surgical categories include specific clues a coder can use to locate a needed code range. A knowledge of appropriate alternative terms that may apply to a procedure, injury, illness, or condition will make the process of locating a code both easier and faster.

Standard general surgical definitions for definitions or therapeutic interventions are as follows:

Anastomosis. Connection between two vessels or an opening surgically created between two organs or spaces normally separated.

Debridement. Removal of contaminated, devitalized tissue or foreign material usually by sharp dissection, until healthy tissue is exposed.

Destruction. Ablation, removal or eradication of tissue.

Dilation. Stretching an orifice or tubular structure beyond its normal dimensions.

Endoscopy. Visual inspection of any cavity by means of an instrument.

KEY POINT

By becoming familiar with the organization of the CPT code book, as well as an understanding of the anatomy of the body, you will find it helpful when the physician's documentation does not readily point toward the main term in the index.

Example of anastomosis

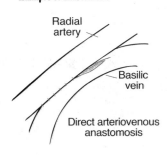

Radial artery

Basilic vein

Direct arteriovenous anastomosis

Excision. Surgical removal, as of an organ.

Exploration. Examination for diagnostic purposes.

Incision. The act of cutting.

Reconstruction. To reassemble or reform from constituent parts.

Repair. Restoration of diseased or damaged tissue.

Resection. Removal of a portion of an organ or tissue.

Shaving. The sharp removal by transverse incision or horizontal slicing.

SURGERY SECTION GUIDELINES

Surgical Procedure Packaged Services

What is a "package?" In terms of surgical care, it includes the basic procedure, topical and local anesthesia, and routine uncomplicated follow-up care for the surgical procedure performed. Each third-party payer may have a definition for a surgical or global surgical package concept. The number of preoperative and postoperative days for procedures will vary among third-party payers.

The CPT code book definition indicates the following are included in the surgical package per se (see "CPT Surgery Guidelines" for the full definition of a surgical package):

- Local anesthesia
- Subsequent to the decision for surgery, one related E/M encounter on the date immediately prior to or on the same date of the surgery (and this includes the history and physical exam)
- Immediate postoperative care
- Writing orders
- Evaluating the patient postanesthesia
- Typical postoperative follow-up care

Medicare, however, has its own definition for global surgical package concept and one should become familiar with Medicare specific guidelines for compliance with their policies.

Follow-up Care for Therapeutic Surgical Services

A therapeutic procedure is one that provides a therapy or treatment for the patient's condition. Such therapy may be surgical or nonsurgical (such as a drug treatment). The CPT coding guidelines discuss specifically the follow-up care for therapeutic procedures. For example, if complications, exacerbations, or the recurrence or presence of other diseases or injuries require additional services during the global period of the original therapeutic surgical service, those services may be reported separately.

Follow-up Care for Diagnostic Procedures

A diagnostic procedure by contrast is one in which the patient is still being diagnosed with consideration for possible treatment. Care related to recovery from diagnostic procedures is included in the appropriate diagnostic procedure code. Care of the condition for which the diagnostic procedure was performed or of other coexisting conditions is coded separately by CPT coding guidelines. In other words, with

 DEFINITIONS

Package. This term refers to a code that includes the basic procedure, topical and local anesthesia and routine, uncomplicated follow-up care.

 KEY POINT

A patient undergoes a diagnostic laparoscopy for severe abdominal pain, Following a diagnosis of abdominal adhesions, the physician, during the same session, lyses the adhesions by laparoscopic technique. The guidelines for laparoscopy (CPT code 58660, in this example), indicate that the surgical laparoscopy always includes diagnostic laparoscopy.

completion of the diagnostic procedure, so ends the reportable postprocedure care and any further "treatment" may be reported separately. Caution however, should be taken in certain guidelines that include the diagnostic portion for a treatment following the diagnostic examination.

Postoperative Follow-up Visit

For documentation purposes, use code 99024 for normal postoperative follow-up visits within the postoperative period. This code is informational and does not increase the reimbursement for a surgical procedure.

Separate Procedures

A "separate" procedure is one that can be performed by itself but is normally performed as part of another procedure. These codes are indicated with the words "separate procedure" at the end of the code description in parentheses. When the separate procedure is performed as part of another related procedure, do not code it. Occasionally a separate procedure will be performed apart from and not related to another surgical procedure. When this occurs, the separate procedure should be identified and coded (done separately).

Multiple Procedures

Sometimes multiple surgical procedures may be performed in combination with other medical and/or surgical procedures. When this occurs, a multiple procedure modifier is necessary to indicate to the payer that more than one procedure took place during the operative session. Clear documentation in the operative report should accompany the claim to ensure appropriate payment consideration.

Add-on Codes

Add-on codes represent procedures commonly carried out in addition to the primary procedure. These add-on codes are not to be assigned multiple procedure modifiers. You may see these procedures identified by the terminology "each additional" in the code narrative. Add-on codes cannot stand alone. They must always be reported with another CPT code. The add-on code will always have notes following the code description to indicate when there is a specific range of codes to which it applies. In all cases the code will state "List separately in addition to code for primary procedure."

+92547 Use of vertical electrodes (List separately in addition to code for primary procedure)
(Use 92547 in conjunction with codes 92541–92546)

AMA Surgical Package Guidelines

The following are the AMA's surgical package guidelines.

- The listed surgical procedures in the CPT manual include the procedure (operation), local, topical, or metacarpal/digital block anesthesia when used and the normal, uncomplicated follow-up care.
- Therapeutic surgical procedures include any usual care relating to the surgical service. Complications or other conditions that occur should be reported using the appropriate code indicating the service or procedure performed.
- Supplies provided by the physician over and above those usually included with the office visit or other services provided may be listed separately.

- Procedures commonly carried out as an integral part of another procedure are identified by the phrase "separate procedure" in the code descriptor. These procedures should not be billed in conjunction with the related procedure. However, these procedures may be billed when done independently or unrelated to the procedures performed during an episode of care.

Unlisted Procedures

The CPT code book contains a number of unlisted procedure codes that are to be used when there are no appropriate codes available that adequately describes the procedure performed. Payers require a special report to be filed when using an unlisted procedure code since the CPT code description does not indicate the procedure performed. The report should contain pertinent information including a description of the procedure, the extent and need for the procedure, as well as the effort, time, and equipment used.

Surgical Coding Methodology

Use a step-by-step approach to determine the correct codes for surgical procedures. Correct coding will generally minimize claim rejection. Turnaround time in processing may decrease, which could increase cash flow and lessen the likelihood of appeals, denials, and audits. Always use the most recent versions of the CPT code book, and the ICD-9-CM and HCPCS Level II manuals for accurate coding. Checking each claim submitted against the guidelines listed below will help improve coding accuracy.

1. Read the surgery guidelines at the beginning of the surgery section.

2. Locate the code in the index that most accurately describes the procedure(s) performed.

3. Read the descriptive nomenclature of the code carefully, and read any information before and after the code that might give directions. Make sure your documentation and/or operative report justifies the use of the code.

4. Page back as necessary to the subheading for the code and read any guidelines, notes or directions for the section that apply to the code(s).

5. Watch for notes or see references that apply to the code you wish to use. Does a note specify the code cannot be used with another code? Does it send you to another area for a more correct code? Does it explain additional procedures that may be billed with the code?

6. Consider the code and what is included in it. Do not unbundle, but do not miss the opportunity to code additional procedures not included in the code.

7. Enter the code correctly on the claim form, always listing the most revenue-intensive code first.

8. When more than one code is used, apply the correct modifiers from the list of modifiers in appendix A of the CPT code book that apply to second and additional codes. Except when using modifier 22, never adjust fees on the claim form. Allow the payer to make the appropriate adjustments. For modifier 22 Unusual services, adjust your fee to take into count additional work or resources for the unusual service provided.

9. On the CMS-1500 claim form, apply the correct diagnostic codes and indicate next to the CPT code in the correct box every diagnosis that applies to the surgery or procedure.

10. Follow any contractual arrangements you may have with the payer.

 KEY POINT

Unlisted procedures are located within or at the end of each section of the CPT code book. Be careful to select the appropriate unlisted code for the anatomic site or intervention for the procedure performed.

Use a step-by-step approach to determine the correct codes for surgical procedures. Correct coding will generally minimize claim rejection. Always use the current versions of CPT, ICD-9-CM, and HCPCS Level II codes.

 KEY POINT

Do not rely on a computerized coding system to give you the correct code. While computer systems are meant to speed up coding, they are not meant to replace the CPT code book or other coding books. The most sophisticated coding programs are incapable of consistently applying the correct codes and rules.

Do not rely on a computerized coding system to give you the correct code. While computer systems are meant to speed up coding, they are not meant to replace the CPT code book or other coding manuals. The most sophisticated coding programs are incapable of consistently applying the correct codes and rules.

ANCILLARY SERVICES

An ancillary service is one that supports another service, usually of a core clinical service. For example, a diagnostic test that determines a need for surgical intervention may be considered ancillary. The ancillary services in the radiology and pathology sections of the CPT code book present quite a different realm of services from those reviewed in the surgery section. Because these services encompass a "technical" component, reporting these services requires an understanding of the technical and professional parts of the services.

TECHNICAL AND PROFESSIONAL COMPONENTS

Radiology procedures are comprised of two components: technical and professional. Laboratory services, on the other hand, have codes that are technical only, a few professional only, and others that are both technical and professional. The technical component includes the provision of the equipment, supplies, technical personnel, and costs attendant to the performance of the procedure other than the professional services. When hospitals report radiology or pathology services, they are reporting the technical portion of the service only. Physicians who are reporting only the technical component should report the service with HCPCS Level II modifier TC Technical component only, appended to the radiology code to indicate that only a technical service was performed.

Professional Component

The professional component encompasses the physician's work in providing the service, including supervision, interpretation, and report of the procedure. Think of this as the brain work and skills provided by the physician. Education, malpractice insurance, and other expenses incident to maintaining a practice are also part of the professional component (see chapter 6 for more information on relative value reporting). When a physician is reporting only for the professional component, modifier 26 Professional component only, should be appended to the radiology code to indicate that only a professional service was performed.

A "global" service would be one in which the provider is reporting for both the technical and professional components of a service. No modifier is necessary for reporting the global service. For example, a physician's office or clinic providing radiology services would not qualify for a PC/TC split because the physician usually owns the equipment and bills the total service. Modifier 26 is usually not needed for these places of service.

Confusion has abounded in coding radiology and pathology services due to the technical component inherent to these areas of medicine. The sophisticated and expensive equipment required for radiology services, as well as pathology services, has been owned by hospitals and large facilities. Hospitals reported the use of the equipment, the specially trained personnel, and related costs associated with the technical component. The advent of freestanding medical facilities including physician offices capable of offering radiological imaging services, catheterizations, and other diagnostic and therapeutic radiology services poses a challenge in securing reimbursement for both components. One should be familiar with which

---

CODING AXIOM

The CPT book describes modifier 26 as the method to report the professional component only of a global service, but makes no such provision for reporting technical services. The technical component of a global radiology service is reported using a HCPCS Level II modifier TC.

DEFINITIONS

Technical component. Includes the provision of the equipment, supplies, technical personnel, and costs attendant to the performance of the procedure, other than the professional services. Professional component encompasses all of the physician's work in providing the service, including interpretation and report of the procedure.

---

component(s) are being billed in order to prevent over-reporting or under-reporting of the technical and/or professional components of radiological services. Most payers now accept modifier TC for the technical component. In addition, payers have developed fee schedules reflecting each component separately and many also have a fee reflecting a global reimbursement rate for the service provided. Reimbursement for each component performed requires the use of the correct modifiers.

Unless instructed otherwise by payers, the professional component should be reported with modifier 26, the technical component with modifier TC. The global service (technical and professional) should be reported once without a modifier unless instructed differently by a specific payer.

Technical Component

The following case study is an example of technical component reporting. When a radiological examination is performed at a hospital or other facility where a radiologist works independently in the hospital and reports his or her services separately, the hospital or other facility reports the technical component.

An elderly patient trips on a sidewalk and the treating physician suspects a fracture of the scaphoid in the patient's left wrist. The physician refers her to the outpatient radiology department of a nearby hospital for diagnostic x-rays. Three radiologic views of the wrist are required.

Let's see how we might code this scenario from the technical as well as professional perspective.

Hospital reports CPT code 73110 for the technical portion of taking the films on a UB-92 claim form with no modifier.

The physician reports CPT code 73110 with modifier 26 for the professional portion of reading the films and preparing a written report of the findings.

814.01   Closed fracture of navicular (scaphoid) of wrist

E885.9   Fall on same level from slipping, tripping, or stumbling

The radiology and pathology sections follow the surgery section of the CPT code book. Because of their uniqueness, the radiology and pathology sections will be reviewed briefly to familiarize you with their nuances.

RADIOLOGY

Radiology Codes and Guidelines

Perhaps no area of medicine integrates technological advancement faster than radiology. The specialty regularly employs imaging, diagnostic, and therapeutic technologies developed only a few decades or even years ago. Consequently, the radiology section (70010–79999) is under constant review to reflect current standards of service.

Radiological procedures are divided into four subsections in the CPT book:

- Diagnostic radiology (70010–76499)
- Diagnostic ultrasound (76506–76999)
- Radiation oncology (77261–77799)
- Nuclear medicine (78000–79999)

CODING AXIOM

A global service may be reported when one physician provides both the professional and technical components of the radiology procedure, such as owning the equipment, employing the technologist, and providing a written interpretation of the examination.

DEFINITIONS

Contrast material. any internally administered substance that has a different opacity from soft tissue on radiography or computed tomography; includes barium, used to opacify parts of the gastrointestinal tract; water-soluble iodinated compounds, used to opacify blood vessels or the genitourinary tract; may refer to air occurring naturally or introduced into the body; also, paramagnetic substances used in magnetic resonance imaging. Substances may also be documented as contrast agent or contrast medium.

DEFINITIONS

The radiology section of the CPT code book contains unique terms. The following list includes those most frequently applied.

Anteroposterior (AP). Front to back.

Anteroposterior and lateral. Two projections are included in this examination, front-to-back and side.

Cineradiography. Real-time image under motion by x-ray.

Contrast material. Radiopaque material that is placed into the body to visualize a system or body structure. Terms include: non-ionic and low osmolar contrast media (LOCM), ionic, and high osmolar contrast media (HOCM), barium, and gadolinium.

Decubitus (DEC). Patient lying on the side.

Interventional radiology. The clinical subspecialty that uses fluoroscopy, CT, and ultrasound to guide percutaneous procedures such as biopsies, draining fluids, inserting catheters, or dilating or stenting narrowed ducts or vessels.

Lateral (LAT). Side view.

Modality. A form of imaging. This includes x-ray, fluoroscopy, ultrasound, nuclear medicine, duplex Doppler, CT, and MRI.

Oblique (OBL). Slanted view of the object being x-rayed.

Posteroanterior (PA). Back to front.

Real-time. Immediate imaging, usually in movement.

Stent. Tube to provide support in a body cavity or lumen.

Subtraction. Removal of an overlying structure to better visualize the structure in question. This is done by imposing one x-ray in a series on top of another.

Tomogram. Specialized type of x-ray imaging that provides slices through a body structure to obliterate overlying structures. This is commonly performed for studies on the kidneys or the temporomandibular joint.

Codes are ordered according to anatomic site (e.g., head, chest, abdomen) and body system (e.g., gynecological and obstetrical, gastrointestinal, aorta, arteries) within each section, except for radiation oncology which is a unique type of service. The codes in the radiology section may be reported when a physician either performs or supervises the services. With regard to supervision, the radiologist would be supervising radiology technicians whose job is to obtain the images for review by the radiologist.

Within each subsection, procedures are described by type of service (modality), the specific body site examined, and are followed by additional information regarding the use of contrast material and the complexity of the procedure.

The CPT code book provides guidelines for radiology codes at the beginning of the radiology section. Some subsections also contain guidelines and those should be reviewed before code selection. Notes clarify the use of codes within the subsections. Code categories, subcategories, and parenthetical phrases also may be presented. The guidelines are arranged similar to other sections of the CPT code book and are unique to the individual code, category, subcategory, or range of codes. You may locate the appropriate code in the index by looking up the specific imaging technology used or the body part imaged.

Some additional procedures frequently performed by radiologists may be found outside the radiology section, such as noninvasive vascular diagnostic studies (93875–93990) found in the medicine section. Services involving the invasive or interventional component of interventional radiology services are found in the surgery section. These include percutaneous biopsies, injection procedures, and transcatheter procedures which are discussed in this chapter.

Types of Radiology Services

Diagnostic Radiology Services

Procedures in the diagnostic radiology section establish a diagnosis or follow the progression or remission of a disease process. However, also included in this section are procedures that are therapeutic in nature. These therapeutic procedures are often referred to as interventional or invasive radiology services. Codes in this chapter of the CPT code book report the radiological supervision and interpretation of these interventional and invasive procedures.

Diagnostic radiology uses different modalities, including x-rays, fluoroscopy, CT, and MRI. Procedures in the diagnostic radiology section are ordered by anatomic site. They are then described by type of service (modality), specific body site, number of views, and use of contrast materials.

Services described in the CPT manual as a "radiological examination" refer to plain films of specific sites. Other terms used to describe plain films include standard or conventional films. Services employing other modalities and/or additional techniques are described by the modality or technique, such as radiography with fluoroscopy, computerized axial tomography (CT), or magnetic resonance imaging (MRI).

CT Scan

Computerized axial tomography (CT) is a type of imaging that employs basic tomographic technique enhanced by computer imaging. Computer enhancement synthesizes the images obtained from different directions in a given plane, effectively reconstructing a cross-sectional plane of the body.

Computerized tomography angiography (CTA) provides multiple rapid thin section CT scans, a series of x-ray beams taken from different angles to create cross-sectional images of organs, bones, and tissues.

MRI

Magnetic resonance imaging (MRI) involves the application of an external magnetic field that forces a uniform alignment of hydrogen atom nuclei in the soft tissue. The nuclei emit radiofrequency signals that are converted into sets of tomographic images and displayed on a computer screen for three-dimensional visualization of the soft tissue structure.

MRA

Magnetic resonance angiography (MRA) has many medical applications, including the diagnosis of artery and vein abnormalities (e.g., aneurysms in the brain). MRA is non-invasive, can be performed without catheterization, and does not require the administration of contrast material; however, to enhance the diagnostic capability of MRA, a contrast agent can be injected prior to the MRA scan and that image data must be acquired at the moment the contrast agent is flowing through the vessels of interest.

Views

Views describe the patient's position in relation to the imaging device. A code may specify a position, as in 71010, which describes a single frontal view of the chest. Other codes do not specify a position, but designate the number of views, as in 73610, which specifies a minimum of three views of the ankle.

Diagnostic Ultrasound

What exactly is ultrasound? Ultrasound technology uses rapidly oscillating crystals that produce the sound waves used in the ultrasound beam. A transducer, which must be in close contact with the skin, transmits the sound waves and receives the echo. A gel conducting agent spread over the skin improves the transmission of sound.

Procedures in diagnostic ultrasound are organized by anatomic site. However, when the ultrasound is part of an interventional radiology procedure for localization purposes, the procedure is listed under "Ultrasonic Guidance Procedures."

Radiation Oncology

Radiation oncology involves the following services: consultation, clinical treatment, planning, medical radiation physics, and treatment delivery and management for the treatment and follow-up of cancer patients. The radiation oncology section is divided accordingly and contains very specific guidelines about the reporting of these services.

Nuclear Medicine

Nuclear medicine relies on radium or other radioelements for either diagnostic imaging or radiopharmaceutical therapy. Radiopharmaceutical therapy destroys diseased tissues, usually malignant neoplasms, using radioelements. This subsection is organized first by the nature of the procedure, diagnostic or therapeutic. The diagnostic codes are organized by body system. Procedures are further defined by the extent or complexity of the service.

Supervision and Interpretation

The radiological supervision and interpretation of many interventional and invasive procedures are reported with codes from diagnostic radiology.

Body Planes

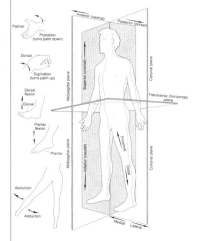

 FOR MORE INFO

See pages 61–62 for more anatomical information.

 DEFINITIONS

Nuclear medicine. Involves radioactive elements for either diagnostic imaging or radiopharmaceutical imaging. A radioactive element, such as uranium, spontaneously emits energetic particles by the disintegration of the nuclei.

Interventional/invasive codes may be used to report procedures diagnostic in nature, such as fluoroscopic localization for percutaneous renal biopsy 76003. Or, the codes may be used to report therapeutic procedures, such as radiologic supervision and interpretation of transcatheter embolization 75894.

PATHOLOGY

Pathology and Laboratory Subsections

The pathology and laboratory (80048–89399) section of CPT is divided into 17 subsections:

- Organ or disease oriented panels (80048–80090)
- Drug testing (80100–80103)
- Therapeutic drug assays (80150–80299)
- Evocative/suppression testing (80400–80440)
- Consultations (clinical pathology) (80500–80502)
- Urinalysis (81000–81099)
- Chemistry (82000–84999)
- Hematology and coagulation (85002–85999)
- Immunology (86000–86849)
- Transfusion medicine (86850–86999)
- Microbiology (87001–87999)
- Anatomic pathology (88000–88099)
- Cytopathology (88104–88199)
- Cytogenetic studies (88230–88299)
- Surgical pathology (88300–88399)
- Transcutaneous procedures (88400)
- Other procedures (89050–89240)
- Reproductive medicine procedures (89250–89356)

Many procedures are performed by various methods and coders must know the methodology used. In many instances, identification of the method used is key to appropriate coding. The codes in the pathology section may be reported when a physician either performs or supervises the services. With regard to supervision, the pathologist would be supervising laboratory technicians who job is to obtain the images for review by the pathologist.

The majority of the codes represent a technical component only, but certain codes represent a global service—a combination of professional and technical components, as discussed previously in the radiology section. If the pathologist must review a test result and/or render an opinion, the appropriate code should be selected and a modifier 26 attached to indicate that only a professional service was provided.

Guidelines that clarify how pathology and laboratory codes should be used are found at the beginning of the section and in notes, and parenthetical phrases throughout the section. The guidelines are in the same arrangement as the other sections of the CPT code book and unique to the section, subsection, subheading, range of codes, or to an individual code.

Inpatient coders are not usually required to code pathology or laboratory tests since they are not necessary in the assignment of DRGs (diagnosis-related groups, which

 KEY POINT

Inpatient coders seldom code pathology or laboratory tests since they are not necessary in the assignment of DRGs. The services are typically reported through the chargemaster or CDM.

Outpatient coders, on the other hand, frequently must code pathology and laboratory tests.

In many instances, identification of the method is key to appropriate coding and reimbursement for pathology and laboratory.

There is no mechanism in the CPT coding system for reporting lab procedures performed on a stat basis. Physician documentation with an order for immediate or "stat" testing must be included in the medical record.

are discussed in chapter 7). However, pathology and laboratory codes are itemized on chargemasters for reporting services and supplies to patients.

Outpatient coders frequently code pathology and laboratory tests. Coding instructions include listing each laboratory procedure separately, unless it is part of a panel. Never use modifier 51 for multiple procedures in pathology or laboratory coding.

Many lab tests can be performed by different methods. To choose the correct code, carefully review code descriptions as well as any notes. When in doubt, request information from the physician or laboratory for clarification, or consult an authoritative reference.

Correct diagnostic coding is extremely important in pathology and laboratory test reimbursement. Many payers will exclude payment if a diagnosis code does not match the list of diagnoses a payer has assigned as payable for a particular test.

Organ or Disease-Oriented Panels

Panel codes are groups of laboratory services that are frequently performed together to assess general health or specific medical conditions. Tests included in each panel are listed by name with the CPT code identified in parentheses. In order report panel code, all test in addition to those listed for the specific panel.

In the CPT book, the panels are described by their CPT name and each test defined by the panel is listed with its name and associated CPT code. It is important to note that the name in the CPT book may not reflect the panel a medical office may have named on its own with a different set of tests. Careful review of the required tests in each panel and the number of times the test must be performed is essential to correct coding. Also watch for the term "and" and "or" in the descriptions of the required tests. Panel codes should only be reported when all tests included in the panel are performed. Performance of additional tests not included in the panel should be reported separately.

Drug Testing

This section reports qualitative screening to detect the presence of specific drugs or classes of drugs. When drugs are detected on the initial screen, they are normally confirmed by a second method, which is reported separately. A qualitative test is one in which the determination is made regarding the nature of the substance.

Drug Assays

Codes listed under therapeutic drug assays or under chemistry are used when a drug is quantitated, or measured. Screening may be used to detect a substance, but it is not a prerequisite for quantitation. For example, screening is not necessary when a known drug has been overdosed. Coding for quantitative assays is based on the substance tested. Unless the code description notes otherwise, the examination material may be from any source.

Evocative/Suppression Testing

Codes in this section report test panels involving the administration of evocative or suppressive agents. Panels include testing baseline levels of specific chemical constituents, as well as subsequent measurements, to assess the effect of the agents administered. These codes report only the laboratory components.

 KEY POINT

Organ or disease-oriented panels are described in the CPT book by their name and tests making up that panel are listed below the CPT code and description.

 KEY POINT

Coding for quantitative assays is based on the substance tested.

 DEFINITIONS

Analyte. Any material or chemical substance subjected to analysis.

✓ QUICK TIP

Look up the substance or analyte being evaluated in the CPT code book index to find the appropriate code(s). For example, "blood," "urine," "calcium," "potassium," etc.

The physician's administration of the agent is reported separately. Supplies and drugs are reported separately. To report physician attendance and monitoring during the testing, one should use the appropriate evaluation and management codes.

Pathology Consultation

Two consultation codes (80500 and 80502) are reserved for the pathologist to indicate a service, not a test. The pathology consultation is performed at the request of an attending physician and requires a written report. Code 80500 is a limited service without review of the patient's history and medical records. Code 80502 is a comprehensive service for a complex diagnostic problem, with review of the patient's history and medical records.

Like consultations in the evaluation and management section of the CPT code book, these consultation codes may only be reported when the pathologist is consulted at the request of another physician or if material from another pathologist or facility has been referred.

Pathology consultation codes cannot be used to report the pathologist oversight of the pathology department.

Urinalysis

The urinalysis section lists only a limited number of tests. Many additional tests can be performed on urine and these are listed in the appropriate section.

Chemistry

Laboratory chemistry examination may be performed on specimens from any source (blood, stool, urine, blood serum) unless a specific source is defined in the narrative description. According to the CPT code book, multiple specimens, including those from different sources or those obtained at different times, are reported separately for each source and each specimen. Chemical tests are assumed to be quantitative unless otherwise specified.

Hematology and Coagulation

The hematology and coagulation subsection lists those laboratory procedures specific to blood and blood-forming organs, including complete blood counts (CBC), clotting factors, clotting inhibitors, prothrombin and thrombin time, platelets, and sickling.

In addition, bone marrow aspiration, biopsy, and smear interpretation are found here.

Immunology

Immunology is the study of the immune system, including sensitivity and allergy. The immunology subsection identifies codes for antigen and antibody studies. Specific tissue typing procedures are also found in the immunology subsection.

Transfusion Medicine

Once listed in immunology, most blood bank codes are now grouped together under the transfusion medicine subsection. These codes report antibody screening and identification, blood typing, autologous blood collection and storage, compatibility test, and preparation of blood and blood procedures. These codes do not, however, report the supply of blood or blood products. Those areas are typically reported using HCPCS Level II codes (see chapter 5).

📖 DEFINITIONS

Antibody. A protein that B cells of the immune system produce in response to the presence of a foreign antigen and reacts to the antigen.

Antigen. A chemical that stimulates cells to produce antibodies.

Qualitative. To determine the nature of the component of substance.

Quantitative. To determine the amount and nature of the components of a substance.

Microbiology

The microbiology codes identify services related to culture, organism identification, and sensitivity studies. Many of the narratives are similar to those in the immunology section, so it is important to pay close attention to technique.

Anatomic Pathology

Anatomic pathology includes postmortem examinations (e.g., necropsy, autopsy), cytopathology (e.g., fluids, washing or brushing, Pap smears, fine needle aspirations, flow cytometry, etc.) and cytogenetic studies (e.g., tissue cultures for chromosome studies, etc.). Postmortem examination procedures are used to report only the physician portion of the service.

Cytopathology

Codes in this range report the examination of body fluids, in particular cervical or vaginal smear, for screening purposes (Pap smears).

Cytogenic Studies

Test in this range of codes involve analysis of DNA, RNA or other genetic materials (e.g., protein and enzymes) to determine probability of an inherited disease such as tests for inborn errors of metabolism and genomic aberrations such as Down syndrome as well as to determine sex in cases where anatomy is inconclusive.

Surgical Pathology

Surgical pathology codes report gross and microscopic examination of tissue, special stains, consultations during surgery, as well as a number of additional special studies.

QUICK TIP

Codes in the pathology section may be reported when a physician either performs or supervises the service.

MEDICINE

The CPT code book medicine section (90281–99600) follows the pathology and laboratory section. The most used codes in the CPT code book are the E/M and medicine codes. Although the Medicine section is one section, it is comprises of many different codes used by varying specialties. Again, it is important to note that these codes like all other codes in CPT are not limited to use by one specialty.

Many of the codes in the medicine section are modifier 51 exempt and are indicated with the ⊘ symbol.

An overview of the subsections within the medicine section include:

- Immune globulins (90281–90399)
- Immunization administration for vaccines/toxoids (90471–90474)
- Vaccines/toxoids (90476–90749)
- Therapeutic or diagnostic infusions (excludes chemotherapy) (90780–90781)
- Therapeutic, prophylactic or diagnostic injections (90782–90799)
- Psychiatry (90801–90899)
- Biofeedback (90901–90911)
- Dialysis (90918–90999)
- Gastroenterology (91000–91299)
- Ophthalmology (92002–92499)
- Special otorhinolaryngologic services (92502–92700)
- Cardiovascular (92950–93799)
- Noninvasive vascular diagnostic studies (93875–93998)
- Pulmonary (94010–94799)

KEY POINT

Many of the codes in the medicine section are modifier 51 exempt and are indicated with the ⊘ symbol.

DEFINITIONS

AAN. American Academy of Neurology, the professional organization that certifies for the specialty of medicine that performs neurology and neuromuscular procedures.

QUICK TIP

There is a significant difference between the procedures described in physician medicine and rehabilitation, osteopathic manipulative treatment, and chiropractic manipulative treatment. Consult the CPT book for the definitions and guidelines for these three disparate forms of treatment.

KEY POINT

In order to become a proficient coder, you must be familiar with the organization of the CPT book.

- Allergy and clinical immunology (95004–95199)
- Endocrinology (95250)
- Neurology and neuromuscular procedures 95805–96004)
- Central nervous system assessments/tests (e.g., neurocognitive, mental status, speech testing) (96100–96117)
- Health and behavior assessment/intervention (96150–96155)
- Chemotherapy administration (96400–96549)
- Photodynamic therapy (96567–96571)
- Special dermatological procedures (96900–96999)
- Physical medicine and rehabilitation (97001–97799)
- Medical nutrition therapy (97802–97804)
- Osteopathic manipulative treatment (98925–98929)
- Chiropractic manipulative treatment (98940–98943)
- Special services, procedures and reports (99000–99091)
- Qualifying circumstances for anesthesia (99100–99140)
- Sedation with or without analgesia (conscious sedation) (99141–99142)
- Other services and procedures (99170–99199)
- Home health procedures/services (99500–99512)
- Home infusion procedures/services (99601–99602)

SUMMARY

Coders are instructed in the medicine codes section of the CPT code book to report each procedure separately. The word "procedure" may also describe a medical and/or E/M service. The medicine section is reviewed in greater detail in the next tier in this series, *Ingenix Coding Lab: Physician Offices.*

In summary, you see that the CPT coding system is a complex compilation of the procedures and services performed by both physicians and other healthcare providers. In order to become a proficient coder, you must be familiar with the organization of the CPT code book, the index, medical anatomy and terminology, and the guidelines that apply to each section and subsection of the CPT code book.

The following discussion questions and issues are for your consideration upon completion of this chapter. A full series of test questions on this chapter are found on the accompanying CD-ROM and in the instructor's manual.

DISCUSSION QUESTIONS

- Contemplate the nature of most physician services and imagine how these codes evolved to report these types of services. Review modifiers and think about their role in leveraging a code's description without changing its basic purpose. As you look at the front pages of a copy of the CPT code book, think about the processes involved to make guideline changes, introduce new codes, or eliminate a description.
- How many additional pages do you think would be added to the CPT code book if the indented codes and semicolon system weren't employed?

- Think about the mental discipline physicians employ to document a visit from a patient with multiple symptoms and a complex diagnosis. Does the SOAP approach offer help to coders in the review and assignment of the E/M coding for the same visit? Think about the development of the E/M coding system. Are the documentation elements required relevant to the evaluation and treatment of a patient?

- Does the concept of global services make sense to you? Practice explaining it to a lay audience. Explain how unbundling of services can be viewed as financially exploitive.

- As you review the sections of the CPT book, consider specialties of medicine that you might see yourself working for.

Chapter 4: Diagnosis Coding and ICD-9-CM

INTRODUCTION

In the medical field, a diagnosis is of extreme importance. In common language, it is what's wrong with the patient, whether disease, injury, or other reason to seek medical care. Diagnosis coding is the method that translates medicine's terminology for diseases, injuries, and the other reasons to seek medical treatment into the alphanumeric digits understood by statisticians, data analysts, and the computers that process insurance claim forms.

The *International Classification of Diseases, Ninth Revision, Clinical Modification, Sixth Edition,* more commonly referred to as ICD-9-CM, is the classification system used by physician offices as well as inpatient and outpatient facilities. ICD-9-CM, volumes 1 and 2 are used to code diagnosis information and are the focus of this chapter. Volume 3 is used to report procedures in the hospital or ambulatory surgery centers and will not be discussed in this chapter. ICD-9-CM books for physicians traditionally contain only volumes 1 and 2.

A prime role of the medical coder is to translate a physician's written diagnoses into codes. In the main, this coded information is used to communicate to commercial and government payers the medical reason for a billed service. That was not the original purpose of diagnosis codes. As a communication tool, ICD-9-CM diagnosis codes relate the disease, condition, complaint, sign, symptom or other reason for medical services provided. In addition to a means to communicate between provider and payer, diagnosis codes are used to gather statistics for purposes such as: number and types of diseases being treated, indexing medical records, financial analysis, standards compliance, and facilitating medical care reviews.

This diagnosis system is based on the World Health Organization's (WHO) International Classification of Diseases (ICD). In the United States, the system has been expanded and modified to meet unique clinical purposes (hence the CM, or clinical modification). The responsibility for maintenance of the classification system is shared between the National Center for Health Statistics (NCHS) and the Centers for Medicare and Medicaid Services (CMS).

WHO developed and extensively tested a new edition of the diagnostic code set, ICD-10. The United States has not yet adopted ICD-10. Anticipated effective dates have been rumored for many years. Recent recommendations for adoption by national associations suggest that ICD-10 may be adopted in the next several years. Coders are encouraged to be aware of all coding changes and to receive training prior to an effective date when finalized.

HISTORY

The current diagnostic coding system originated in 17th-century England as a statistical study of diseases entitled the London Bills of Mortality. By 1937, this

OBJECTIVES

In this chapter, you will learn:

- About the nature of diagnosis coding both historically and currently
- The conventions and format of ICD-9-CM
- The basics of the index and tabular listings
- The rules and guidelines
- About the organization of ICD-9-CM and how to recognize general categories

DEFINITIONS

Indexing. Refers to listing diseases and conditions according to classification system.

QUICK TIP

ICD-9-CM is often shortened to the terms "ICD-9" and even "I-9."

information had evolved into the International List of Causes of Death. Addition revisions were made and the study became the International Classification of Causes of Death. This information was very important to the statistically oriented WHO, which in 1948, published lists for tracking morbidity as well as mortality. The combined list was renamed the ICD, the name it retains.

In 1978 the WHO published its ninth revision of this list (ICD-9). Once ICD-9 became internationally recognized, the United States NCHS moved to create a more precise clinical picture of the patient than was needed for statistical groupings and trend analyses. NCHS modified ICD-9 with clinical information that allows a more thorough indexing of medical records, medical case reviews, and ambulatory and other medical care programs. This version was appended the term "clinically modified," or CM.

In the United States, ICD-9-CM codes are often referred to simply as ICD-9. It is updated every year with new codes, as well as revisions to the current codes. The director of NCHS and the administrator of CMS make final decisions concerning any revisions to the system. Once determined, the final decisions are published in the *Federal Register* and become effective October 1 of each year.

ICD-9-CM DIAGNOSIS CODING

The ICD-9-CM coding system is a method of translating medical terminology for diseases and procedures into codes. Codes within the system are made up of three, four, or five characters. All characters are either numeric or alphanumeric. "Coding" involves using numeric or alphanumeric characters to describe a disease or injury. For example, the diagnosis of "pneumonia, organism unspecified," is translated into code "486."

The advent of computerized claims processing has forced the medical community to learn the common language of coding, and ICD-9-CM volumes 1 and 2 provide the diagnostic half of that language. Care must be taken to select the correct code. Computer software applications can link diagnoses to the services provided and automatically reject claims when ICD-9-CM codes do not justify the service performed. For government claims, the correct use of ICD-9-CM codes is required by law. In 1988, Congress passed the Medicare Catastrophic Coverage Act. Although the act itself was later repealed, the mandate was maintained to require ICD-9-CM codes on all physician-submitted Part B claims. Medicare's rules tightened in 1996 when it began to reject any claim that did not assign the most specific ICD-9-CM code available.

By looking over the ICD-9-CM volumes I and II, you will see that diagnostic codes from 001.0–V83.89 are used to:

- Identify symptoms, conditions, problems, complaints, or other reasons for the medical service or procedure being billed
- Report medical necessity by indicating the severity and emergent nature of the condition or complaint
- Translate written information into a numeric/alphanumeric system that can be stored and retrieved for use in medical education, research, reimbursement, and statistics
- Translate written information in the patient's chart onto a form that can be submitted electronically for reimbursement
- Another section reports external causes of injury and poisoning, which are collectively referred to as E codes.

 KEY POINT

Insurance payers use "medical necessity" to decide whether or not to pay a claim. Medical necessity is determined by whether the ICD-9-CM code reflects a medical reason that warrants the need for a procedure.

ICD-9-CM is published in three volumes. Volumes 1 and 2 contain diagnostic information used by physicians, outpatient facilities and inpatient hospitals, freestanding ambulatory surgical centers, and others. Volume 3 contains procedural information that is generally reserved for inpatient and outpatient facility coding. See chapter 7 for more information on volume 3 and inpatient procedure coding.

ORGANIZATION

The ICD-9-CM contains an introduction, along with an "Alphabetic Index to Diseases" (volume 2), which is presented first by most publishers. Many coding books also list the coding guidelines in the front of the book.

ICD-9-CM volume 2 is also called the "Alphabetic Index to Diseases." It lists diseases in alphabetical order with their the corresponding codes. This logical placement of the alphabetic index allows for quick location of terms for verification in the tabular list.

The "Tabular List of Diseases" (volume 1) contains a numerical listing of all the codes, as well as codes that begin with a V (V codes) and codes that begin with an E (E codes). The tabular listing is divided into 17 chapters based on disease and is commonly presented second, listing information from volume 2 in numeric order along with other pertinent coding conventions.

CODING GUIDELINES

The basis of accurate coding is in following the coding guidelines. These "official" guidelines are presented by the Public Health Service and the Centers for Medicare and Medicaid Services, both under the U.S. Department of Health and Human Services. The guidelines are considered a companion document to the official versions of the ICD-9-CM. These guidelines are developed and approved by the cooperating parties for ICD-9-CM: the American Hospital Association, CMS, the American Health Information Management Association, and the NCHS.

The guidelines were developed to assist coders in situations where the manual does not provide direction. However, coding and sequencing instructions in the three volumes of ICD-9-CM, take precedence over the guidelines.

The guidelines do not cover every situation. The guidelines are continuously under review and are revised and updated as needed. Make sure whenever you are reviewing coding guidelines for ICD-9-CM, that you are using the "official" version of the guidelines.

The Public Health Services and CMS maintain the official coding guidelines for coding and reporting using the ICD-9-CM classification system. These guidelines are used as a companion to the official version of ICD-9-CM.

The guidelines for coding and reporting have been developed and approved by the cooperating parties for ICD-9-CM, which are:

- American Hospital Association (AHA)
- American Health Information Management Association (AHIMA)
- Centers for Medicare and Medicaid Services (CMS)
- National Center for Health Statistics (NCHS)

The guidelines are published by the AHA in the *Coding Clinic for ICD-9-CM*.

QUICK TIP

The guidelines in ICD-9-CM do not cover every situation. You should use *AHA Coding Clinic* as a supplement to the guidelines.

DOCUMENTATION AND DIAGNOSIS CODING

Many types of source documents (e.g., medical records, encounter forms, superbills, operative reports, etc.) are used to identify a patient's diagnosis and the services provided to the patient. The source document furnishes information such as the diagnostic statement and the procedural statement. Analyzing the diagnostic statement is the first step in assigning an ICD-9-CM code.

Coding a diagnosis is difficult when the physician's terminology does not match the descriptions in the ICD-9-CM code book or when the diagnosis cannot be found in the code book.

Understanding the definitions of medical terms and the intricacies of the coding system allows any diagnosis to be coded.

If you cannot locate the diagnosis in the ICD-9-CM code book, do not assume that a code for the diagnosis does not exist. It is just a matter of tracking down the "clues."

For example, the physician documents the patient's diagnosis as strep throat. Even though the alphabetic index lists both "Streptococcus" and "Throat" as main terms, no code is provided for either term. The cross-reference "see also condition" is given. Strep throat, which is the patient's condition, is an infection. Locate "Infection," subterms "throat" and "streptococcal," in the index. Code 034.0 is the correct code to use for strep throat.

Consult with a physician, or refer to medical resource materials, to determine the meaning of unfamiliar terms. Ignoring unfamiliar terms reduces coding accuracy.

Following is a summary of the steps to follow to identify the appropriate code for a diagnostic statement:

1. Note all main terms in the diagnostic statement that describe the patient's condition.

2. Use the alphabetic index to locate each main term identified.

3. Identify words that modify the main term.

4. Carefully review subterms listed under the main term.

5. Review notes and/or cross-references.

6. Select a tentative code from those provided in the alphabetic index.

7. Turn to the tabular list to verify the accuracy of the code. Be sure to use four- or five-digit codes, when available.

8. Carefully review any instructional notes.

9. Assign the code selected from the tabular list.

ICD-9-CM VOLUME 2

Volume 2, the alphabetic index, is covered first because it is presented first in most publications. It is referenced first in selecting a diagnosis code. Volume 2 is divided into section 1, "Alphabetic Index to Diseases," section 2, "Table of Drugs and Chemicals," and section 3, "Alphabetic Index to External Causes of Injury and Poisoning." These sections are covered here.

> ✓ **QUICK TIP**
>
> When the statement in the record contains both the patient's complaints (e.g., shortness of breath, dizziness, frequent headache, and nosebleeds) and the physician's diagnoses explaining those symptoms (e.g., hypertension and obesity), code only the diagnosis. If no diagnosis was made, code the complaints or symptoms.
>
> Remember, always use the alphabetic index first, then verify the code in the tabular list.

Alphabetic Index to Diseases

The first step to finding the correct ICD-9-CM code is to correctly identify the main term in a diagnostic phrase. For example, the main term in the diagnostic phrase "closed fracture of femoral shaft" is "fracture." Therefore, "fracture" is the term referenced in section 1 of volume 2. Next the modifying terms should be identified. In this case three modifying terms can be found: femur, shaft, and closed. If the main term had been incorrectly identified as "femoral," volume 2 provides instructions on selecting the correct code, in this case a note to "see condition."

Section 1, "Alphabetic Index to Diseases," lists conditions alphabetically by these commonly used medical terms called "main terms" or "main entries." Main terms are shown in bold type. Main terms are medical conditions not anatomical sites. Main terms may have a specific code assigned to them or may be modified by one or more terms which are indented and listed alphabetically below the main term.

A common difficulty for new coders is to become familiar with identifying the main term. As in the example above, there are usually many terms associated with a clinical diagnosis. The additional words add to the specificity of the diagnosis. For a physician to say someone has a broken bone, is very general indeed. We would want to know, what bone was broken. How did it break? Were multiple bones in the area broken? What type of fracture occurred? Codes exist for general statements, but these are known as nonspecific codes, meaning, "we didn't have enough information to get a more specific code." As we have mentioned previously, codes can only be derived from what is documented. So how do we get to the main term? The main term should be the general statement of what the illness or injury is. In the above example, it is a fracture. "Fracture" would be the main term. The additional information derived from what is documented regarding the illness or injury, adds more specific information to the diagnosis.

For example, the patient has a fracture. The main term is "fracture." If the physician, however, documents, "The patient has a closed fracture of the distal portion of the tibia," the main term is still "fracture." The other words "closed" and "distal" add more specific information about the type and exact location of the fracture, thus adding specificity to the code selection.

Try to identify the main terms in the following examples for practice:

> Facial spasm
>
> Muscle weakness
>
> Drug dependence
>
> Sebaceous cyst of the breast
>
> Brief loss of consciousness due to concussion
>
> Psychogenic bladder retention

If you practiced these, the main terms are underlined below:

> Facial <u>spasm</u>
>
> Muscle <u>weakness</u>
>
> Drug <u>dependence</u>
>
> Sebaceous <u>cyst</u> of the breast
>
> Brief loss of <u>consciousness</u> due to concussion
>
> Psychogenic bladder <u>retention</u>

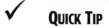

QUICK TIP

The first step to finding the correct ICD-9-CM code is to correctly identify the main term in a diagnostic phrase.

DEFINITIONS

Etiology. The science and study of the causes of disease.

DEFINITIONS

Nosology. The science of disease classification. A nosologist is the professional who performs this function.

DEFINITIONS

Ca in situ. A malignant neoplasm arising from the vessels, glands, and organs that has not spread to the neighboring tissues.

CODING AXIOM

Neoplasms are coded only after review of the pathology report.

The other words in these examples add more specific information to the patient's diagnosis and make to code selection more specific as well.

It may take a while for you to become proficient with the main term, but the ICD-9-CM book is good at referring you to the correct term if you have problems.

Tables

Two main terms are presented in volume 2 as tables. The hypertension and neoplasm tables are found in their proper alphabetical place in the index. The "Table of Drugs and Chemicals," another table, follows the alphabetical listing. Knowing how to use these tables correctly is essential to determine proper codes.

Hypertension Table

The complications, etiology, and clinical manifestations of hypertension are listed alphabetically under the bold heading **Hypertension, hypertensive**.

Clinical manifestations are the display or disclosure of signs and symptoms of an illness.

Look up the table in your ICD-9-CM book. You will see there are three subcategories for each listing in this category: malignant, benign and unspecified.

The table includes categories 401–405 plus additional codes, such as hypertension, that may complicate pregnancy, childbirth, or the puerperium. Read the diagnostic statement carefully, watching for the words "due to" and "with." These terms supply information necessary for accurate coding. Remember, the index table is only the beginning. Verify your code by looking it up in the tabular section. Also note that categories 402–405 require fifth digits.

Neoplasm Table

The neoplasm table lists neoplasms alphabetically by location and further identifies them by behavior as malignant, benign, uncertain behavior, or unspecified.

Malignant indicates a tumor has the potential to spread. Malignant neoplasms must be further defined as primary, secondary, or carcinoma in situ. When a neoplasm has metastasized (spread to a new location) the new growth is secondary to the primary (original) site.

Benign identifies neoplasms that are noncancerous but have neoplastic characteristics (e.g., fibromas and lipomas).

Uncertain behavior identifies tissue that is beginning to exhibit neoplastic behavior, but cannot yet be categorized as benign or malignant. Further testing by the physician is required. Watch pathology reports for information such as "further examination is necessary." If unsure about choosing the uncertain behavior category, query the physician.

Neoplasms should be coded following review of the pathology report. Pathology report information should also be documented by the physician in the medical record.

Unspecified identifies neoplasms of unspecified morphology and behavior, based on documentation in the medical record (i.e., the provider did not document enough information to code the neoplasm specifically).

Table of Drugs and Chemicals

The "Table of Drugs and Chemicals" appears after the alphabetical listing. It contains an extensive list of drugs, industrial solvents, corrosives, gases, noxious plants, pesticides, and other toxic agents in a six-column format. The first column identifies the substance. The second column identifies the corresponding poisoning code. The next five columns, grouped under the heading "External Cause" (E code), identify the circumstances of the poisoning or adverse effect as accidental, therapeutic use, suicide attempt, assault, or cause "undetermined." The "Table of Drugs and Chemicals" comes after the letter Z in the index to diseases.

The E codes in columns 2 through 5 in this table are defined as follows:

Accident codes. Identify accidental overdose of a drug, a wrong substance given or taken, a drug taken inadvertently, accidents that occur in the usage of drugs and biologicals in medical and surgical procedures.

Assault codes. Indicate situations where drugs or substances are "purposely inflicted" by another person with the intent to cause bodily harm, injure, or kill.

Suicide attempt codes. Identify the effects of drugs or substances taken to cause self-inflicted injury or to attempt suicide.

Therapeutic use codes. Indicate an adverse effect or reaction to a drug that was administered correctly, either therapeutically or prophylactically.

Undetermined codes. Apply when the intent of the poisoning or injury cannot be determined as intentional or accidental.

Index to External Causes

Section 3, "Index to External Causes" (E codes), is an alphabetic list of terms, which classify the causes of injury and other adverse effects. Think of these codes as ones used to indicate "how" something happened—the cause of the illness or injury.

It is organized by main terms, which describe the accident, circumstance, event, or specific agent causing the injury or other adverse effect. This index identifies codes that are supplemental and should never be listed as the primary reason for medical care.

 DEFINITIONS

Adverse effect or reaction. Occurs when a drug is administered correctly, either therapeutically or prophylactically, but causes an adverse response in the patient.

ICD-9-CM Volume 1

ICD-9-CM volume 1, also referred to as the tabular list, is a numerical list of the same diseases and conditions found in volume 2. The tabular list contains codes and their narrative descriptions. It is divided into three sections:

- "Classification of Diseases and Injuries" (chapters 1–17)
- "Supplementary Classification" (V codes and E codes)
- Appendixes

The first section of the tabular list contains 17 chapters. Ten chapters are devoted to major body systems. The main section, "Classification of Diseases and Injuries," groups code numbers primarily by body system and secondarily by etiology. Seven chapters describe specific injuries or illnesses that affect the body. These chapters contain only numeric codes, from 001.0–999.9.

 KEY POINT

ICD-9-CM volume 1 is also referred to as the tabular list.

Chapter Number and Title	Category
1. Infectious and Parasitic Diseases	001–139
2. Neoplasms	140–239
3. Endocrine, Nutritional and Metabolic Diseases, andImmunity Disorders	240–279
4. Diseases of the Blood and Blood-forming Organs	280–289
5. Mental Disorders	290–319
6. Diseases of the Nervous System and Sense Organs	320–389
7. Diseases of the Circulatory System	390–459
8. Diseases of the Respiratory System	460–519
9. Diseases of the Digestive System	520–579
10. Diseases of the Genitourinary System	580–629
11. Complications of Pregnancy, Childbirth and the Puerperium	630–677
12. Diseases of the Skin and Subcutaneous Tissue	680–709
13. Diseases of the Musculoskeletal System and Connective Tissue	710–739
14. Congenital Anomalies	740–759
15. Certain Conditions Originating in the Perinatal Period	760–779
16. Symptoms, Signs and Ill-defined Conditions	780–799
17. Injury and Poisoning	800–999

Category—three-digit codes. Three-digit codes and their titles are called "category codes." Some three-digit codes are very specific and are not subdivided. These three-digit codes can stand alone to describe the condition being coded. The following is an example of a three-digit category code that is not subdivided and can stand alone. This is considered a valid code.

    075   Infectious mononucleosis

Subcategory—four-digit codes. Most three-digit categories have been further subdivided with the addition of a decimal point followed by another digit. The fourth digit provides specificity or more information regarding such things as etiology, site, and manifestation.

Four-digit codes are referred to as "subcategory codes" and take precedence over three-digit category codes.

In the following example, the category code 461 is invalid and cannot stand alone to describe sinusitis. However, the subcategory code 461.9 Acute sinusitis, unspecified, can stand alone.

    461   Acute sinusitis
           Includes: abscess
                     empyema
                     infection acute, of sinus (accessory) (nasal)
                     inflammation acute, of sinus (accessory) (nasal)
                     suppuration
         Excludes: *chronic or unspecified sinusitis (473.0–473.9)*

    461.0 Maxillary
           Acute antritis

    461.1 Frontal

    461.2 Ethmoidal

461.3 Sphenoidal

461.8 Other acute sinusitis
Acute pansinusitis

461.9 Acute sinusitis, unspecified
Acute sinusitis NOS

Note: The four-digit subcategories "8" and "9" usually, but not always, are reserved for "other" specified conditions and "unspecified" conditions, respectively. The "Other" subcategory is referred to as "residual subcategory." Residual subcategory codes are used to classify conditions that have not been assigned a separate code within the classification system.

For an example of a residual subcategory refer to category 461 Acute sinusitis. The subcategory 461.8 Other acute sinusitis, is used for coding sinusitis that is fully described in the medical record, but ICD-9-CM does not provide a code specific to the sinusitis described, such as pansinusitis. Pansinusitis is the inflammation of all the paranasal sinuses on one side. This condition of pansinusitis cannot be classified to any of the other available acute sinusitis codes. This is the same as "not elsewhere classified (NEC)," which is addressed later in the chapter covering ICD-9-CM conventions.

The subcategory 461.9 is used when the medical record does not specify the paranasal sinuses involved in the acute sinusitis. This is the same as "not otherwise specified (NOS)," which is also addressed later in the chapter covering ICD-9-CM conventions. An example of when it is appropriate to use this code would be when the medical record documentation indicates only "acute sinusitis."

Subclassification—five-digit codes. Greater specificity has been added to the ICD-9-CM system with the expansion of four-digit subcategories to the fifth-digit subclassification level. Five-digit codes are the most precise subdivisions in the ICD-9-CM system.

The following are examples of fifth-digit subclassifications:

427.4 Ventricular fibrillation and flutter

427.41 Ventricular fibrillation

427.42 Ventricular flutter

Codes are arranged in numerical order in both this section and in the supplementary classification. Three-digit category codes are generally subdivided by adding a fourth and/or fifth digit after the decimal point to further specify the nature of the disease or condition. Again, codes with fourth digits are called subcategory codes, and those with fifth digits are referred to as subclassifications.

Knowing the three-digit category usually is not enough for accurate ICD-9-CM coding. In fact, there are only a few three-digit codes that are considered valid. The rest require the addition of further digits. See appendix E in ICD-9-CM for a list of valid three-digit ICD-9-CM categories.

SUPPLEMENTAL CLASSIFICATION: V CODES

This section contains two supplementary classifications:

"Classification of Factors Influencing Health Status and Contact with Health Services" (V codes). This classification, otherwise known as V codes, are

 DEFINITIONS

Fibrillation. Small localized and involuntary contraction of muscles; flutter.

 CODING AXIOM

Code to the highest level of specificity (three, four, or five digits) allowed by the diagnostic information.

alphanumeric and begin with the letter "V." These codes are used to describe circumstances, other than a disease or injury, that are the reason for an encounter with the health care delivery system or that have an influence on the patient's current condition.

> V70.0   Routine general medical examination at a health care facility

V codes are sequenced depending on the circumstance or problem being coded. Some V codes are sequenced first to describe the reason for the encounter, while others are sequenced second because they identify a circumstance that affects the patient's health status but is not in itself a current illness. Assignment of V codes will be discussed in depth in a separate section.

The V codes immediately follow the injury and poisoning codes of chapter 17. Only in very specific circumstances are these alphanumerical codes listed as a principal diagnosis for inpatient coding or as a primary diagnosis for outpatient coding based on coding guidelines.

The "Supplementary Classification of Factors Influencing Health Status and Contact with Health Services" (V01–V82), also known as V codes, describes circumstances that influence a patient's health status and identifies reasons for medical encounters resulting from circumstances other than a disease or injury classified in the main part of ICD-9-CM.

V codes are divided into three main classifications:

Problem-oriented V codes. Identify circumstances that could affect the patient in the future but are neither a current illness nor injury. Use these codes to describe an existing circumstance or problem that may influence future medical care or a patient's health status. Usually, problem-oriented V codes are not listed first on the medical claim form because they represent supplemental information.

> V10.04   Personal history of malignant neoplasm of stomach
>
> V15.3   Personal history of exposure to radiation
>
> V17.3   Family history of ischemic heart disease

Service-oriented V codes. Identify or define examinations, aftercare, ancillary services, or therapy. Use these V codes to describe when a person with a known disease or injury, whether it is current or resolving, encounters the health care system for a specific treatment of that disease or injury. Follow the outpatient coding guidelines carefully to determine if these codes can be used as the primary diagnosis.

> V25.2   Sterilization
>
> V54.89   Other orthopedic aftercare
>
> V56.0   Encounter for extracorporeal dialysis
>
> V65.5   Person with feared complaint in whom no diagnosis was made
>
> V67.2   Follow-up examination following chemotherapy
>
> V76.2   Special screening for malignant neoplasm of cervix (Pap smear)

Fact-oriented V codes. Do not describe a problem or a service; they simply state a fact. These generally do not serve as an outpatient primary or inpatient principal diagnosis. Again it is important to check whether the code is listed as an acceptable inpatient principal diagnosis. Codes V30–V39 are applied to all live births (fourth and fifth digits) and always the principal diagnosis if the birth occurred during this

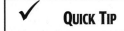

QUICK TIP

V codes describe circumstances other than a disease or injury that are the reason for an encounter with the health care delivery system.

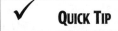

QUICK TIP

V codes are sequenced depending on the circumstances or problem being coded.

admission. Code V40–V49 classify conditions that may influence a patient's health status, such as the presence of a cardiac pacemaker or colostomy.

V21.1   Constitutional state in development: puberty

V27.2   Outcome of delivery: twins, both live born

V61.41   Alcoholism within family

V71.1   Observation for suspected malignant neoplasm

APPENDIXES TO VOLUME 1

The appendixes to volume 1 are provided in ICD-9-CM for reference purposes only. They are:

- Appendix A: Morphology of Neoplasms
- Appendix B: Glossary of Mental Disorders
- Appendix C: Classification of Drugs by American Hospital Formulary Service List Number and Their ICD-9-CM Equivalents
- Appendix D: Classification of Industrial Accidents According to Agency
- Appendix E: List of Three-digit Categories

Below is a brief description of each appendix:

- Appendix A—Morphology of Neoplasms: This appendix is an adaptation of the International Classification of Diseases for Oncology (ICD-O), a coded nomenclature of the morphology of neoplasms. These codes are alphanumeric and begin with the letter "M." An example is code M8000/0 Neoplasm, benign.
- Appendix B—Glossary of Mental Disorders: This glossary consists of psychiatric terms that are used in ICD-9-CM chapter 5, titled, "Mental Disorders." This glossary can be used to ensure that their terminology is consistent with the ICD-9-CM coding system.
- Appendix C—Classification of Drugs by American hospital formulary Service List Number and Their ICD-9-CM Equivalents: The ICD-9-CM classification of adverse effects is keyed to the code structure of the hospital formulary of the American Hospital Formulary Service (AHFS). Published under the direction of the American Society of Hospital Pharmacists, the AHFS list is updated continuously to include newly released drugs.
- Appendix D—Classification of Industrial Accidents According to Agency: This appendix is a classification of machines and other agents that might cause accidents in an industrial setting.
- Appendix E—List of Three-digit Categories: This appendix lists all three-digit categories of the classification of diseases and injuries.

 KEY POINT

Pay special attention to Industrial Accident classifications when coding a workers' compensation claim. Many states require extra information about how the accident occurred only reportable through ICD-9-CM codes.

CONVENTIONS

Just as road signs guide us along the highway, each space, type face, indentation, and punctuation mark determines how you must interpret ICD-9-CM codes. These "conventions" were developed to help you match correct codes to the diagnoses you encounter.

Format

The ICD-9-CM coding system has an indented format. Subterms are indented two spaces to the right of the term to which they are linked. Continuations of lines that are too long to fit the column are indented four spaces.

> Hernia, hernial
>   inguinal (direct) (double) (encysted) (external) (funicular) (indirect)
>   (infantile) (internal) (interstitial) (oblique) (scrotal) (sliding) 550.9 ✓5ᵗʰ

Typeface

Bold type identifies all codes and main terms in the tabular list (volume 1), separating them from subordinate information or notes.

From volume 1:

> **237.3 Paraganglia**
>   Aortic body
>   Carotid body
>   Coccygeal body
>   Glomus jugulare

Italicized type identifies those categories that cannot be reported as a primary diagnosis and also for all exclusion notes. The italicized words in the following entry indicate that 580.81 Acute glomerulonephritis, is not a primary diagnosis versus 580.9, which is not italicized and may be reported as a primary diagnosis as also shown below:

From volume 1:

> *580.81*   *Acute glomerulonephritis in diseases classified elsewhere*
>   *Code first underlying disease, as:*
>   infectious hepatitis (070.0–070.9)
>   mumps (072.79)
>   subacute bacterial endocarditis (421.0)
>   typhoid fever (002.0)
>
> **580.9**   **Acute glomerulonephritis with unspecified pathological lesion in kidney**

Punctuation

Brackets enclose synonyms, alternative wordings, or explanatory phrases. The brackets may be regular type [ ] or italicized *[ ]*. See the example below:

From volume 1:

> **460**   **Acute nasopharyngitis [common cold]**

Parentheses enclose supplementary (nonessential) modifiers that do not affect the code number. Think of a nonessential modifier as one that could possibly make the diagnosis more specific for clinical reasons, but does not change the code assignment. Modifying terms enclosed in parentheses need not be present in the diagnostic statement. Parentheses also enclose many "see also" references.

From volume 2:

Diarrhea, diarrheal (acute) (autumn) (bilious) (bloody) (catarrhal) (choleraic) (chronic) (gravis) (green) (infantile) (lienteric) (noninfectious) (presumed noninfectious) (putrefactive) (secondary) (sporadic) (summer) (symptomatic) (thermic) 787.91

The code for diarrhea if described with any of these nonessential modifiers is still 787.91.

A colon indicates a term that is incomplete without one or more of the modifiers following it. They are used in volume 1 to help assign a given category.

From volume 1:

695.4 Lupus erythematosus
    Lupus:
        erythematodes (discoid)
        erythematodes (discoid), not disseminated

A brace encloses a series of terms modified by the statement appearing to the right of the brace.

From volume 1:

560.2 Volvulus

    Knotting
    Strnagulation
    Torsion } of intestine, bowel, or colon
    Twist

Symbols and Color Coding

√4ᵗʰ   This symbol in the Ingenix ICD-9-CM indicates that a code requires a fourth digit.

√5ᵗʰ   This symbol in the Ingenix ICD-9-CM indicates that a code requires a fifth digit.

From volume 1:

√5ᵗʰ **640.8**   **Other specified hemorrhage in early pregnancy**
[0,1,3]

The Ingenix edition of ICD-9-CM, volumes 1 and 2 uses color to identify unspecified, other specified, and manifestation codes. A yellow bar over the code description indicates a code is not specific. These codes capture conditions that are not specified in other codes, and are sometimes the best option available. Other times, however, these codes don't give payers enough information and reimbursement may be delayed while queries are made. A gray bar indicates a specific condition for which a unique code is not available. A blue bar indicates that a code represents a manifestation and is not to be used as a primary diagnosis. These codes should always be presented secondarily to the primary diagnosis.

DEFINITIONS

Nonspecific code. A catch-all code that specifies the diagnosis as "ill-defined," "other," or "unspecified." A nonspecific code may be a valid choice if no other code closely describes the diagnosis.

Notes

Notes are found in ICD-9-CM volumes 1 and 2 and have no fixed length. They give coding instructions.

From volume 1:

> 344   **Other paralytic syndromes**
>
>> Note: This category is to be used when the listed conditions are reported without further specification or are stated to be old or long standing but of unspecified cause. The category is also for use in multiple coding to identify these conditions resulting from any cause.

Notes also list five-digit choices or define terms to give additional information.

From volume 1:

> 574   **Cholelithiasis**
>
>> The following fifth-digit subclassification is for use with category 574:
>> 0   without mention of obstruction
>> 1   with obstruction

From volume 2:

> **Cyst** (mucus) (retention) (serous) (simple)
>
> *Note—In general, cysts are not neoplastic and are classified to the appropriate category for disease of the specified anatomical site. The generalization does not apply to certain types of cysts which are neoplastic in nature, for example, dermoid, nor does it apply to cysts of certain structures, for example, brachial cleft, which are classified as developmental anomalies.*

Notes in volume 1 are indented and printed in plain type, while those in volume 2 are boxed and printed in italics. The placement of these notes is as important as their content. Notes at the beginning of a chapter apply to all categories within the chapter. Those at the beginning of a subchapter apply to all categories within the subchapter. Likewise, notes preceding three-digit categories apply to all four- and five-digit codes within that category.

Instructional Notes

To assign diagnosis codes at the highest level of specificity, you must follow four additional kinds of notes:

Includes notes: "Includes" appears at the beginning of a chapter or section to provide further definition or to give an example of the category contents. The code includes those term listed under "includes," for example:

From volume 1:

> 633   **Ectopic pregnancy**
>
>> Includes: ruptured ectopic pregnancy

Excludes notes: "Excludes" indicates terms that are not to be coded under the referenced term, as they are listed elsewhere in ICD-9-CM. A code reference directing the reader to the term or area is listed in parentheses. For example:

From volume 1:

> 711   **Arthropathy associated with infections**
>
>> *Excludes: rheumatic fever (390)*

Code first notes: "Code first underlying disease" identifies diagnoses that are not primary and are incomplete when used alone. In such cases the code, its title, and instructions appear in italics. This type of instructional note appears only in volume 1. A code with this instructional note is referred to as the manifestation code and

---

☸ CODING AXIOM

When a single code does not fully describe a given condition, use multiple codes to identify all components of the diagnosis.

---

should be recorded second, with the underlying cause recorded first. Italicized brackets identify this situation in volume 2.

From volume 1:

595.4 Cystitis in diseases classified elsewhere
Code first underlying disease, as:
actinomycosis (039.8)
amebiasis (006.8)
bilharziasis (120.0–120.9)
Echinococcus infestation (122.3, 122.6)

Use additional code: "Use additional code" appears in volume 1 in those categories where an additional code is available to provide further information and to give a more complete picture of the diagnosis or procedure. The additional code should identify other aspects of the disease, including manifestation, cause, associated condition, and nature of the condition itself.

From volume 1:

358.2 Toxic myoneural disorders
Use additional E code to identify toxic agent

Abbreviations

NEC is an abbreviation for Not Elsewhere Classifiable. NEC is found only in volume 2. The index will direct you to the codes in this category when no other specific code has been created for the particular diagnosis. Therefore, codes followed by "NEC" should only be used when the available information specifies a condition, but no separate code for that condition is provided. "NEC" codes report "other specified" diagnoses which do not have a more specific code.

From volume 2:

Infestation
cestodes 123.9
specified type, NEC 134.8

NOS is an abbreviation for "not otherwise specified." NOS is found only in volume 1. Codes designated as "NOS" are to be used only when the information available is not sufficient to allow assignment of a more specific code.

From volume 1:

420.90   Acute pericarditis, unspecified
Pericarditis (acute):
NOS
infective NOS
sicca

Assigning Diagnosis Codes

Step 1: Determine the Main Terms

Analyze encounter forms, operative reports, and diagnostic statements for those words or main terms that identify the patient's condition or symptoms. Think of the main term as a common denominator—a total disease classification. Once you've located this general term, follow the alphabetic lists to the specific condition. The main terms in the following diagnoses are printed in bold type.

 DEFINITIONS

NEC. Denotes "not elsewhere classifiable" and directs you to codes when no other code has been created for that diagnosis.

NOS. Denotes "not otherwise specified" and should only be used when information available does not allow you to assign a specific code.

 KEY POINT

Analyze encounter forms, operative reports, and diagnostic statements for words or terms that identify the patient's condition or symptoms.

Acute **otitis** media
Upper respiratory **infection**
Infectious **mononucleosis**

Step 2: Look up the Main Term in Volume 2

There are exceptions to this guideline. For example, complications of medical and surgical procedures are listed under the main term complication. Late effects of certain conditions are found under the terms "Late" and "Status (post)."

> **Complications**
>> surgical procedures 998.9
>>> burst stitches or sutures 998.32
>
> **Late**
>> effect(s) (of)
>>> wound, open
>>>> head, neck, and trunk (injury classifiable to 870–879) 906.0

Step 3: Follow Cross-References

Volume 2 uses cross-references to possible modifiers for a term or its synonyms. Follow the cross-references to the correct code when the diagnosis is not located under the first term you find. There are three types of cross-references:

"See" indicates that you must reference the condition listed instead of the term you've found. You must follow the instruction to assign the correct diagnosis code.

> **Glomerulonephritis**
>> desquamative—see Nephrosis
> **Elbow—see condition**

"See also" indicates that additional information is available. This cross-reference provides you with an additional diagnosis and code when the main term or subterm is insufficient. The additional information helps select the correct code. Always follow this instruction to ensure appropriate coding.

> **Tuberculoma**—*see also* Tuberculosis
>> brain (any part) 013.2

"See category" directs you to an additional three-digit category in volume 1, tabular list. You cannot assign an appropriate code unless you follow this instruction and read the applicable notes in volume 1.

> **Laceration**
>> vagina
>>> with
>>>> molar pregnancy (*see also* categories 630–632) 639.2

General adjectives such as acute and hereditary, and references to anatomic sites such as arm and face, appear as main terms, usually with a cross-reference to see condition or see also condition.

Don't skip any of these directional steps when referring to volume 2. The notes are there to direct you to the correct code assignment and you must follow all the necessary directions to ensure proper coding.

When a single code does not fully describe a given condition, use multiple codes to identify all components of the diagnosis. However, medical record documentation must mention the presence of all the elements for each code to be used. If uncertain, query the physician.

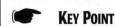

KEY POINT

"See also" indicates that additional information is available.

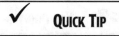

QUICK TIP

The medical record tells a written story of what has occurred with a patient The numeric and alphanumeric codes assigned by the medical coder must tell the same story in code.

Step 4: Review Subterms or Modifiers

A main term may be followed by one or more subterms that further describe the patient's condition. These supplemental words, called modifiers, may describe the severity, location, or symptoms of the condition. There are two types of modifiers, essential and nonessential.

Nonessential Modifiers

These subterms are listed immediately to the right of the main term and are enclosed in parentheses. They serve as examples to help you translate written terminology into numeric codes and do not affect the selection of the diagnostic code.

> **Goiter** (adolescent) (colloid) (diffuse) (dipping) (due to iodine insufficiency) (endemic) (euthyroid) (heart) (hyperplastic) (internal) (intrathoracic) (juvenile) (mixed type) (nonendemic) (parenchymatous) (plunging) (sporadic) (subclavicular) (substernal) 240.9

Essential Modifiers

These subterms are listed below the main terms and are indented two spaces. They are generally presented in alphabetical order, with the exceptions of with and without, which appear before the alphabetized modifiers. Each additional essential modifier clarifies the previous one and is indented two additional spaces to the right. These descriptive terms affect your code selection and describe essential differences in site, etiology, and symptoms.

> **Goiter**
>   simple 240.0
>   toxic 242.0
>   adenomatous 242.3
>   multinodular 242.2

When a main term in volume 1 has only one essential modifier, it appears on the same line as the main term, separated by a comma.

> 240.9   Goiter, unspecified

Step 5: Verify Code Selection in Volume 1

Although it may be tempting to code strictly from the volume 2 index, volume 1 is the authoritative ICD-9-CM coding reference. It contains diagnostic codes, full descriptions, additional instructional notes, and examples of terms assigned to each code. These are intended to enhance the verification process and ensure proper code selection. There are times, however, when a descriptive term listed in volume 2 is not found in volume 1. In these instances trust the index as the volume most often updated to reflect current usage, check to verify the tabular entry is not contradictory to the term, and use the index code.

When choosing diagnostic codes, you must code to the highest level of specificity; in other words, use four- and five-digit codes when they are available. The first three digits make up the category and identify the main condition or disease. Fourth and fifth digits further specify the diagnosis and are required when available. Based on the information found in the following example, an initial episode of care for acute myocardial infarction of the anterolateral wall is coded 410.01.

KEY POINT

Volume 1 is the authoritative ICD-9-CM coding reference.

CODING AXIOM

When choosing diagnosis codes, you must code to the highest level of specificity.

From volume 1:

410   Acute myocardial infarction

The following fifth-digit subclassification is for use with category 410:

0   episode of care unspecified

1   initial episode of care

2   subsequent episode of care

410.0   Of anterolateral wall

410.1   Of other anterior wall

410.2   Of inferolateral wall

410.3   Of inferoposterior wall

410.4   Of other inferior wall

410.5   Of other lateral wall

410.6   True posterior wall infarction

410.7   Subendocardial infarction

410.8   Of other specified sites

410.9   Unspecified site

If no five-digit code exists, code to the fourth digit if one is available. The following category includes only four digits:

From volume 1:

413   Angina pectoris

413.0   Angina decubitus

413.1   Prinzmetal angina

413.9   Other and unspecified angina pectoris

Three-Digit Diagnosis Codes

Three-digit diagnosis codes are used only when no fourth or fifth digit is available. There are approximately 100 codes at the highest level of specificity in the three-digit form. See appendix 3 for a list of these three-digit codes. Many payers, including Medicare, do not accept three-digit codes when higher levels of specificity exist. Never use 0 or 9 as "fillers" to add fourth or fifth digits to codes.

From volume 1:

Correct:

412   Old myocardial infarction

Incorrect:

412.0 or 412.00

CLINICAL APPLICATIONS OF CODING GUIDELINES

Diagnostic coding has guidelines that must be applied to a broad variety of diseases and conditions. The medical record tells a written story of what has occurred with a patient. The numeric and alphanumeric codes assigned by the medical coder must tell the same story in code. Although diagnosis coding rules for inpatient and outpatient services are similar in some areas, they are very different in others. In some cases the rules directly contradict each other. The areas where inpatient and

---

✓   **QUICK TIP**

There are approximately 100 codes at the highest level of specificity in the three-digit form.

⌇   **CODING AXIOM**

All coders must learn how to correctly sequence and report diagnosis codes in accordance with the accepted guidelines.

---

outpatient services differ become familiar as you use the official coding guidelines. The most important factor in ICD-9-CM coding, whether outpatient or inpatient, is an understanding of the rules. Knowing how to correctly sequence and report diagnostic codes must be the goal for all coders. For official coding guidelines consult the *Official ICD-9-CM Guidelines for Coding and Reporting*, ICD-9-CM coding book instructional notes, and the *AHA Coding Clinic for ICD-9-CM*. The following sources are secondary resources that should be considered:

- Federal notices such as Medicare and Medicaid program memorandums
- *Federal Register* notices
- Medicare carrier and fiscal intermediary provider bulletins
- CMS online manual system (Pub. 100 manuals)

SUMMARY

We have learned that the diagnosis coding information has more uses than just as a means for reimbursement. Diagnosis coding should be accurate and reflect only what has been documented in the medical record. Understanding the format of ICD-9-CM and being able to use the official coding guidelines and coding conventions are mandatory for proper code assignment. Whenever you have a question regarding conflicts in the documentation, always consult with the practitioner for clarification before assigning the code. In the next book in this series, Ingenix Coding Lab, much more detail is offered into the specifics for each coding guideline.

The following discussion questions and issues are for your consideration upon completion of this chapter. A full series of test questions on this chapter are found on the accompanying CD-ROM and in the instructor's manual.

DISCUSSION QUESTIONS

- Historically, diagnosis codes were used to compile morbidity and mortality statistics. Do you think this function is still important today? Weigh in your mind the relative value of diagnosis codes to statisticians, outcomes researchers, financial managers, and insurance underwriters. Why do you think it is necessary for medical coders to use a version of ICD-9-CM that is "clinically modified"?
- Smallpox has been eradicated for more than 20 years, yet diagnosis codes still exist for this disease. Why do you think it is necessary to either maintain or eliminate the listing? Think about the role that diagnoses play in the world of medicine and examine the consequences of misdiagnosis. Examine the consequences of assigning an incorrect ICD-9-CM code.
- ICD-9-CM features codes for healthy individual seeking routine health check-ups. Why do you think diagnosis codes are necessary (or unnecessary) for this purpose?
- Can you successfully differentiate diagnosis codes by sight? What comes to mind when you hear the term "V codes"? How about "E codes"? Are you comfortable with the conventions of both volumes of ICD-9-CM?

Chapter 5: HCPCS Level II Coding

INTRODUCTION

As we have discussed in the previous two chapters, medical coders have tools to report medical procedures and services and the diagnoses that justify the treatment. But another area of medical coding has yet to be addressed: nonphysician services, specific supplies, and the administration of drugs. HCPCS Level II codes are the tools to report these types of services and supplies.

The term HCPCS can be confusing. HCPCS (pronounced "HICK-picks") is most accurately used as the acronym for the entire three-level Healthcare Common Procedure Coding System. The federal government refers to all procedure codes as the HCPCS system. But HCPCS is also commonly used to specifically identify HCPCS Level II national codes, the topic of this chapter. The *Physicians' Current Procedural Terminology* (CPT) codes are Level I of the system. The HCPCS Level II codes are published by the Centers for Medicare and Medicaid Services (CMS) and are updated annually, effective on the first of each year. Because the Level I CPT coding system does not include codes for nonphysician services and specific supplies, CMS created a series of codes to supplement and complement the CPT coding system. In addition, a specific category was created for the administration of certain drugs.

To see how HCPCS fits within the entire CMS coding system, we offer the following overview of each of the three levels, their official names, and their popular, commonly used names.

HCPCS LEVEL I /CPT CODING SYSTEM

Level I is the American Medical Association's (AMA) CPT coding system, which was developed and is maintained and copyrighted by the AMA. The CPT book provides five-digit codes with descriptive terms to report services performed by healthcare providers and is the country's most widely accepted procedure coding reference. The CPT book was first published in 1966 and is updated annually. Code changes become effective January 1st of each year. (Further information about the CPT book can be found in chapter 3.)

In the CPT book, procedures are grouped within six major sections: evaluation and management (E/M), anesthesia, surgery, radiology, pathology and laboratory, and medicine. They are then broken into subsections according to body part, service, or condition (e.g., mouth, amputation, septal defect).

HCPCS LEVEL II NATIONAL CODES

More than 2,800 codes make up the HCPCS Level II national codes. The code set may be known informally as national codes, supply codes, or just as HCPCS.

OBJECTIVES

In this chapter, you will learn:

- About the nature and uses of Level II of the HCPCS
- The role of HCPCS in billing and reimbursement
- About DMEPOS, DMERCs, and basic Medicare requirements
- About Level II modifiers and their conventions and guidelines

FOR MORE INFO

Maintenance and modification of HCPCS Level II codes are duties of the alpha-numeric coordinator, Center for Medicare Management, Centers for Medicare and Medicaid Services (CMS), located in Baltimore, MD.

These codes are updated annually but new codes may be introduced throughout the year as necessary. Codes may also be changed or deleted throughout the year. The alphanumeric codes represent groups of services or supplies. HCPCS codes are now required to report most medical services and supplies provided in outpatient settings to Medicare and Medicaid patients. And recent federal rules pertaining to HIPAA (Health Insurance Portability and Accountability Act of 1996) formally mandate Level II codes for standardized electronic claims. Most of the larger national payers, including workers' compensation payers, recognize HCPCS codes. The codes are available from CMS, the regional Medicare carrier, or from commercial publishers such as Ingenix. If an appropriate HCPCS Level II code exists, it takes precedence over a CPT code in Medicare billing. Many private payers, however, prefer Level I codes or National Drug Codes (NDCs) over their counterpart HCPCS Level II codes.

THE HCPCS NATIONAL CODES IN DETAIL

According to the CMS, literally millions of medical products are described by Level II codes. Nonetheless, no actual products are named in the descriptions or endorsed through assignment of the codes. Furthermore, development of the codes occurs independently of issues surrounding reimbursement. Consequently, the presence of a Level II code is only an indicator that the product or service is available within the larger medical system, rather than an indicator that reimbursement is warranted.

HCPCS Level II national codes may be used throughout the United States in all Medicare regions. And as a component of HIPAA legislation, the codes will be required to report and bill supplies by electronic transaction.

National codes consist of one alpha character (A through V) followed by four digits (A0000–V9999). The letter "I" is not used because of its high likelihood of being mistaken for the numeral "1." Several other letters are not currently represented. Each letter category embraces an area, or several areas, of similar products and services.

HCPCS Level II provides specific codes for supplies, services, injections and certain drugs, durable medical equipment (DME), orthotics, prosthetics, and similar supplies. HCPCS Level II codes are designed to provide more specificity than CPT codes. The codes are public domain and are maintained by CMS.

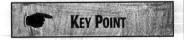

KEY POINT

The presence of a Level II HCPCS code is only an indicator that the product or service is available within the larger medical system, rather than an indicator that reimbursement is warranted by its use.

HCPCS CODES

Each section of codes is designated by a letter code except for the last section, "Table of Drugs."

A codes. Include ambulance and transportation services, medical and surgical supplies, administrative, and miscellaneous and investigational services and supplies.

B codes. Include enteral and parenteral therapy.

C codes. Used exclusively for services paid under the outpatient prospective payment system (PPS) and are not used to bill services paid under other Medicare payment systems.

D codes: Include diagnostic, preventive, restorative, endodontic, periodontic, prosthodontic, prosthetic, orthodontic, and surgical dental procedures. These codes are supplied to CMS by the American Dental Association, which holds copyright for this category. The association maintains the code set and develops new ones as needed. The D codes have recently been removed from the official HCPCS listing but remain available from the ADA.

E codes. Include durable medical equipment such as canes, crutches, walkers, commodes, decubitus care, bath and toilet aids, hospital beds, oxygen and related respiratory equipment, monitoring equipment, pacemakers, patient lifts, safety equipment, restraints, traction equipment, fracture frames, wheelchairs, and artificial kidney machines.

G codes. Include temporary procedures and professional services that are under review prior to inclusion in the CPT code book.

J codes. Include drugs that cannot ordinarily be self-administered, chemotherapy drugs, immunosuppressive drugs, inhalation solutions, and other miscellaneous drugs and solutions.

K codes. Temporary codes for durable medical equipment and drugs. Once these codes are approved for permanent inclusion in HCPCS, they typically become A, E, or J codes.

L codes. Include orthotic and prosthetic procedures and devices, as well as scoliosis equipment, orthopedic shoes, and prosthetic implants.

M codes. Include office services and cardiovascular and other medical services.

P codes. Include certain pathology and laboratory services.

Q codes. Miscellaneous temporary codes.

R codes. Diagnostic radiology services codes.

S codes. Replaced many of the Level III (local) codes. Local codes are being phased out as a provision of HIPAA.

T codes. Established for state Medicaid agencies and are not valid for Medicare.

V codes. Include vision, hearing, and speech-language pathology services.

The "Table of Drugs" lists all drugs found in HCPCS by their generic name, with amount, route of administration, and code number. Brand name drugs are also listed in the table with a reference to the appropriate generic drug.

KEY POINT

The HCPCS D codes, commonly known as dental codes, have been removed from the official listing. The codes are supplied and maintained by the American Dental Association, which holds copyright to this category. A full listing of D codes is available from the ADA.

DEFINITIONS

Enteral. Pertaining to the intestines and parenteral pertains to other than the alimentary canal. Enteral is often used in the context of nutrition management: formulas, jejunostomy tubes, nasogastric devices, etc. Parenteral is usually used in a method of delivery context: total parenteral nutrition (TPN) and parenteral nutrition therapy (PNT) formulas, kits, and devices.

USE OF HCPCS

The following points summarize why practices use HCPCS codes:

- HCPCS codes are mandated by CMS for use on Medicare claims and are also required by most state Medicaid offices. The codes are becoming a standard component of electronically transmitted claims.
- HCPCS codes improve a provider's ability to communicate services or supplies correctly without resorting to narrative descriptions.
- The codes reduce resubmission of claims for correction or review.
- Up-to-date and accurate HCPCS codes on office routing slips allow office staff to assign fees quickly and efficiently to services and supplies, saving both time and money.
- Consistent submission of "clean claims" (claims having all correct information necessary to process) helps avoid audits by carriers due to lack of specificity.
- Use of HCPCS is essential for accurate and complete reimbursement from Medicare.
- Supplies billed to Medicare as "other than incidental to an office visit" (CPT code 99070) are not reimbursed unless identified with Level II/HCPCS.

HOW TO USE HCPCS

The various publishers of HCPCS may have differing instructions on use of the codes. The Ingenix *HCPCS Level II Expert* uses CPT code book conventions to indicate new and revised codes. A black circle (●) precedes a new code to be used only for services or supplies provided on or after January 1 of the given year; a black triangle (▲) precedes a code with revised terminology. Codes deleted from last year's active list appear with a strikethrough

Other pertinent information is given with each HCPCS code. Codes that are not covered by—or valid for—Medicare are so noted. When "Carrier Discretion" is indicated, contact the carrier for specific coverage information on those codes. "Special Coverage Instructions" keys coders to refer to the CMS online manual system Pub. 100 reference manuals. Some codes are cross-referenced to other Level II/HCPCS codes, specific CPT codes, or to the CPT book in general.

COLOR-CODED COVERAGE INSTRUCTIONS

The Ingenix *HCPCS Level II Expert* provides symbols and color bar indicators for each coverage and reimbursement instruction. A legend to these symbols is provided on the bottom of each page.

Codes that are not covered by or valid for Medicare are indicated. Refer to the appropriate CMS Pub. 100 reference manual chapters and sections.

When carrier discretion is noted, the carrier can be contacted for specific coverage information on those codes.

When special coverage instructions are indicated and apply to a code, they are typically found in Pub. 100 reference manual chapter and sections, which are listed in an appendix to the book.

The Ingenix *HCPCS Level II Expert* provides a quantity alert because many codes report quantities that may not coincide with quantities available in the marketplace.

For instance, a HCPCS code for a disposable syringe reports one syringe, but the syringe is generally sold in boxes of 100, and "100" must be indicated in the quantity box on the CMS claim form to ensure proper reimbursement.

Codes applicable only to males or only to females are also indicated in the Ingenix *HCPCS Levell II Expert.*

MODIFIERS

Modifiers should, or in some cases must, be used to identify circumstances that alter or enhance the description of a service or supply. There are also three levels of CMS coding system modifiers—one for each level of codes.

Level I/CPT modifiers are two numeric digits (e.g., 22 Unusual procedural services) and are described in detail in the CPT book. They are also maintained and updated on an annual basis by the AMA.

Level II/HCPCS modifiers are two alphabetic or alphanumeric digits (e.g., AA–VP). There are also several one-digit modifiers that must be used in the two-digit combinations. They are recognized by carriers nationally and are updated annually by CMS.

The complete listing of modifiers is found in the HCPCS manual. Some notable ones include:

AA	Anesthesia services performed personally by anesthesiologist
AS	Physician assistant, nurse practitioner, or clinical nurse specialist services for assist at surgery
GM	Multiple patients on one ambulance trip
GZ	Item or service expected to be denied as not reasonable and necessary
NU	New equipment
Q5	Service furnished by a substitute physician under a reciprocal billing arrangement
Q6	Service furnished by a locum tenens physician
QB	Physician providing service in a rural HPSA
QM	Ambulance service provided under arrangement by a provider of services
QN	Ambulance service furnished directly by a provider of services
QP	Documentation is on file showing that the laboratory test(s) was ordered individually or ordered as a CPT-recognized panel other than automated profile codes 80002–80019, G0058, G0059, and G0060
QU	Physician providing service in an urban HPSA
QW	CLIA waived test
QX	CRNA service: with medical direction by a physician
QZ	CRNA service: without medical direction by a physician
SA	Nurse practitioner rendering service in collaboration with a physician
SB	Nurse midwife
SC	Medically necessary service or supply
SE	State and/or federally-funded programs/services
SG	Ambulatory surgical center (ASC) facility service
TC	Technical component.
TD	RN

 DEFINITIONS

HPSA. Health professional shortage area. Medicare and other federal health programs offer incentives to physicians to practice in these designated areas.

TE	LPN/LVN
TF	Intermediate level of care
TG	Complex/high tech level of care
TH	Obstetrical treatment/services, prenatal or postpartum

Under certain circumstances, a charge may be made for a technical component alone. Under those circumstances adding modifier TC to the usual procedure number identifies the technical component charge. Technical component charges are institutional charges and not billed separately by physicians.

Unlisted HCPCS Codes

Unlisted HCPCS codes are unique to a section or a subsection of codes. Third-party payers designate as unlisted all HCPCS codes that include the term unlisted in the definition. In addition, payers often apply the unlisted codes to services and supplies that are described in indefinite terms, do not have a precise meaning, and/or have language open to differing interpretations. Terms and phrases commonly found in the descriptions of these unlisted HCPCS codes include the following:

- Miscellaneous
- NES (not elsewhere specified)
- NOC (not otherwise classified)
- Unclassified
- Unspecified

Definitions

Medicare carrier. An organization that contracts with the Centers for Medicare and Medicaid Services (CMS) to process Medicare claims under Part B, the supplemental medical insurance program. Medicare carriers are responsible for daily claims processing, utilization review, records maintenance, and dissemination of information based on CMS regulations. In addition, the carrier determines the eligibility status of beneficiaries, determining whether the services are covered and whether the payments for those services are appropriate.

Practicing the Principles

Now you can begin the process of locating codes and modifiers that apply to services and procedures.

To locate a HCPCS Level II code, follow these steps:

1. First identify the services or procedures the patient received. For example, a patient rents a nonprogrammable ambulatory infusion pump for chemotherapy treatment.

2. Look up the appropriate term in the index. For example: Pump, Implantable infusion.

3. Assign a tentative code(s).

   Codes E0782 and E0783 are tentatively assigned.

   Note: To the right of the terminology, you find a single code, or multiple codes, or a cross-reference. Tentatively assign all codes listed.

4. Locate the code(s) in the appropriate section of the alphanumeric list.

   E0782   Infusion pump, implantable, nonprogrammable

   E0783   Infusion pump system, implantable, programmable

5. Check for symbols, notes, and footnotes.

6. Review the footnote definitions and other guidelines for coverage issues that apply.

7. Determine whether any modifiers should be used.

8. Assign the code.

To report a specific drug, use a Level II code from the J section rather than a CPT code.

When a CPT code includes the word "specify" as part of its description, check for a HCPCS Level II. See CPT code 90788 as an example.

HOSPITAL OUTPATIENT SERVICES

The Omnibus Budget Reconciliation Act (OBRA) of 1986 requires hospitals to report claims for outpatient services using the HCPCS code system, including the CPT coding system and HCPCS Level II. This requirement applies to acute care hospitals, long-term care hospitals, rehabilitation hospitals, psychiatric hospitals, and hospital-based rural clinics. End-stage renal disease (ESRD) claims for both hospitals and free standing facilities require HCPCS coding.

HCPCS must be used when submitting claims to Medicare Part A and B for:

- ESRD drugs and supplies
- Chemotherapy drugs
- Ambulance services
- Outpatient medical and clinical services
- Emergency services
- Laboratory services
- Radiology and other diagnostic services
- Orthotic/prosthetic devices and DME
- Evaluation and management services

PHYSICIAN OFFICE SERVICES

As stated in *Medicare Claims Processing Manual*, Pub. 100-04, chap. 15, sec. 50, HCPCS codes must be used to submit claims to Medicare Part B for:

- ESRD drugs and supplies
- Chemotherapy drugs
- Ambulance services
- Certain drugs and biologicals which cannot be self-administered
- Laboratory and pathology services
- Radiology and other diagnostic services
- Orthotic/prosthetic devices and DME
- Evaluation and management services
- Services of nonphysician practitioners
- Services incident to physician services

DMEPOS

An individual or entity (group medical practice, medical equipment company, or franchised vendor) that dispenses, sells, or rents certain durable medical equipment and supplies to Medicare patients is known as a DMEPOS. Many physician practices, multi-specialty clinics, and certain facilities are registered as suppliers. Coding and billing duties, therefore, are handled by the medical coding staff. The treating provider and the DMEPOS supplier may be under the same roof.

DEFINITIONS

Medicare Part A. Coverage includes hospital, nursing home, hospice, home health, and other inpatient care. Claims are submitted to intermediaries for reimbursement. Ten regional offices provide the Centers for Medicare and Medicaid Services (CMS) with decentralized administration and delivery of Medicare programs. Each regional office manages private insurance companies that contract with the government to process and make payment for Medicare services.

DEFINITIONS

Fiscal intermediary (FI). An organization, usually an insurance company, that Medicare contracts with to handle claims for services provided to Medicare patients for Part A coverage. Fiscal intermediaries process the claims sent in by providers according to Medicare guidelines. Providers can sign a participating provider agreement (PAR) with the FI to accept assignment on all claims submitted to Medicare. Accepting assignment simply means that the provider has agreed to accept the amount Medicare pays for a service or product and will not bill the patient the difference between the provider's ordinary charge and the Medicare allowable.

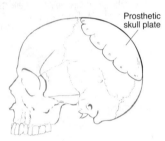

Example of skull prosthesis

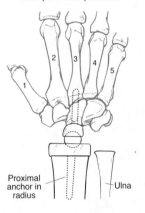

Example of wrist prosthesis

 DEFINITIONS

Prosthesis. A device that serves as an artificial substitute for any of a broad range of missing or defective body parts. A prosthesis may be applied to a limb, an eye, or an internal organ such as a heart valve. The device may be functional, such as a palate device, or cosmetic, such as a facial device. Prosthetic is a term that generally pertains to the use or application of such devices.

Durable medical equipment, prosthetics, orthotics, and supplies (DMEPOS) embrace a full range of medical products. According to CMS, durable medical equipment must meet specific criteria to be eligible for Medicare coverage. These criteria are shown here in the form of questions.

DME Criteria

The provider or supplier must answer yes to all questions for the equipment or device to be eligible for reimbursement under the Medicare program:

- Can the medical equipment withstand repeated use?

- Is the medical equipment primarily and customarily used for medical purposes?

- Is the medical equipment not of use to a person without illness or injury or in need of improvement of a malformed body part?

- Is the medical equipment appropriate for home use?

If the above listed criteria in the second and third items is not met, payment for the DME item may still occur if the therapeutic purpose of the equipment or device is clearly distinguished.

DMEPOS Definitions

Prosthetic devices, as recognized by CMS and many third-party payers, are those devices that replace all or part of an internal body organ, or replace all or part of the function of a permanently inoperative or malfunctioning internal body organ or body part. This category of devices includes:

- Artificial limbs
- Breast and eye prostheses
- Maxillofacial devices
- Joint implants
- Devices that replace all or part of the ear or nose
- Ostomy and colostomy bags
- Irrigation and flushing equipment directly related to ostomy/colostomy care

Orthotics are devices used for the correction or prevention of skeletal deformities. This includes braces for the neck, shoulder and arm, forearm, wrist and hand, hip, leg, ankle, and foot, as well as spinal or back devices. Supplies are generally considered items or accessories needed for the effective use of durable medical equipment, or prosthetic, or orthotic devices, appliances, or items.

Administration

Medicare claims for DMEPOS are contracted by CMS to four insurance companies for processing and payment. The companies are known as durable medical equipment regional carriers (DMERC) and the regions are designated by letters A, B, C, and D.

Suppliers of durable medical equipment and supplies register with a DMERC and are issued a supplier number through the National Supplier Clearinghouse. Part of the enrollment process involves a Medicare assignment agreement similar to those offered to providers. By accepting assignment, the supplier agrees to accept Medicare approved amounts as payment in full. Suppliers who choose not to accept assignment are known as nonparticipating and must accept payment through the patient.

Participating suppliers agree to cover the costs of a claim should it not meet Medicare's coverage criteria for that item. Nonparticipating providers can choose to accept assignment on a claim-by-claim basis.

Documentation

Suppliers in many instances must document a written dispensing order, a certificate of medical necessity (CMN), and diagnosis information to support medical need and uses for the product. The treating physician's signature and identification number must be documented. Patient authorization and proof of delivery documentation is also demanded upon audit.

Payment Categories

The DMERCs feature payment categories for supplies. Coders should be familiar with the categories used most frequently in their facilities. The categories are:

- Capped rental
- Frequent and substantial service DME
- Customized DMEPOS
- Prosthetics/orthotics
- Inexpensive and routinely purchased DME
- Oxygen and oxygen equipment
- Parenteral/enteral nutrients
- Parenteral/enteral supplies and kits
- Parenteral/enteral pumps
- Immunosuppressive drugs
- Ostomy, tracheostomy, and urologicals
- Surgical dressings
- Supplies
- Not otherwise classified
- Nebulizer drugs
- Therapeutic shoes for diabetics
- Individual consideration
- Epoetin
- Dialysis supplies and equipment
- Oral antiemetic drugs

Some HCPCS codes may not be designated by category.

THE HCPCS LEVEL II CODES

As previously mentioned, the range of medical products and services described by Level II codes is enormous. The following is a commentary on the nature of some Level II code categories.

A Codes

The A codes embrace a variety of services and products ranging from ambulance and transportation to blood glucose reagent strips. Many of the A codes are supplies related to ostomies, tracheostomies, and urologicals. Inexpensive DME for the A codes is defined as equipment priced not higher than $150 and quite a number of these codes qualify, particularly nebulizer replacement components. Modifiers include RR for rental, NU for new equipment, and UE for used equipment.

DEFINITIONS

Orthosis. This term derives from a Greek word meaning "to make straight." It is an artifical appliance that supports, aligns, or corrects an anatomical deformity or improves the use of a movable body part. Orthotic is a term that pertains generally to such devices. Unlike a prosthesis, an orthotic device is always functional in nature.

DEFINITIONS

Nebulizer. This term is derived from a Latin word meaning "mist." It is a device that converts liquid into a fine spray. These devices are commonly used to deliver medicine to the upper respiratory, bronchial, and lung areas.

B Codes

These codes largely describe products related to enteral and parenteral nutrition. Enteral nutrition is formula delivered by tube into the intestines. Parenteral is delivery by other means, typically intravenous. Stomach tubes, kits, and pumps are also coded from this category. These codes are usually assigned through facilities with clinical protocols to govern the administration of enteral and parenteral nutrition.

E Codes

The E codes embrace equipment such as canes, crutches, walkers, wheelchairs, and many of the items that come first to mind when durable medical equipment is mentioned. But also included is a variety of compressors, pumps, and oxygen-related products.

J Codes

The J codes stand aside from the rest of the Level II codes because of their function in reporting drugs and pharmaceuticals.

The J codes were developed to report drugs that cannot ordinarily be self-administered, and most are delivered by intramuscular, intravascular, or by skin injection. Chemotherapy drugs, immunosuppressive drugs, inhalation solutions, and other miscellaneous drugs and solutions are also listed. Proprietary names are not part of the official listing, although publishers such as Ingenix do offer brand references.

KEY POINT

The J codes stand aside from the rest of the Level II codes because of their function in reporting drugs and pharmaceuticals.

SUMMARY

Clearly, HCPCS level II codes comprise an important aspect of medical coding. The sheer volume of products, supplies, and pharmaceuticals reported by these codes is astounding. And accurate, conscientious code selection from this level is imperative. Good coding practices do not stop at the procedural and diagnosis levels. The third leg of the stool is HCPCS and when this area of medical coding is as strong as the other two, financial and regulatory success is almost guaranteed.

The following discussion questions and issues are for your consideration upon completion of this chapter. A full series of test questions on this chapter are found on the accompanying CD-ROM, and in the instructor's manual.

DISCUSSION QUESTIONS

- Consider the differences in coding methodology for procedural, diagnostic, and medical supply purposes. Does the system seem sensible to you? Do you think this level of coding could be constructed differently? Why aren't all codes alphanumeric? Or five-digit numeric? Or bar-codes?
- Why do you think a HCPCS Level II code should take precedence over a matching CPT code for Medicare purposes?
- Can you identify the categories of HCPCS codes by sight? What comes to mind when you hear the term J code? How about E code?
- Are you comfortable using Level II modifiers? Compare them to CPT modifiers.

Chapter 6: Medical Coding and Practice Management

INTRODUCTION

As has been presented in previous chapters, medical codes and the people who work at the job of assigning them are at the center of this training. However, many other aspects of a health care practice affect the assignment of medical codes. The finance, and billing departments, medical records, the legal department, front office, and of course, the health care providers themselves.

In many practices and smaller clinics, billing duties and medical coding may be performed by the same individual. In others a reimbursement specialist will oversee a coding staff as well as insurance billing clerks. Some clinics employ a Medicare reimbursement specialist. Inpatient facilities usually feature close interaction between coders and the medical records staff. Variations in operations structure and type of service offered to patients greatly influences how medical coding fits into the larger management picture. But coders-in-training should be familiar with some of the duties of their colleagues in health care settings. This chapter only touches upon a broad variety of practice management areas and is not intended as formal training in these fields of health care.

In the first part of this chapter we provide you with a broad overview of the following areas of medical management:

- Registration
- Preauthorization and precertification
- Claim submission and processing
- Problem claims
- Charge amounts

OBJECTIVES

In this chapter, you will learn:
- Basic management and front-office procedures and duties
- About the concepts behind fee schedules and relative values
- About inpatient reimbursement methodologies
- The elements of medical documentation and components
- Basic tenets of legal and compliance issues

REGISTRATION

The registration process begins when the patient schedules an appointment and continues to when the patient arrives for the medical visit. Registration is the gathering of pertinent information such as the patient's address, emergency contact, insurance information, and payment responsibility. This is often when a medical record number is assigned, which may follow a patient throughout a lifetime. Accurate registration information insures timely payment from insurers and decreases the chances for claim rejection.

In hospital settings, an admissions clerk usually fills out the admission information for the medical record, called a face sheet. It contains hospital specific patient and billing information, including admission diagnosis. But it does not contain information such as allergies, current medications, or previous medical history and pertinent family history.

While it may seem that the registration of a patient may have nothing to do with coding, it does in fact play an important role in code selection. Some payers have their own "payer specific" coding rules and knowing what type of insurance the patient has may affect code selection. Where payer specific coding rules apply, they take precedence over the general CPT or ICD-9-CM coding rules. For example, Medicare will not pay for administration of an injection (90782–90784) when reported with an office visit code. Only the office visit code is reported for coding purposes.

ENCOUNTER FORMS

The encounter form is an internal tool to transmit information from the physician or medical staff to the billing staff. It is not part of the medical record. However, it is important to mention encounter forms briefly.

	New	Established	Fee	DX
❑ Level 1	99201	99211	_____	____
❑ Level 2	99202	99212	_____	____
❑ Level 3	99203	99213	_____	____
❑ Level 4	99204	99214	_____	____
❑ Level 5	99205	99215	_____	____

An encounter form, sometimes referred to as a superbill or charge ticket, is a preprinted form that lists select procedure and diagnosis codes. The form may also contain standard CPT nomenclature (terminology) for services commonly performed in a practice. Several categories of charge tickets may be used by one office: office services, out-of-office services, ancillary services, etc. HCPCS Level II codes may also appear on charge tickets. During the patient encounter, the physician checks off procedures and diagnoses applicable to the patient visit. The information from the encounter form is transferred to a billing system. The billing system will then generate electronic or paper claims for submission to payers.

Due to the checklist format, encounter forms are not considered a documentation tool. Coders rely mainly on the patient record to make coding decisions, although encounter forms are used as a source of comparison. The encounter form should be reconciled to the patient list each day to assure that charges are captured for all patients seen.

Because some practices use encounter forms for charge capture, the form should be reviewed each year when the CPT, HCPCS, and ICD-9-CM code sets are updated to verify the codes are still current for use in the coming year.

PRECERTIFICATION AND PREAUTHORIZATION

Many insurance company contracts require precertification prior to performance of certain procedures or they will not reimburse for the procedure. With a precertification, the payer states that it covers that procedure for that patient, but this does not guarantee payment. Precertification authorizes the service to be performed, based on medical information about the patient's signs, symptoms, injury, or illness.

To preauthorize a service is to find out from a payer if it is a covered benefit under the medical circumstances. It gives authorization for an admission or to set a time for the initial review of the hospital stay. Insurance companies authorize a service prior to performance in order to make certain it is necessary. Medical necessity is the determining factor for reimbursement based on the codes submitted for the procedure and its relationship to the diagnosis code. To predetermine a procedure is to ask a payer if and how much it will pay for that service. However many insurance companies do not disclose payment information until they have received an actual claim. All of these requests should include a brief narrative clearly describing the procedure and its anticipated CPT code, documentation regarding medical necessity, sometimes with a diagnosis code, and, if requested, estimated charges.

Preauthorization Form
Physician Name
Address
Phone

PATIENT INFORMATION

Insurance Company _____ Phone _____

Address _____

Patient Name _____

Address _____

Phone _____ Date of Birth _____

Subscriber/Policy Holder _____

Address if Different_____

Member # _____ Group # _____

PHYSICIAN INFORMATION

Physician/Surgeon _____ Provider # _____

Diagnosis/ ICD-9 code(s)	Procedure(s)—CPT code(s)

Pre-Cert for ❏ Admission and/or ❏ Surgery

Hospital/Facility _____ ❏ IP ❏ OP _____ Date _____

Estimated Length of Stay _____Requires Second Opinion ❏ NO ❏ YES

Insurance Contact Person _____ Ext. _____

Approval ❏ YES – Certification # _____ Denial ❏ NO

Why Denied _____

Any special qualifiers _____

All preauthorizations should supply and organize the information relevant to a procedure's insurance coverage.

CLAIMS SUBMISSION AND PROCESSING

What is a claim? A claim is a request to the responsible third party payer for the payment for services rendered. As soon as possible after providing the service, a claim should be submitted to the insurance company. Submitting the claim is the next step toward receiving payment. Claims may be submitted electronically or on paper. Medicare and other payers are mandating that more claims be submitted electronically rather than in paper format. With today's technology, claims submitted

 KEY POINT

All preauthorizations should supply and organize the information relevant to a procedure's insurance coverage.

electronically are processed more quickly and the claim's status and payment response are received more promptly. However, the claim must be completed properly to assure payment. Prompt payment helps with cash flow for the practice or facility.

Coders for a small office, may also be responsible for entering the data into the software system for transmission to the insurance company. Anyone entering claims data should be educated on the importance of linking the appropriate CPT codes, modifiers, as well as diagnosis codes appropriately during entry. A misplaced code or modifier may mean the claim does not pass edits or is denied because the codes cannot be paid as submitted.

Once received by the payer, claims go through a series of important steps as they are processed. The form or electronic transfer is duplicated and any attachments such as operative reports, cover letters, or pathology reports are separated from the claim.

The data are then transferred into the payer's computer system. A claim must pass through a series of electronic "edits" that verify completeness and accuracy. It goes through computer edits that verify the patient's coverage or eligibility and check for medical necessity. Coding errors (invalid or nonexistent codes) and other invalid data is also checked. A claim also passes through a series of edits to verify that the procedure is appropriate for the age or sex of the patient. If the claim is "clean" (meaning it has passed all of these edits), it is paid.

When a claim fails the edits, it is returned to the provider for correction of the data submitted. A claim that fails edits is said to be "rejected." A claim that passes the edits but requires additional information is known as a denied claim. The insurer requests the additional information, which is usually sent back through electronic transmission or by paper. Many times the payer simply puts an encoded message on the payment voucher to let the provider know what additional information is needed or why the claim was not paid.

Even clean claims can be delayed if they are complicated. Although a claim may contain all the information needed for payment, it may require examination by the payer's medical review department, which usually delays payment.

When the payer sends a check for payment, it will also send an explanation of benefits (EOB) to enable to provider to reconcile the payment against the bill submitted for the patient's services. The EOB may also indicate the status of unpaid claims that have been denied.

 KEY POINT

Claims are edited prior to evaluation for payment. A "clean" claim passes the edits.

 DEFINITIONS

Remittance or voucher. A statement or notice that a provider of services receives from a payer to reflect finalized claims, either paid or denied (commonly called the EOB—explanation of benefits or EOMB—explanation of Medicare benefits). It usually, but not always, accompanies payment.

CLAIMS SERVICE CENTER

THE ADVANTAGE INSURANCE SOCIETY
OF THE UNITED STATES

Date: February 3, 1994

David Johns MD
1220 South Street
Any town, USA 00000

Employee Name ....Jon Richards
Employee ID/Soc Sec 500-00-0000
Policy/Group ID 7891
Branch..57X   Office 2X
Location ....ABCD

Below is an Explanation of Benefits of the Employee's Group Medical Benefits with WESTERN AUTO SUPPLY CO.

a Patient: JON		Rel: CHILD (CH)		Claim Cntrl: 9104250929590-821322				Document #: 9110701173300-5		
b Type of Service	Service Date(s)	Total Charges	c Excluded	c See Remarks	d Covered Amount	e Deductible Amount	f Balance	Pay At	Benefit	
Office Visits	03/12/91	50.00			50.00	50.00		75%		
Surgery Out-patient	03/13/91	595.00			595.00	50.00	545.00	75%	408.75	
	03/22/91	46.00			46.00		46.00	75%	34.50	
Totals		691.00			691.00	100.00	691.00		443.25	

PAYMENT SUMMARY
Patient Account #: Joseph Richards   Amount Paid: **443.25**   Draft #:460303181

··**PLEASE REFER TO REVERSE SIDE FOR YOUR RIGHTS OF REVIEW AND APPEAL** ··
Detach and retain this statement for your records

Payers use codes on the explanation of benefits to explain reasons for nonpayment or payment reduction. For example, Medicare puts encoded messages on the remittance to explain the reason for nonpayment or denial. For those types of EOMBs, or explanation of medicare benefits, billers refer to the last page of the voucher for an explanation of the code. Medicare might add remarks to a CPT code on the EOMB to show that the payment was reduced because the appropriate diagnosis information is not present. It is possible to see a "CC" following the code, meaning Medicare has changed the submitted code to a more appropriate one (CC is a Level II modifier from the HCPCS coding system).

Care should be taken when payment is received to verify the amount is consistent with fee schedules and contracted amounts.

Postpayment review is discussed later in this chapter.

PROBLEM CLAIMS

The process of monitoring payments also involves dealing with problem claims. When payment is not received in 30 days, an inquiry is usually made by the provider's office about the status of the claim. Many payers require written inquiries, sometimes on the insurance company's specific forms. Other inquires can be made by phone.

An attached copy of the claim may be required for written inquiries unless use of the payer's specific claim inquiry form is used. Phone conversation notes and written correspondence are filed by hard copy or electronic backup by the insurance company.

Submission of a deleted or invalid code may trigger a review.

Challenges to code adjustments are often made by a provider's billing staff. Similarly, mistakes happen and a corrected claim is resubmitted. Medicare and most private payers also have appeals processes.

ADVANCE BENEFICIARY NOTICE

Medicare designated some procedures as noncovered services. These procedures, however, may still be recommended treatment for the patient. In these instances certain steps must be taken PRIOR to the performance of the procedure. The patient should be verbally notified of the procedure's noncovered status. The procedure, its risks and benefits should be explained to the patient. If the patient agrees to continuing with the procedure an advance beneficiary notice (ABN) should be completed.

The ABN includes the patient's name, the procedure to be performed, a statement indicating that the service in not covered by Medicare but is being performed at the patient's request. The ABN also assigns financial responsibility to the patient for the procedure. Any amounts paid by the patient for the procedure do not apply to the patient's deductible. In addition, Medigap payers may not cover the service.

Medicare regulations state that signing an ABN must be specific to that procedure. The ABN cannot be routinely signed for all services rendered by a provider or type of provider.

Additional information regarding ABNs and their usage may be obtained from the Medicare website www.hhs.cms.gov or the Medicare learning site, Medlearn.

DEFINITIONS

Resubmitted claim. One that has been sent more than once to the payer for a response.

DEFINITIONS

Chargemaster. A file, usually in an electronic billing system, where charge amounts are kept for all procedures, services, and supplies in a hospital for use with billing software in claims submission.

CHARGE AMOUNTS

Fees or charges are determined based on a number of factors such as the expenses of operating an office or hospital, the cost of malpractice insurance, staffing costs. Care analysis and profit margin are also typical factors. The fee schedule of a medical practice—or the chargemaster of a hospital—is where the fees are listed, usually according to procedure code.

Insurance companies have their own fee schedules or payment amounts by which they pay a claim when submitted. Commercial insurance companies typically keep their payment and allowable information as confidential before payment of a claim. Medicare, however, publishes its fee schedule and it is available to the general public. All of this information is important to the development of a fee schedule for a practice or hospital. Fees are often developed according to the rationale that they always be at least as much as the lowest paying insurance allows.

PHYSICIAN REIMBURSEMENT METHODOLOGIES

Procuring reimbursement for health care services is one of the most complex processes of the system. Since the cost of health care has risen dramatically in recent years, the federal government has taken the lead in cost containment through a number of legislative enactments affecting the reimbursement system.

On December 19, 1989, the Omnibus Budget Reconciliation Act of 1989 provided for replacing the previous "reasonable charge" mechanism (actual, customary, and prevailing charges) with a resource based relative value scale (RBRVS) fee schedule. The intent of this physician payment reform, which began in 1992, was to establish consistent payment policies as well as payment equity.

The RBRVS system was created to accurately reflect the skill, time, and resources required for each procedure or office visit. Revisions are made annually to the payment policies and adjustments are made to the relative value units. The Medicare physician fee schedule data base (MPFSDB) is released in the fall with changes effective January 1st of each year.

The major factors for computing the payment amount under the RBRVS system are:

- Relative value units (RVUs)
- Conversion factor (CF)
- Geographical practice cost indices (GPCIs)

Other factors that can affect the payment amount for services under the physician fee schedule are the use of modifiers, the site of service, global surgery periods, and payment status.

Relative Value Units

The total relative value unit (RVUt) of a service or procedure has three components:

- **Work (RVUw).** This element reflects the physician resources of skill, time, and intensity of effort to furnish the service.
- **Practice expense (PE-RVU).** Practice RVU reflects the overhead expenses (space, equipment, supplies, and support personnel) incurred to provide the service.
- **Malpractice (RVUm).** Malpractice RVU reflects the cost of professional liability insurance as a percentage of physician revenue.

With implementation of the RBRVS system, uniform payment policies and procedures by all carriers became increasingly important. This launched the Correct Coding Initiative (CCI). The goal of this initiative is to develop correct coding methodologies based on conventions in the American Medical Association's CPT book. The initiative applies to national and local policies and edits, coding guidelines developed by national societies, analyses of standard medical and surgical practices, and to review of current coding practices. Initiated in January 1996 and updated quarterly as an ongoing refinement process, the CCI develops correct coding edits designed to ensure uniform payment for the same rendered services, regardless of carrier jurisdictions.

> **QUICK TIP**
>
> The Correct Coding Initiative (CCI) is updated quarterly. Providers should use the most current version of the CCI.

INPATIENT REIMBURSEMENT METHODOLOGIES

Inpatient reimbursement is somewhat different. There are three basic inpatient reimbursement methodologies, although many variations exist within these three broad categories. One method is to reimburse based on cost or billed charges. The second is to reimburse a fixed amount per day, also called a per diem reimbursement. The third method is the prospective payment system (PPS).

Fee-for-Service/Cost/Billed Charge Reimbursement

Fee-for-service, also referred to as cost or billed charge, is based on the actual expenses a hospital incurs for a specific patient during a single admission, plus an added amount to cover administrative costs and profit. Under this method of reimbursement, all costs for documented services are covered, including: room, meals, nursing care, procedures, pharmaceuticals, supplies, etc. However, given that all billed charges are allowed or covered, hospitals have little incentive to contain costs.

Per Diem Reimbursement

A per diem reimbursement is a fixed amount paid per day for hospital care. Usually payers allow varying per diem amounts based on type of service. For example, an intensive care bed day is paid at a higher rate than a medical/surgical bed day or a newborn bed day. This method of reimbursement does not provide for a fixed rate for each admission. It does provide hospitals with an incentive to provide cost effective care by limiting the amount paid for each day of service.

Prospective Payment System

Under a PPS, the amount paid for services is determined prospectively. Prospective payment was not a new concept for payers when it was introduced to reimburse inpatient services. Payers had applied this methodology to reimbursement of physician services for some time by setting maximum allowables for various services, including office visits, surgical procedures and maternity care. In other words, the insurance companies set in advance the amount they will pay for a given service.

In order to develop a prospective payment system for inpatient services, a method of categorizing inpatient services needed to be developed. This was accomplished by the system of diagnosis-related groups (DRG) as described in the next section. The DRGs categorize the patient by type of case (a case being defined as a single admission for a single patient). Cases with similar characteristics are grouped together and a fixed reimbursement amount is calculated for each type of case.

The goal behind a prospective payment system is to contain the ever-increasing cost of health care. By setting a fixed, predetermined payment rate for each type of case, payers felt better able to control healthcare costs.

> **DEFINITIONS**
>
> **Prospective payment system (PPS).** System of paying for services at a predetermined rate for each type of discharge or for services based on a standard type of case. For inpatients, the Medicare PPS of diagnosis-related groups (DRG) was implemented in 1983 to hold down the rising cost of health care.

DIAGNOSIS-RELATED GROUP

The prospective payment system for inpatient services used today by the federal government (Medicare) and many other third-party payers is called the DRG system.

A diagnosis-related group (DRG) is a grouping of similar diagnoses and/or procedures. The groups are clinically cohesive and demonstrate similar consumption of hospital resources and length of stay patterns. In 1983, Congress mandated a national hospital PPS for all Medicare inpatients. The following types of hospitals are excluded from the PPS:

- Psychiatric hospitals or units
- Rehabilitation hospitals and units
- Children's hospitals
- Long-term care hospitals
- Cancer hospitals

DRGs provide the basis for payment to hospitals for Medicare, Medicaid, and an increasing number of commercially insured patients. The federal government adopted DRGs more than a decade ago to curb rising hospital costs associated with reasonable cost and line-item reimbursement methods.

The ICD-9-CM classification system is used to determine the DRGs. DRGs are assigned using the principal and secondary diagnosis codes, the principal and secondary procedure codes, age, sex, and discharge status. One DRG is assigned to each inpatient stay. The codes are reported to the Medicare fiscal intermediary (FI) for processing and reimbursement electronically using 837i format or on the Uniform Bill-92 (UB-92) claim form. The UB-92 claim form accepts up to nine diagnosis codes and six procedure codes.

Through DRGs, hospitals are reimbursed a flat rate based on a patient's diagnosis and treatment. The model assumes patients with similar illnesses undergo similar procedures and require similar care. Consequently, each category of illness/treatment is assigned a DRG that is the main factor in determining reimbursement.

Before DRGs, hospitals were paid based on itemized services following treatment and release. The payer and provider tallied the costs in retrospect, after the care was provided. Because DRG payments are standardized by diagnosis and treatment, DRGs allow payers and providers to predict reimbursement prospectively—before the care is provided. This type of reimbursement is called a PPS. Hospitals still itemize bills for their patients, but today, reimbursement now falls largely under the umbrella of the DRG assignment.

Personnel in medical record departments now influence the financial health of hospitals, as DRGs are based upon the ICD-9-CM codes assigned to diagnoses and procedures. Provider documentation is crucial to appropriate code assignment.

Evolution of DRGs

The implementation of a DRG-based payment system was prompted by Medicare administrators, who in the 1960s identified significant differences among hospitals in the costs incurred to care for patients with similar profiles. Intuitively, administrators knew that the more complex a hospital's patient mix, the higher its cost of doing business. For example, tertiary care facilities and teaching hospitals tend to admit patients referred from other facilities because they are too sick or injured to treat in a smaller facility. Although these sicker patients clearly contributed to higher costs,

---

 KEY POINT

Diagnosis-related groups (DRG) provide the basis for payment to hospitals for Medicare, Medicaid, and an increasing number of commercially insured patients. The federal government adopted DRGs more than a decade ago to curb rising hospital costs associated with reasonable cost and line-item reimbursement methods.

 DEFINITIONS

Case mix. The categories of patients (type and volume) treated by a hospital that represents the hospital's case load.

Tertiary care. Those health care services provided by highly specialized providers such as neurosurgeons, thoracic surgeons, and intensive care specialists. These services often require highly sophisticated technologies and facilities.

---

there was no established method to define the case mix and its exact association with the higher costs. For this reason, a methodology to closely define and measure hospital's patient case mix was undertaken.

Case Mix Complexity

Hospital executives closely evaluate case mix since the nature and severity of overall patient illnesses play heavily in budget projections. Researchers at Yale University developed the early application of the ICD-9-CM version of DRGs on the concept of patient case mix complexity. The researchers identified patient attributes that contributed most to resource demands. Key among them were the following:

- Severity of illness
- Prognosis
- Treatment difficulty
- Need for intervention
- Resource intensity

Patient Classifications

The next step was to classify patients based on information routinely collected in hospital medical records. The result was 25 major diagnostic categories (MDC). A distinction was then made to further separate MDCs into categories of medical or surgical cases.

The picture that began to emerge for the Yale researchers was a decision-making tree for DRG assignment. Once a surgical category had been established for a patient, further specification was based on the type of procedure performed—the surgical hierarchy. Medical patients were further defined according to principal diagnosis when admitted to the hospital. Both the medical and surgical classes within an MDC are organized by principles of anatomy, surgical approach, diagnostic approach, pathology, etiology, or treatment process.

Complications and Comorbidities

The medical and surgical classes were further tested to determine whether complications or comorbidities (CC) would affect consumption of hospital resources. For example, patients admitted for congestive heart failure may exhibit numerous CCs, such as kidney failure or urinary retention, which affect their length of stay in the hospital as well as their use of other services.

A comprehensive list of diagnoses generally associated with complications and comorbities was generated. It soon became apparent, however, that the validity of CCs is dependent upon the principal diagnosis. Over time, government and private parties developed a list of CC exclusions for inappropriate associations with the principal diagnoses.

The presence of a CC meant increased reimbursement should the CC be deemed valid in relation to the principal diagnosis.

Other Variables

A patient's age was determined to be a defining factor in DRG assignment. Pediatric patients and patients over age 70 were often assigned a DRG that evaluated age. The patient's status upon discharge from the hospital was also considered a variable in the definition of a DRG. Burn patients transferred to another facility, for example, were designated a separate DRG. Similarly, separate DRGs were designated for patients who leave the hospital against medical advice.

Following extensive testing, the DRG system was launched nationwide in 1983 with implementation of the Medicare prospective payment system.

POSTPAYMENT PROCESS

Once reimbursement is received the following procedures should be performed to complete the process:

- Read the explanation of benefits (EOB)
- Post the payment to the account
- Audit the payment for correct amount
- Conduct write-offs
- Review denials
- Balance bill where appropriate
- Process overpayments

It is as important to receive the correct payment and credit the correct patient account as it is to report the correct services and bill correctly. Payments not correctly reported may result in needless rebilling, confusion and ultimately may result in lost revenue.

Read the Explanation of Benefits (EOB)

Attached to the payment check or electronic funds transfer notification is a document explaining the reimbursement. This is called the explanation of benefits (EOB) or explanation of Medicare benefits (EOMB). The EOB usually contains the following information:

- Provider name
- Patient name
- Date(s) of service
- Procedure code(s) billed
- Amount billed

The EOB will usually indicate the amount allowed for a procedure, the amount paid, patient responsibility and any amounts to be written-off.

For any service reduced or not paid there must be an explanation, which is usually done by an appended code explained within the EOB.

The postpayment process is based on the information contained on the EOB. The EOB should be retained for a period of time for reference and in case of an audit.

Post the Payment to the Account

Payments must be posted in the accounting system. Just as a checking account is reconciled to verify the funds deposited and withdrawn from an account, patient accounts need to be reconciled.

Ideally the payment amounts will be reconciled to each billed code for each patient. Applying a lump-sum payment to a date of service does not allow quick access to valuable information obtained from the accounting system. Many payment systems allow identification of the origin of remittance made toward each code.

Patient payment amounts must also be posted appropriately. Payers may request verification that the patient has paid for the claim and/or their co-pay. If a patient pays for the service and subsequently an insurance company also pays it is important to be able to identify the sources of all payments to determine if and where an overpayment occurred and who should receive the payment refund.

Audit the Payment for the Correct Amount

The payment amounts need to be reconciled to each service. Medicare and many payers have a designated fee schedule or allowable amount. When you have a contract with a payer it is important to know how much to expect for that service.

The allowable amount should agree with the contracted arrangement. The portion paid by the payer and the patient responsibility should be verified that they match the allowed amount. Any patient deductibles can be noted.

The amount reimbursed must be verified as correct. A payer may have different reimbursement amounts based upon participation and contracts negotiated. If payment is not correct the provider may have been reimbursed based upon incorrect information that may result in continued incorrect payment. Over time, this may result in the overpayment or loss of a significant amount that may be even more difficult to reconcile. It may also result in discounting or writing off more than the contract states or additional lost revenue.

During the audit process, note any procedures not allowed by Medicare and why. If Medicare disallowed a billed secondary procedure, ensure its correctness. Medicare denies procedures for a variety of reasons. The billed procedure may be a noncovered procedure or an unbundled procedure, or there may be a conflict with a CCI edit.

Conduct Write-offs

When a provider has a contract with payer or Medicare, any amounts that exceed the allowed amount are usually subtracted from the patient account. This amount is called a write-off because the amount is written off from the account.

Write-offs may also occur due to denied services. Medicare and other payers may require that the patient is not notified before the procedure that the service may not be covered. Medicare requires an ABN if the patient is to be responsible for the procedures reimbursement.

Another type of write-off may occur for accounts sent to collections such as bad debt or even financial hardship. The provider should have an established policy for this type of write-off to apply the same guidelines to all patients.

Review Denials

It is estimated that as many as 20 percent of claims are denied. By reviewing the denied services lost revenue may be recovered. Reading the EOB to determine why a service was denied is the first key to recovery.

For example, if a claim is denied for incorrect patient information including patient name, policy number, insurance company, or employer the corrections can be made and the claim resubmitted. If an incorrect procedure code number was entered, a modifier not appended or incorrect diagnosis code corrections may be made and the bill can be resubmitted.

Some denials are the result of an incorrect billing practice. Making the correction on this claim and applying the correction to future claims can avoid additional denials. This is an opportunity for communication with the provider, billers and coders to effectively communicate and submit correct claims.

Balance Bill Where Appropriate

After the payer has reviewed and paid its portion of the claim and contractual write-offs have been made there may be a portion still not paid. Determine who is responsible for this additional amount. Billing for the remainder of the fee is called balance billing.

For example secondary payers such as Medigap will often cover the unpaid balance. When billing a secondary payer, a copy of the EOB may be required. If the EOB lists more than one patient copy, use only the portion related to that patient.

If the patient has a deductible or co-pay amount, then the patient may be billed for the balance billed for this portion.

One notable exception to balance billing is workers' compensation claims. Most states prohibit billing the patient for amounts that exceed the state designated allowable. These amounts must be written off.

Process Overpayments

Whenever the amount received for a claim exceed the amount billed or allowed by contractual agreement the overage needs to refunded. It is important to be able to track where each payment originated, who was responsible by reviewing the EOB, and determine who is entitled to the refund.

Keeping overpayments is illegal in most states and is considered fraudulent by Medicare and other payers. Some states do not allow the amount over from once claim to be applied to other outstanding claims. Knowledge of your state guidelines will be essential in the postpayment process.

THE MEDICAL RECORD AND DOCUMENTATION

The patient's medical record is a compilation of all the information that is gathered and recorded as a result of patient care. The record contains information about the patient's history of illnesses and treatments in a variety of locations, including office, inpatient, and outpatient settings. It also contains opinions from consultations provided by other healthcare providers and ancillary findings such as lab and x-ray results.

A well organized, accurate, and comprehensive chart is essential to quality patient care and enables the physician and other healthcare professionals to quickly access needed information.

Much of what the physician documents in the medical record is translated by medical coding specialists into diagnosis and procedure codes, as well as the DRGs used by hospitals and ambulatory payment classifications (APCs) used in outpatient settings.

As these codes are submitted for reimbursement, they become part of the statistics that are used for quality assurance, research, grants, studies (medical, revenue, etc.), vital statistics (births, infectious disease, morbidity and mortality), tumor registry, utilization review, and case management.

The medical record is also a legal document, and as such may be subpoenaed as evidence in professional liability or criminal action against healthcare providers. One way providers can help prevent liability claims is to keep well documented, organized, and unaltered records, and maintain clear and effective chart documentation. When malpractice claims do arise, a sound medical record is often a physician's best defense.

☞ **KEY POINT**

The medical record is also a legal document, and as such may be subpoenaed as evidence in rofessional liability or criminal action against health care providers.

Protecting the Medical Chart

The inpatient, outpatient, clinic or office medical record is a legal document that contains personal and confidential patient information. In all cases the record is protected and secured. Access to medical records is strictly limited to personnel who legitimately need access to the record.

More facilities and practices are moving towards electronic medical records (EMR). Commercially produced EMR programs are required to include security procedures for access and the need to make changes to the medical record. Security must also include electronic signatures of the medical record to be appended and essentially freeze the document from additional editing or changes. Archiving a patient's EMR without compromising security when accessing records is an important concern.

Reimbursement records and claim forms are also protected. Any document that links a patient's name with information such as diagnoses and procedures is considered protected and requires a release from the patient to share the information.

One of the most publicized portions of HIPAA is protected health information (PHI). This includes keeping the medical record confidential. It includes release of information only for reimbursement purposes or by signed patient consent. This includes protecting confidentiality in conversations and communications in and out of the health care setting.

Chart Format

There are a variety of formats used to organize charts. Inpatient and outpatient facility charts are organized in accordance with policies established by the individual hospital or facility. In general, office charts have all related information sorted and filed together, such as all lab information, medical history information, insurance data, etc.

Chart Monitoring

Because patient care is dependent on a complete medical record, hospital nurses and other specialized medical records personnel work together to ensure all areas of the hospital medical records are clearly labeled and complete within a specified period of time. Patient charts in a physician's office or in a clinic may be more of an ongoing activity with one person overseeing the entire process. Medical coding of the chart may take place during the hospital stay, after discharge, or at the end of a visit whether or not the chart has been completed. As stated previously, however, all code selection should be based on completed documentation.

Components of the Medical Record

A complete and accurate patient information sheet is usually the first component of the medical chart or record.

Patient information falls into two categories—general medical information and billing information. Because people may see more than one provider or they may move, change jobs, and switch insurance plans, patient information forms are updated on a regular basis.

The following shows the information gathered in the office.

Patient Medical Information

A patient medical information form should contain the following:

- Patient's full name
- Current address and telephone number

 KEY POINT

Never allow any information from a patient record to be inadvertently or deliberately exposed to unauthorized individuals.

- Date of birth
- Sex
- Occupation, employer's name, address, and telephone number
- Reason for visit
- Allergies (must be documented at each patient encounter)
- Current medications
- Previous medical history and pertinent family history
- Referring physician name, address, and telephone number
- Name and telephone number of person to contact in an emergency

Patient Billing Information

A patient billing form is separate from the medical record and contains the following pertinent information:

- Patient's full name
- Current address and telephone number
- Date of birth
- Sex
- Social security number
- Driver's license number
- Occupation, employer's name, address, and telephone number
- Responsible party (insured), address, and telephone number
- Reference: a relative or friend not living with the patient including address and telephone number
- Medical insurance information including address, contract or policy number, group number, and effective dates for coverage

Preprinted Patient History Forms

One of the most important elements in a patient's medical record is the health history. Preprinted checklist-style forms are often used to obtain a patient's history. Different types of forms are used in hospitals, although various departments sometimes use preprinted patient history forms as a screening tool. The physician should make pertinent comments, and date and sign the history form as part of the medical record.

Preprinted Patient Exam Forms

Preprinted exam forms are similar in concept to preprinted patient history forms. Exam forms are available by specialty and usually list anatomical sites with check-offs for normal or abnormal findings. An alternative to the exam checklist is a form with anatomical headings followed by ample room for the physician to fill in information revealed by the examination. This style of form allows more explanation of the areas checked. The physician dates and signs the form after documenting the exam.

Summary Sheets

As charts become thicker, particularly with long-term office patients who have significant medical histories, reviewing the patient's history before a medical service can be time consuming. To increase efficiency while at the same time preserving access to important medical information, a cover or "problem" sheet summarizing the patient's history and allergies may be placed at the front of the chart. Physicians then have a snapshot view each time the patient is seen. A good summary sheet is brief but still presents the most important facts. A summary sheet however, does not replace

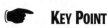

KEY POINT

One of the most important elements in a patient's medical record is the health history.

the physician's documentation of the patient's visit and coder's should never code from a problem sheet.

CLINIC CHART SUMMARY SHEET

Patient _____ ID# _____
Date _____ Time _____

Date	Medical Problem	Treatment/Resolution
	Surgical Procedures	**Significant Findings**
	Medications	**Dose/Route/Interval**
	Allergies	**Reaction**
	Tests	**Results**
	Hospital Admissions	**Treatment/Resolution**
	Miscellaneous	**Miscellaneous**

Physician Signature _____

INPATIENT CHARTING

Inpatient charts may contain volumes of information. All volumes are treated according to an individual hospital's rules and regulations. The hospital may require that all volumes be available to physicians, nurses, and other health care professionals on the patient's unit or floor. Hospital departmental policy, especially in a teaching hospital, may dictate how much of the history must be reviewed. Accreditation guidelines set forth by the Joint Commission on Accreditation of Healthcare Organizations (JCAHO) call for stringent standards for inpatient charting. Documentation must be entered, transcribed when necessary, and on file usually within 24 hours. Guidelines require that an operative progress note must be entered in the medical record immediately after surgery to provide pertinent information to anyone attending to the patient.

 DEFINITIONS

Joint Commission on Accreditation of Healthcare Organizations (JCAHO). The primary accrediting body for hospitals, outpatient facilities, and other facilities. This nonprofit organization audits these facilities and was previously known as the Joint Commission for the Accreditation of Hospitals.

Each inpatient medical event is documented as soon as possible after its occurrence. The records of discharged patients are completed within 30 days following discharge. Noncompliance with these regulations is taken very seriously by hospitals and their accreditation agencies. Physicians who consistently fail to keep proper records risk disciplinary actions as severe as the suspension of staff privileges.

Within each inpatient record are a variety of forms or reports. Many of these are vital to coding the patient's inpatient record and you should become familiar with them. The chart may contain any or all of the following:

Admission/Discharge Summary

The admission/discharge summary is a compilation of the facts summarized by the discharging physician regarding the patient's hospital stay. It includes the reason for the admission, any surgeries performed during the admission, tests, progress and current status of the patient at the time of discharge.

Special Consents

The patient or guardian may sign certain consent forms prior to or during admission such as a Consent for Treatment or Consent of Release of Information (such as for billing purposes). These consents remain in the chart for legal reasons.

History and Physical Examination Report

Upon admission to the hospital, it is a requirement of JCAHO that the patient have a history and physical examination (H&P) report for every hospital admission. The H&P contains information regarding the patient's past medical, social and family history, including previous surgeries, illness, injuries and childhood disease. It also contains the patient's current physical condition based on a comprehensive examination, and a plan for treatment based on the patient's condition and physical exam.

Physician's Orders

The orders placed by physicians to nursing and ancillary services, whether verbal or written, are all placed on the patient's chart during the hospital stay. The orders contain information about what treatments, medications, or tests were requested by the physicians responsible for the patient's care during the admission. Each order is signed by the ordering physician.

Progress Notes

Progress notes offer a brief summary of care given by all health care providers during the hospital stay and the patient's response to the treatment or care. Each provider will make entries daily for any services or interventions performed during the admission. Each entry is dated and signed by the author. Nurses, physicians, therapists, anesthesiologists and so on, all make entries into the progress notes.

Operative Reports

The operative report is a summary of what occurred during the patient's surgical episode and includes all interventions, anesthesia care, techniques, equipment, devices, and complications and pathology information concerning the patient's surgery.

 KEY POINT

The operative report is a summary of what occurred during a patient's surgical episode.

OPERATIVE REPORT

Patient _____ ID# _____

Date _____ Time _____

Preoperative Diagnosis(es) _____
_____
_____

Postoperative Diagnosis(es) _____
_____
_____

Procedure(s) _____
_____
_____

Surgeon(s) _____

Assistant Surgeon(s) _____

Anesthesia _____

Anesthesiologist _____

Indications _____
_____

Findings _____
_____
_____

Procedure in Detail _____
_____
_____
_____

Disposition _____
_____

Sutures/Drains _____

Estimated Blood Loss _____

Fluids _____

Complications (if any) _____
_____
_____
_____

Physician Signature _____

Obstetric Records

For maternity patients, the obstetric record logs all events prior to delivery, during the labor, leading up to and including the delivery, as well as post-partum (after delivery) care.

Newborn Care Data

Newborn records contain a few special forms such as a birth history, identification form and examination information.

Anesthesia Reports

Anesthesia care is provided in support of surgery by another physician. The anesthestic record is actually a log of the care the patient received while under anesthesia. It documents the patient vital sign statistics, surgery performed and the patient's status prior to and following the anesthesia and surgery.

Pathology Reports

All tissues, organs and body parts excised during surgery are reviewed by a pathologist. The pathology report is a summary of the findings once the tissue has

 KEY POINT

The anesthestic record is actually a log of the care the patient received while under anesthesia.

 DEFINITIONS

Pathology. The medical science, and specialty practice, concerned with all aspects of disease, but with special reference to the essential nature, causes, and development of abnormal conditions, as well as the structural and functional changes that result from the disease processes.

been examined either by gross examination (visually) or microscopically (through a microscope).

Radiology Reports

The reports for all types of radiologic imaging are called radiology reports. They provide the physical findings for studies performed and reviewed by radiologists.

Consultation Reports

A consultation occurs when one physician requests another physician's participation in the care of the patient. The consulting physician completes the consultation report to provide documented clinical information back to the requesting physician.

Nurse's Notes

Nurses are comprehensive documenters. A significant element of their nursing education deals with "charting." Nurses document every day, all day, regarding the patient's care, medications, requests, and problems that occur while hospitalized. They also document on graphs that report the patient's vital statistics such as pulse, respirations, blood pressure, etc

COMPLIANCE AND LEGAL CONSIDERATIONS

As pointed out previously, proper code assignment is closely linked to the financial and legal well-being of a practice. Not surprisingly, then, risk management analysts in health care facilities often take special interest in the activities and policies of coders. Health care providers can be prosecuted for consistently assigning medical codes having higher dollar values than are justified by the medical record documentation.

Many of the legal considerations and compliance issues in health care settings are beyond the scope of this publication. However, even the beginning coder should know some basic tenets.

Fraud Issues

Over the past decade, Medicare has bolstered its enforcement capabilities. The Medicare Anti-Fraud Unit is charged with preventing and detecting fraudulent activities in both Part A and Part B programs. A primary focus is to protect the interest of Medicare beneficiaries.

The CMS defines fraud as an intentional deception or misrepresentation that results in an unauthorized benefit, usually money. Fraud in the Medicare program takes such forms as, but is not limited to:

- Claiming costs for noncovered or nonchargeable services, supplies, or equipment (disguised as covered items)
- Incorrect reporting of diagnosis or procedures to maximize payments
- Billing that appears to be deliberate application for duplicate payment for the same services or supplies. This includes billing the program twice, billing both Medicare and Medicaid, billing both Medicare and another insurer, or billing both Medicare and the beneficiary, in an attempt to be paid twice
- Misrepresentation of dates and descriptions of services furnished

Because the forms of fraud mentioned above bear on coding and billing, one can easily see the importance of correct code assignment. But verification that the medical record documentation supports the code assignment is also of great importance.

Abuse Issues

The CMS defines abuse as action inconsistent with accepted sound medical practices. The abusive action may result in unnecessary costs to the Medicare program. The actions may involve improper payment, payment for services that fail to meet professionally recognized standards of care, or payments that are medically unnecessary.

Abuse differs from fraud in that the provider does not knowingly and intentionally misrepresent facts to garner improper payment for items or services. Examples of abuse include, but are not limited to:

- Billing for services that are not medically necessary
- Billing for services at a higher level than what is supported by documentation (commonly known as upcoding)

As one can see, a fine line distinguishes fraud from abuse, and under certain circumstances federal authorities will develop an abuse case into a charge of fraud. A provider or staff member who is educated about proper billing practices, but who continues improper billing activities may see initial charges of abuse increased to fraud. As a coder, a level of professionalism is expected and professional materials should be regularly consulted, particularly those published by official sources such as Medicare carriers, the AMA, the American Academy of Professional Coders and the American Health Information Management Association.

Records Management

All case records must be considered sensitive and confidential. Never allow any information from a patient record to be inadvertently or deliberately exposed to unauthorized individuals.

Medical records can be altered only under very special circumstances. Never attempt to obliterate or erase an entry in a medical record. If an alteration is warranted, existing material should be stricken but remain legible. The change should be dated and initialed, preferably by the attending physician. Facilities always have strict protocol in these matters and accreditation hinges on closely following these rules.

Preserve the medical records and keep all components intact. Lost documentation holds extreme legal implications and is a blotch on the integrity of any health care setting. Proper archiving is important and many settings now store records in digital files on CD-ROMs.

SUMMARY

In summation, we can see more clearly how medical coding fits into the bigger picture of health care management. Front-office duties, financial office functions, and clinical work dovetail together in the coding office. None can function well when one does function properly.

The following discussion questions and issues are for your consideration upon completion of this chapter. A full series of test questions on this chapter are found on the accompanying CD-ROM and in the instructor's manual.

QUICK TIP

The Centers for Medicare and Medicaid Services (CMS) defines abuse as action inconsistent with accepted sound medical practices.

KEY POINT

Front-office duties, financial office functions, and clinical work dovetail together in the coding office. None can function well when one does function properly.

DISCUSSION QUESTIONS

- Mentally track perhaps one of your own medical encounters, from the registration process through to the final explanation of benefits and physician and/or facility reimbursement:
  — Do you remember the registration process? Did you fill out a detailed patient history?
  — Do you remember seeing a charge ticket? How about your medical record?
  — Did you decipher the codes on your EOMB?

- Consider medical fees:
  — Have you ever wondered how doctors figure out their charges? How about hospitals and other facilities?
  — Do you hold a better understanding of medical costs and fees?

- Imagine you must teach the DRG system to someone with little knowledge of health care reimbursement. Does the logic of the system come through?

- Consider the differing needs that facility and physician office staff have of medical records. How, too, are they similar?

- Imagine a scenario where you accidentally upcode a major procedure and garner a windfall in unearned revenue for your setting. Imagine a similar scenario that results in a significant downcoding:
  — How would you handle each situation?
  — How would you handle both on the same day?
  — How would you justify your decisions to the physicians whose services you miscoded?

Chapter 7: Inpatient Coding

INTRODUCTION

Coding accuracy of inpatient services is an important factor to establish medical necessity and for research and statistical data, as well as for the financial health of the hospital. The coder's role is pivotal to the success of a hospital's inpatient reimbursement.

This chapter focuses on inpatient coding. Inpatient diagnosis coding as well as procedure coding using ICD-9-CM volume 3, inpatient reimbursement methodologies, and diagnosis-related groups (DRG) assignment are reviewed.

Previous discussions have focused on coding and insurance basics, as well as practice management issues that touch on coding. Much of the emphasis and most of the examples have been directed toward physician office and group practice settings. Hospitals, or inpatient facilities as they are known, have a somewhat different coding structure.

Inpatient coding is different because the entire admission is actually assigned codes. An admission occurs when the patient has an order by a physician for the patient to become an "inpatient." All encounters from the time of admission and up to the patient's discharge must be reviewed to assure that nothing is overlooked in code assignment. The source document for the coding is the patient's medical record. As mentioned in chapter 6, various documents may contain pertinent information for code assignment. The record should be carefully reviewed because of the financial impact to the hospital if procedures, services, or supplies are missed in the coding process.

THE CODING PROCESS

There are two main arteries that feed to the final codes in the charge capture process of a facility. The first system, called a charge description master, or CDM, is actually a schedule of fees and their descriptions for services rendered in all settings in a hospital. When services, procedures or supplies are consumed, personnel at the point of the utilization make entries into a computer system, or document them on a charge ticket for entry at a later time. The charge amount for that service or supply goes through to the patient's account and the charge is posted for billing to the payer. The CDM is useful in identifying what resources or how many resources have been used and aids in the budget process for the facility.

The other method of capturing services and supplies is through the health information management's coding department or a separate coding service for the facility. The department receives reports about patients who have been discharged and this prompts the department to recognize a chart needs to be coded for billing. The chart is then reviewed for all services, supplies, and procedures performed and for documentation by medical personnel for the reason for the hospitalization.

Both avenues are vital to the charge capture process for the facility and are necessary for appropriate reimbursement. Financial loss may occur if one of the processes fails.

OBJECTIVES

In this chapter, you will learn:
- The basics of inpatient coding
- About hospital billing
- Conventions of ICD-9-CM volume 3
- How diagnosis coding relates to the DRG system of facility reimbursement
- About software features for inpatient DRG assignment

Complete and detailed documentation by the physician is essential so that the coder can code appropriately. Source documents (progress notes, procedure/surgery reports, histories and physicals, and discharge summaries) provide the coder with much of the information necessary to select the most appropriate codes. Physicians must be encouraged to submit specific documentation to facilitate the coding and billing process. It is also necessary to try to work with facilities where the physician performs services so that reports are obtained as soon as possible after services are performed.

INPATIENT REIMBURSEMENT OVERVIEW

Proper assignment of ICD-9-CM diagnosis codes is the basis for reimbursement for inpatient facilities. (Inpatient reimbursement is the payment to a hospital for the facility costs incurred to treat a patient while in the hospital.) The method used to calculate payments are known as diagnosis-related groups or DRGs. The DRGs are used to classify patients with similar diagnoses and treatments because statistically their lengths of stay in the hospital should be similar. This allows insurance companies to project how much they will pay for each condition treated. The principal diagnosis is one factor that determines which DRG group a patient's stay will be in. This final diagnosis is determined at the end of the patient's stay when all tests and studies have been completed.

In general, the principal diagnosis of a case determines the major diagnostic category (MDC) to which the case is assigned. Each MDC is organized into one of two sections—surgical or medical. The surgical section classifies all surgical conditions based upon operating room procedures (ICD-9-CM volume 3). The medical section classifies all diagnostic conditions based upon diagnosis codes (ICD-9-CM Volume 1). Diagnoses and procedures are designated by ICD-9-CM codes, with procedures being coded from volume 3 of ICD-9-CM. The MDCs are mutually exclusive, meaning only one category applies for each procedure or diagnosis. The majority are organized by major body system and/or are associated with a particular medical specialty.

Finally, the case is analyzed for presence of complications and comorbidities. The case is then assigned to the appropriate surgical or medical DRG based upon: the principal diagnosis, up to eight additional diagnoses, the principal procedure and up to five additional procedure codes, and age, sex, and discharge status. One DRG is assigned to each in patient stay and this is the basis for payment.

DRGs serve three main purposes: to determine hospital reimbursement based on severity of illness, to evaluate the quality of care, and to evaluate the utilization of services consumed. Each DRG represents the average resources needed to treat patients grouped to that DRG. The relative weight (or value) for each DRG is relative to the national average of resources used to treat all patients within that DRG.

A collaborative approach to coding for DRG assignment is the key to successful accuracy and reimbursement of DRG payment. The relationship between the health information coding staff and all clinical staff documenting in the medical record must be interactive and complementary to engage more complete, compliant, and accurate medical record documentation of each patient's condition.

NEW MEDICAL SERVICES AND TECHNOLOGIES

Beginning October 1, 2002, a new mechanism to recognize costs of new services and technologies under the hospital inpatient prospective payment system was implemented. The annual update to the ICD-9-CM volume 3 codes for 2003

DEFINITIONS

Principal diagnosis. The condition established after study for being chiefly responsible for the patient's admission to the hospital. "After study" refers to results of diagnostics performed to determine the final diagnosis.

DEFINITIONS

Comorbidity. A preexisting condition that causes an increase in length of stay by at least one day in about 75 percent of cases (e.g., chronic obstructive pulmonary disease, diabetes).

Complication. Additional diagnosis that describes a condition arising after the beginning of observation and treatment and that modifies the course of the patient's illness or the medical care required. It may be an undesired result or misadventure in medical care (e.g., bed sore, postoperative infection, hemorrhage, adverse effect of medicinal agent, infection, pneumonia, etc.). Together they are referred to as "CC" and both are used in DRG assignment.

---

provides a limited expansion of codes for assigning new technology categories. A series of code categories have been identified and can be found in a new chapter with the category of code range 00.00–00.99.

A medical service or technology will be considered new and appropriate for additional payment if it represents an advance in medical technology that substantially improves, relative to technologies previously available, the diagnosis or treatment of Medicare beneficiaries. A panel of federal clinical and outside experts will provide oversight to adequately review the services and assist in the assignment of new codes.

The following is an example of a new technology ICD-9-CM code effective for inpatient coding use October 1, 2002:

> Brain Wafer Chemotherapy
>
> New code 00.10 Implantation of chemotherapeutic agent

GLIADEL Wafer received FDA approval in 1996 and is used as an adjunct to surgery to prolong survival in patients with recurrent glioblastoma multiforme (GBM) for whom surgical resection is indicated. Implanted directly into the cavity that is created when a brain tumor is surgically removed, GLIADEL Wafer (proliferosan 20 with carmustine implant) directly delivers antitumor medication to the site of the removed tumor. It is the only implantable drug that delivers chemotherapy directly to the tumor site, thereby avoiding the side effects of systemic agents.

ICD-9-CM VOLUME 3

The third volume of ICD-9-CM is a tabular listing of procedure codes specifically used for inpatient settings. Like the CPT coding system, the codes are used to report services and procedures provided to patients. The diagnosis codes in conjunction with the volume 3 procedural codes are used in this DRG classification system under which the facilities are reimbursed by Medicare and many private payers.

As an extension of the proposed ICD-10, procedure codes are contained in ICD-10 PCS. National health care organizations are recommending the adoption of ICD-10 PCS, even if adopted prior to ICD-10. Coders are encouraged to be aware of coding changes and to receive training prior to the effective dates of any changes.

Some payers require both CPT procedure codes and volume 3 ICD-9-CM procedure codes before considering a review of a facility claim. In addition, some hospitals provide billing services for physician employees (e.g., emergency department physicians, pathologists), specialty clinics, and centralize the coding and medical records for all of these services in one area of the hospital. In these settings, CPT codes are assigned in the usual manner for the various outpatient services.

However, volume 3 ICD-9-CM procedure codes are widely accepted as the reporting mechanism for inpatient hospital diagnostic, therapeutic, and surgical procedures.

Volume 3 consists of both a tabular listing and an alphabetic index.

The procedure classification parallels the diagnosis classification in that it is organized by body systems. All surgical procedures on a single body system appear together (e.g., operations on the nervous system are classified in categories 01–05, operations on the digestive system are classified in categories 42–54, etc.). The one major exception to this arrangement is the last chapter of the classification, "Miscellaneous

DEFINITIONS

Diagnostic procedures. The procedures performed to evaluate the patient's complaints or symptoms. These procedures help the physician establish the nature of the patient's disease or condition so that definitive care can be provided. Diagnostic procedures include endoscopy, arthroscopy, injection procedures, and biopsies.

Therapeutic procedures. Treatment of a pathological or traumatic condition through the use of activities performed to treat or heal the cause or effect change through the application of clinical skills or services that attempt to improve function.

KEY POINT

The procedure classification parallels the diagnosis classification in that it is organized by body systems. All surgical procedures on a single body system appear together.

Diagnostic and Therapeutic Procedures," which lists nonsurgical procedures on all body systems.

The procedure classification is based on a two-digit defined category set, or rubric, (subdivided to three- and four-digit codes) for each chapter.

> √3ʳᵈ   10   Operations on conjunctiva
>
> > 10.0   Removal of embedded foreign body from conjunctiva by incision
> >
> > > *Excludes:*   *removal of:*
> > > *embedded foreign body without incision (98.22)*
> > > *superficial foreign body (98.21)*
> >
> > 10.1   Other incision of conjunctiva
> >
> > √4ᵗʰ   10.2   Diagnostic procedures on conjunctiva
> >
> > > 10.21   Biopsy of conjunctiva
> > >
> > > 10.29   Other diagnostic procedures on conjunctiva

Tabular Listings

The tabular list contains 16 chapters, 15 of which are arranged by anatomical site. The 16th chapter provides categories for miscellaneous diagnostic and therapeutic procedures generally not considered surgical. The volume 3 tabular listing classifies groups of procedures by body system and then by miscellaneous diagnostic and therapeutic procedures like x-rays, tests, or monitoring:

Chapter Number and Title	Category
Procedures and Interventions, Not Elsewhere Classified	00
1. Operations on the Nervous System	01–05
2. Operations on the Endocrine System	06–07
3. Operations on the Eye	08–16
4. Operations on the Ear	18–20
5. Operations on the Nose, Mouth, and Pharynx	21–29
6. Operations on the Respiratory System	30–34
7. Operations on the Cardiovascular System	35–39
8. Operations on the Hemic and Lymphatic System	40–41
9. Operations on the Digestive System	42–54
10. Operations on the Urinary System	55–59
11. Operations on the Male Genital Organs	60–64
12. Operations on the Female Genital Organs	65–71
13. Obstetrical Procedures	72–75
14. Operations on the Musculoskeletal System	76–84
15. Operations on the Integumentary System	85–86
16. Miscellaneous Diagnostic and Therapeutic Procedures	87–99

The alphabetic index to procedures is presented first. It is an alphabetical index of operative and diagnostic procedures and the corresponding codes. The tabular list of procedures is presented second, listing information from the index in numeric order along with other pertinent coding conventions. This logical placement of the alphabetic index allows for quick location of procedural terms for verification in the tabular list. Unlike volume 2, this alphabetical index is not a separate volume, but is part of volume 3.

Coding Specificity

In ICD-9-CM volume 3, the procedures are cataloged in a series of two-digit category codes. For example, all operations on the external ear are found under category 18, and operations on valves and septa of the heart are found under category 35. Knowing the two-digit category is not enough for accurate ICD-9-CM procedure coding because all two-digit codes require further specificity, by the addition of a third digit subcategory, and frequently a fourth digit subclassification.

√3rd **18 Operations on external ear**
        Includes: operations on:
                   external auditory canal
                   skin and cartilage of:
                     auricle
                     meatus

√4th **18.0 Incision of external ear**
        Excludes: removal of intraluminal foreign body (98.11)

   18.01 Piercing of ear lobe
           Piercing of pinna

   18.02 Incision of external auditory canal

   18.09 Other incision of external ear

√4th **18.1 Diagnostic procedures on external ear**

   18.11 Otoscopy
           DEF: Exam of the ear with instrument designed for visualization.

   18.12 Biopsy of external ear

   18.19 Other diagnostic procedures on external ear
           *Excludes: microscopic examination of specimen
                        from ear (90.31–90.39)*

√3rd **35 Operations on valves and septa of heart**
        Includes: sternotomy (median)
                     (transverse)   } as operative approach
                   thoracotomy

        Code also cardiopulmonary bypass [extracorporeal circulation] [heart-lung machine] (39.61)

√4th **35.0 Closed heart valvotomy**
        Excludes: percutaneous (balloon) valvuloplasty (35.96)

   35.00 Closed heart valvotomy, unspecified valve

   35.01 Closed heart valvotomy, aortic valve

   35.02 Closed heart valvotomy, mitral valve

   35.03 Closed heart valvotomy, pulmonary valve

   35.04 Closed heart valvotomy, tricuspid valve

Third and fourth digits in volume 3 provide coding specificity by clarifying an anatomical site or kind of procedure (e.g., plastic repair, open or closed procedure). For example, the two-digit code 45 identifies incision, excision, and anastomosis of intestine. Add a third digit 0 after the decimal point (45.0) and an enterotomy is

KEY POINT

In ICD-9-CM volume 3, the procedures are cataloged in a series of two-digit category codes. Knowing the two-digit category is not enough for accurate ICD-9-CM procedure coding because all two-digit codes require further specificity, by the addition of a third-digit subcategory, and frequently a fourth-digit subclassification.

KEY POINT

Third and fourth digits in volume 3 provide coding specificity by clarifying an anatomical site or kind of procedure.

specified. A fourth digit (45.01) identifies a specific site, an incision of the duodenum.

> ☑3ʳᵈ   **45   Incision, excision, and anastomosis of intestine**
>> Code also any application or administration of an adhesion barrier substance (99.77)
>
>> ☑4ᵗʰ **45.0 Enterotomy**
>>> *Excludes: duodenocholedochotomy (51.41–51.42, 51.51)*
>>>> *that for destruction of lesion (45.30–45.34)*
>>>> *that of exteriorized intestine (46.14, 46.24, 46.31)*
>>
>>> **45.00   Incision of intestine, not otherwise specified**
>>>
>>> **45.01   Incision of duodenum**
>>>
>>> **45.02   Other incision of small intestine**
>>>
>>> **45.03   Incision of large intestine**
>>>> *Excludes: proctotomy (48.0)*

The index of procedures contains many diagnostic descriptors not appearing in the tabular section of volume 3. Many terms in the index cross-reference to different terms that may be used to identify a procedure, for example, Doppler flow study, which may be found under Ultrasonography and under Dopplergram. The tabular section main term is only listed under diagnostic ultrasound. Consequently, when assigning diagnosis codes, consult the index first.

> **Dopplergram, Doppler flow mapping**—*see also* Ultrasonography
>> aortic arch 88.73
>> head and neck 88.71
>> heart 88.72
>> thorax NEC 88.73
>
>> ☑4ᵗʰ **88.7 Diagnostic ultrasound**
>>> Includes:echography
>>>> ultrasonic angiography
>>>> ultrasonography
>>> *Excludes: therapeutic ultrasound (00.01–00.09)*
>>
>>> **88.71   Diagnostic ultrasound of head and neck**
>>>> Determination of midline shift of brain
>>>> Echoencephalography
>>>> *Excludes: eye (95.13)*
>>
>>> **88.72   Diagnostic ultrasound of heart**
>>>> Echocardiography
>>>> Intravascular ultrasound of heart

Conventions

Many of the coding conventions in volume 3 are the same as those for diagnosis coding in volumes 1 and 2. Each space, typeface, indention, and punctuation mark determines how to interpret ICD-9-CM volume 3 codes. These conventions were developed to help match correct codes to the procedures encountered. The major difference is the types of notes. These additional types of notes are described here along with a review of the conventions detailed in chapter 1.

Format

The ICD-9-CM alphabetic index has an indented format as is used in volume 2. Subterms are indented two spaces to the right of the term to which they are linked.

☞ **KEY POINT**

Many of the coding conventions in volume 3 are the same as those for diagnosis coding in volumes 1 and 2. Each space, typeface, indention, and punctuation mark determines how to interpret ICD-9-CM volume 3 codes.

When indentions for the main term are too numerous to fit the column, they will continue with the same indention to the next column. Use care when following the indentions from column to column to ensure you are still under the same main term reference.

Operation
Abbe
    construction of vagina 70.61
    intestinal anastomosis—see Anastomosis, intestine
abdominal (region) NEC 54.99
abdominoperineal NEC 48.5
Aburel (intra-amniotic injection for abortion) 75.0
Adams
    advancement of round ligament 69.22
    crushing of nasal septum 21.88
    excision of palmar fascia 82.35
adenoids NEC 28.99
adrenal (gland) (nerve) (vessel) NEC 07.49
Albee
    bone peg, femoral neck 78.05
    graft for slipping patella 78.06
    sliding inlay graft, tibia 78.07
Albert (arthrodesis, knee) 81.22

Typeface
Bold type identifies all codes and main terms in the tabular list of volume 3, separating it from subordinate information or notes.

43.9   Total gastrectomy

Punctuation
[ ] Brackets enclose synonyms, alternative wordings, or explanatory phrases. The brackets may be regular [ ] or italicized *[ ]*.

52.14   Closed [endoscopic] biopsy of pancreatic duct

( ) Parentheses enclose supplementary (nonessential) modifiers that do not affect the code number (even if they are absent). Parentheses also enclose many *see also* references.

71.21   Percutaneous aspiration of Bartholin's gland (cyst)

} A brace encloses a series of terms modified by the statement appearing to the right of the brace.

07.64   Total excision of pituitary gland, transfrontal approach

Ablation of pituitary by implantation
    (strontiumyttrium)   } transfrontal approach
Cryohypophysectomy, complete

Notes
As in volume 2, instructional notes lead to accurate code assignment. To assign procedure codes at the highest level of specificity, you should follow the instructional notes. These include:

Category notes provide instructions specific to all codes in the category.

The following fourth-digit subclassification is for use with appropriate categories in section 77 to identify the site. Valid fourth digits are in [brackets] under each code:

0 unspecified site
1 scapula, clavicle, and thorax [ribs and sternum]
2 humerus
3 radius and ulna
4 carpals and metacarpals
5 femur
6 patella
7 tibia and fibula
8 tarsals and metatarsals
9 other

These fourth-digit subclassifications are followed by the three-digit codes for category 77.

"Includes" notes appear immediately under a code title to provide further definition or to give an example of the category contents. The note may include synonyms or alternative names similar procedures included in the code. The word is indented 10 spaces, in plain typeface, and is followed by a colon. The code includes those terms listed under "includes."

   √3ʳᵈ   **18**   **Operations on external ear**
               Includes: operations on:
                          external auditory canal
                          skin and cartilage of:
                             auricle
                             meatus

"Excludes" indicates terms that are not to be coded under the referenced term. These notes appear following "includes" notes, if applicable, and the corresponding note appears in italics with the code reference for the procedure this is excluded. The exclude note does not prevent reporting of the excluded procedure if the procedure was also performed.

   33.27   **Closed endoscopic biopsy of lung**
               Fiber-optic (flexible) bronchoscopy with fluoroscopic
                    guidance with biopsy
               Transbronchial lung biopsy
               Excludes: brush biopsy of "lung" (33.24)
                          percutaneous biopsy of lung (33.26)

"Omit code" is found only in the alphabetic index of volume 3 and is an instruction to omit codes that are not separately reported because they are included in the surgical or diagnostic procedure or approach.

For some operative procedures it is necessary to record the individual components of the procedure. In these instances, the "Alphabetic Index to Diseases" lists both codes, of which one appears between brackets [ ]. Record these codes in the same sequence as they appear in the index. You may see "code also" instructions regarding "synchronous" procedures in the tabular indicating that procedures performed in concert with the procedure listed should also be coded. This is similar to "code also" in volume 1 indicating additional codes are required.

   √4ᵗʰ   **48.6 Other resection of rectum**

KEY POINT

"Excludes" indicates terms that are not to be coded under the referenced term.

Code also any synchronous anastomosis other than end-to-end
(45.90, 45.92–45.95)

48.61   Transsacral rectosigmoidectomy

48.62   Anterior resection of rectum with synchronous colostomy

48.63   Other anterior resection of rectum
           Excludes: *that with synchronous colostomy (48.62)*

REVIEWING THE OPERATIVE REPORT

Coding a procedure involves reading and interpreting an operative report. A good understanding of the procedure classification conventions, coding guidelines, and clinical aspects of the specific procedure performed is necessary to identify the correct code.

Understanding the definitions of medical terms and the intricacies of the coding system allows any procedure or service to be coded. If you cannot locate the procedure in volume 3, do not assume that a code does not exist. It may be just a matter or tracking down the "clues." The clues are in the medical terms used to describe procedures.

Some of the more frequently used operative terms are listed here with their definitions to help you gain a knowledge of the terminology used in procedure coding.

Amputation. The surgical removal of a limb or appendage.

Arthrodesis. The surgical fixation of a joint, usually by bone fusion.

Excise. To cut out or cut off.

Explore. A surgical investigation for diagnostic purposes.

Incision. A surgical cut.

Insert. A surgical introduction or implant.

Manipulation. Treatment by hand.

Repair. Surgical restoration of diseased or damaged tissue.

In addition to these main terms, many procedures are really a combination of the anatomic site where the procedure is performed with a suffix indicating what was done. Some of the more common suffices with their meanings are:

-centesis. Puncture.

-ectomy. Excision, removal.

-tomy. Incision.

-stomy. Forming an opening.

-rraphy. Suture.

-pexy. Fixation (of an organ).

-plasty. Surgical repair.

-tripsy. Crushing.

When combined with the anatomical term, the combination is actually a procedure.

A sample operative report is included her to demonstrate the link between the actual documentation and key terms for code selection. Read the following operative report and note the key words have been underlined.

 DEFINITIONS

Mastectomy. Removal of the breast. From "mast" (breast) and "-ectomy" (excision, removal).

Operative Report

Preoperative Diagnosis: Occluded thrombosed arteriovenous (AV) fistula, left forearm, and chronic renal failure.

Postoperative Diagnosis: Same

Operation(s): Fogarty thrombectomy of Gor-Tex fistula, left forearm, and revision of the venous end.

Description of Operation: With the patient on the operating table in the supine position after adequate axillary block anesthesia had been administered, his left forearm and upper arm were sterilely prepared and draped in the usual fashion.

An incision was made through the old incision just distal to the antecubital fossa and carried through skin and subcutaneous tissue. Hemostasis was obtained with electrocautery. The venous and arterial ends of the graft were exposed. The venous end appeared to be occluded from thrombosed vein. There was another excellent basilic vein medial to it and quite large. This was a branch going off laterally.

The venous end of the graft was transected and no bleeding was seen from the venous end, and the vein was totally thrombosed. The entire portion of the graft connected to this vein was removed and the veins ligated with stick ties of 4-0 Prolene suture. The graft was thrombectomized with the 4 Fogarty catheter and the arterial line thrombectomized with excellent inbleeding into the graft. The graft was injected with heparinized saline solution and the vascular clamp applied. The basilic vein was dissected proximally towards the distal end of the forearm and I was able to get plenty of vein to anastomose it end-to-end to the existing graft. The vein was ligated with 2-0 silk suture distally and transected and there was a valve right at this area. The valve was removed under direct vision and the vein spatulated to fit to the 6 mm. Gor-Tex graft and it was anastomosed to it with a running suture of 6-0 Gor-Tex. The clamp was removed with an excellent thrill palpable and excellent flow through the graft. No leaks were seen.

The wound was irrigated with antibiotic solution and subcutaneous tissue closed with running suture of 3-0 Vicryl and the skin with a running subcuticular suture of 4-0 Dexon. Steri strips were applied and sterile dressing applied. The patient went to the recovery room in stable condition. He tolerated the procedure well. He was given Phenaphen #3 one to two every four to six hours as needed for pain and to return in two weeks for a follow-up evaluation.

SEQUENCING PROCEDURE CODES

The rules for procedure coding must be applied to a broad variety of procedures. Just as the medical record tells a written story of procedures that occurred during the hospitalization of the patient, the numerical codes assigned by the medical coder must tell the same story in code. The most important factor in ICD-9-CM procedure coding is an understanding of the rules. Knowing how to correctly sequence and report procedures must be the goal for all coders. The entire record of the current admission must be reviewed before selecting a principal procedure.

The Uniform Hospital Discharge Data Set (UHDDS) as published in 1985, provides reporting instructions for diagnoses and significant procedures. An understanding of the definitions of a significant procedure is necessary to decide the appropriate sequence of the procedure codes. Procedures not considered significant are coded and reported according to hospital policy.

What is a significant procedure? According to the UHDDS, for a procedure to be considered significant it must include a procedure that:

- Is surgical in nature (i.e., incision, excision, amputation, introduction, endoscopy, repair, destruction, suture, and manipulation)
- Carries a procedural risk
- Carries an anesthetic risk
- Requires specialized training

> **☞ KEY POINT**
>
> The most important factor in ICD-9-CM procedure coding is an understanding of the rules. Knowing how to correctly sequence and report procedures must be the goal for all coders.

Codes for significant procedures are found in all chapters of the procedure classification, most in chapters 1–15 and a few in chapter 16, "Miscellaneous Diagnostic and Therapeutic Procedures."

Principal Procedure

The definition in the UHDDS for a principal procedure is the procedure "that was performed for definitive treatment rather than for diagnostic or exploratory purposes or for treatment of a complication." If the patient has more than one procedure that meets the definition of a principal procedure, select the one most related to the principal diagnosis as the principal procedure. The most resource intensive or complex is chosen when more than one procedure is related to the principal diagnosis.

Example:

A patient admitted under the diagnosis of unstable angina undergoes a left heart catheterization with left coronary angiography followed by left internal mammary artery to left anterior descending coronary artery bypass.

Principal procedure: 36.15 Single internal mammary coronary artery bypass

Significant procedures: 37.22 Left heart catheterization, and 88.53 Angiography the left heart

Significant Procedures

All secondary procedures that meet the definition of "significant" as stated above and that are performed after the assignment of the principal procedure also should be reported. They are to be sequenced as follows:

- Other definitive procedures, related or unrelated to the principal diagnosis, matching complications and secondary diagnoses codes, when applicable
- Therapeutic procedures
- Diagnostic procedures

Other procedures, such as tests, measurements, or procedures that may be part of another procedure are usually not coded for hospital inpatients (However, the facility may require coding of additional services for statistics, research, grants, or studies.)

When a definitive procedure and a diagnostic procedure, both related to the principal diagnosis, are performed, the definitive procedure is sequenced as the principal procedure regardless of the order in which the procedures were performed or listed in the medical record.

When a definitive, or therapeutic procedure is not performed for the principal diagnosis but is performed for a complication code, the principal procedure is the one performed for the complication.

When a definitive operating room procedure is not performed, but a therapeutic procedure is, the therapeutic procedure is listed as the principal procedure.

Diagnostic procedures are sequenced as the principal procedure only when no definitive or therapeutic procedure is performed.

Request a list from the facility for any other procedures that must be coded and reported according to the facility's policies.

 KEY POINT

The principal procedure is usually reported first. Significant procedures are reported in addition.

QUICK TIP

Procedures. "Biopsy," "bronchoplasty," "Bypass"

Eponyms. "Bischoff operation," "Brock operation," "Burch procedure"

Adjectives. "Balloon," "blood," "bone"

USING THE INDEX

A procedural statement may be a single term or multiple terms. These terms provide the coder with the necessary information about the procedure performed on the patient.

Main terms, which describe the type of procedure performed and not the anatomical site, are in boldface type. Main terms may be procedures, eponyms, or adjectives that describe a procedure.

Modifiers are words listed with the main term providing the coder with additional information that may or may not be used in code selection. The alphabetic index places certain modifiers relevant to classifying the procedure in parentheses or indents them under the main term. When words are indented, they are also known as subterms.

Indentation in the alphabetic index follows the same specific rules as those for the "Alphabetic Index to Diseases" (i.e., each new level of terms is indented one standard indent space, or two character spaces). Any text that is too long for a single line, called a continuation line, is indented two standard indent spaces.

(Main Term) **Bypass**
(Sub Terms)   abdominal-coronary artery 36.17 (Subterms)
             aortocoronary (catheter stent) (with prosthesis) (with
                   saphenous vein graft) (with vein graft) 36.10
               one coronary vessel 36.11
               two coronary vessels 36.12
               three coronary vessels 36.13
               four coronary vessels 36.14

Alphabetizing Rules for the Procedure Index

As in the disease alphabetic index, letter-by-letter alphabetizing is used throughout the procedure index. Letter-by-letter alphabetizing ignores single spaces and single hyphens resulting in sequences such as the following:

**Injection (into) (hypodermically) (intramuscularly) (intravenously) (acting
      locally or systemically)**
   antibiotic 99.21
   anticoagulant 99.19
   anti-D (Rhesus) globulin 99.11
   antidote NEC 99.16
   anti-infective NEC 99.22
   antineoplastic agent (chemotherapeutic) NEC 99.25

Numbers, whether Arabic, Roman, or adjective versions of numbers (i.e., first, second, etc.) are positioned in numerical sequence before alphabetic characters.

Operation
   Beck I (epicardial poudrage) 36.39
   Beck II (aorta-coronary sinus shunt) 36.39
   Beck-Jianu (permanent gastrostomy) 43.19

The prepositions "as," "by," and "with" immediately follow the main term to which they refer. In the case where multiple prepositional references are present, they are listed in alphabetic sequence.

> **Laminectomy (decompression) (for exploration) 03.09**
>> with
>>> excision of herniated intervertebral disc (nucleus pulposus) 80.51
>>> excision of other intraspinal lesion (tumor) 03.4
>> as operative approach-omit code
>> reopening of site 03.02

Other prepositions, such as "for" and "through," indicating a relationship between the main term and subterms, are treated according to standard alphabetizing rules.

> **Cystoscopy (transurethral) 57.32**
>> with biopsy 57.33
>> for
>>> control of hemorrhage
>>>> bladder 57.93
>>>> prostate 60.94
>>> retrograde pyelography 87.74
>> ileal conduit 56.35
>> through stoma (artificial) 57.31

Anatomical sites are not used as main terms. Consequently, eyelid reconstruction would be found under the term for the procedure, "reconstruction," not under the term for the anatomical site, "eyelid."

The alphabetic index supplements the tabular list because it contains many procedure terms that do not appear in the tabular list. Terms listed in the categories of the tabular list are not meant to be exhaustive; they serve as examples of the content of the category. In such cases, the instruction given in the procedure index is to be followed.

CODING AXIOM

Never code directly from the alphabetic index. After locating a code in the index, look up that code in the tabular listing for important instructions.

QUICK TIP

The procedure alphabetic index contains the entry, "Estes operation (ovary) 65.72," but the tabular list does not include "Estes operation" under code 65.72. The coder should follow the instruction of the index and assign code 65.72.

USING THE TABULAR LISTING

The tabular list contains codes and their narrative descriptions. Unlike the "Tabular List to Diseases," which is divided up into three sections, the "Tabular List to Procedures" contains only one section. All procedures, both surgical and diagnostic, are included in one list.

Each of the chapters in the ICD-9-CM "Classification of Procedures" is divided into two-digit categories based on anatomical site. There are no subchapters in the procedure coding system. The two-digit categories are subdivided with a decimal point followed by a third digit and in some cases a fourth.

Category (two digits). Each chapter begins with a two-digit category. In order for the category to be a valid code at least one additional digit must be assigned.

Subcategory (three digits). All two-digit categories have been further subdivided with the addition of a decimal point followed by another digit. The third digit provides more specificity with regard to type of operative procedure or site.

31 Other operations on larynx and trachea
    31.0   **Injection of larynx**
            Injection of inert material into larynx or vocal cords
    31.1   **Temporary tracheostomy**
            Tracheostomy for assistance in breathing

In the above example, the category code 31 cannot stand alone to describe other operations on larynx and trachea. However, the subcategory code 31.0 Injection of larynx, can stand alone.

Subclassification (four digits): Greater clinical detail with regard to surgical technique or diagnosis has been added with the expansion to four-digit subclassifications. Four-digit codes are the most precise subdivisions in the procedure classification.

43 **Incision and excision of stomach**
    43.0 **Gastrotomy**
            gastrostomy (43.11–43.19)
            that for control of hemorrhage (44.49)
    43.1 **Gastrostomy**
        43.11   **Percutaneous [endoscopic] gastrostomy [PEG]**
                Percutaneous transabdominal gastrostomy
        43.19   **Other gastrostomy**
                Excludes: percutaneous [endoscopic] gastrostomy [PEG]
                   (43.11)

In many cases, terminology used in a medical record cannot be found in the procedure index. The coder must look for synonyms in order to classify the procedure. Often, this will result in obtaining the code for the residual category or "other."

Example:

Statement in the medical record: Re-exploration of thorax through recent incision

The main term "Re-exploration" does not appear in the procedure index. The coder must look for synonyms in order to code this procedure. One method of finding a code for this would be to look at the main term "Thoracotomy" since an incision into the thorax would be performed before exploration could be done.

Thoracotomy (with drainage) 34.09

The next step is to refer to the tabular list and look at code 34.09, remembering to scan the previous codes within that category.

CODING AXIOM

Code to the highest level of specificity (three or four digits) allowed by the procedural information. All two-digit categories have been further subdivided.

✓4th **34.0 Incision of chest wall and pleura**
   Excludes: that as operative approach—omit code

   34.01 Incision of chest wall
   Extrapleural drainage
   Excludes: incision of pleura (34.09)

   34.02 Exploratory thoracotomy

   34.03 Reopening of recent thoracotomy site

   34.04 Insertion of intercostal catheter for drainage
   Chest tube
   Closed chest drainage
   Revision of intercostal catheter (chest tube) (with lysis of
      adhesions)

   34.05 Creation of pleuroperitoneal shunt

   34.09 Other incision of pleura
   Creation of pleural window for drainage
   Intercostal stab
   Open chest drainage
   Excludes: thoracoscopy (34.21)
   *   thoracotomy for collapse of lung (33.32)*

By scanning the categories, one discovers that code 34.03, not code 34.09, should be used for re-exploration of thorax through recent incision.

When a term cannot be found in the procedure index, come up with synonyms and try locating them in the index. Then, look up the code listed after the synonym in the procedure tabular. Scan all codes in the category to see if any apply and choose the most appropriate code.

For those procedures that have not been assigned a specific code, the procedure classification provides an "other" listing. This code usually is found at the end of a group of codes for specific procedures.

   14.4 Repair of retinal detachment with scleral buckling and implant

     14.41 Scleral buckling with implant

     14.49 Other scleral buckling
   Scleral buckling with:
      air tamponade
      resection of sclera
      vitrectomy

In the above example, code 14.49 would be assigned if the medical record documentation stated the patient had a scleral buckling with vitrectomy for repair of retinal detachment.

Conventions Shared by the Alphabetic Index and Tabular List of Procedures

Typefaces

The two typefaces used in ICD-9-CM are bold and italic. Bold typeface is used for all codes and titles in the tabular list and all main terms in the Alphabetic Index. Italicized typeface is used for the second code in a synchronous procedure situation, notes in the alphabetic index, and "excludes" notes in the tabular list.

KEY POINT

When a term cannot be found in the procedure index, come up with synonyms and try locating them in the Index. Then, look up the code listed after the synonym in the procedure tabular. Scan all codes in the category to see if any apply and choose the most appropriate code.

Abbreviation

The abbreviation NEC, not elsewhere classifiable, is used with ill-defined terms as a warning that specified forms of the procedures are classified differently. The NEC code only should be used when further information regarding the procedure is available but the classification does not provide a specific code for the procedure.

PUTTING ICD-9-CM PROCEDURE CODING TO WORK

Coding a procedure involves reading and interpreting an operative report. A good understanding of the procedure classification conventions, coding guidelines, and clinical aspects of the specific procedure performed is necessary to identify the correct code. To assist in this process, follow the steps below.

1. Identify the main term (i.e. the type of procedure performed).

2. Use the alphabetic index to find the main term selected.

3. Note any modifiers of the chosen main term.

4. Locate any essential modifiers (i.e., subterms).

5. Read any notes and follow any cross-references.

6. Choose a tentative code from the alphabetic index.

7. Look up the selected code in the tabular list.

8. Review any notes found.

9. Select the final code from the tabular list.

The five-step process to assign procedure codes can be summarized as follows:

Step 1: Determine the Main Terms

Analyze the operative report and procedure statements for those words or main terms that identify the procedure. Think of the main term as a common denominator—a total procedure classification. Once you've located this general term, follow the alphabetical list to the specific condition. Examples of main terms include:

- Excision
- Fixation
- Lysis
- Manipulation
- Reduction
- Repair

Step 2: Look up the Main Term In the Index

Main terms in the index of procedures appear in bold type. Some procedures have more than one listing. If the term describing a condition can be expressed in more than one form, all forms appear in the main entry.

Pneumogram, pneumography

Step 3: Follow Cross-references

Follow cross-references to the alternate term when the procedure is not located under the first term you find. There are three types of cross-references:

"See" indicates that you should see the procedure listed instead of the term found. You must follow the instruction to assign the correct term.

Ankylosis, production of—*see* Arthrodesis

 KEY POINT

A surgical procedure may be identified through the use of an eponym, which generally identifies the person responsible for developing the procedure. An eponym is listed as a main term in the appropriate alphabetic sequence and under the main term "Operation" in the alphabetic index. A description of the procedure or anatomic site usually follows the eponym. For example:

Alexander operation

  prostatectomy

  perineal 60.62

  suprapubic 60.3

  shortening of ligaments 69.22

Alexander-Adams operation (shortening of round ligaments) 69.22

"See also" indicates that additional information is available. This cross-reference provides an additional procedure and code when the main term or subterm is insufficient, or when there is an alternate term. The additional information helps select the correct code.

> Closure—*see also* repair

When a single code does not fully describe a given procedure, use multiple codes to identify all components of the procedure. However, the procedure statement must mention the presence of all the elements for each code to be used.

"See category" directs you to a category, not just a single code. Again, do not assign an appropriate code unless you follow this instruction.

> Apheresis, therapeutic—*see* category 99.7

Step 4: Review Subterms or Modifiers

A main term may be followed by one or more subterms that further describe the patient's condition. These supplemental words, called modifiers, may describe the method, type of closure, or synonyms. There are two types of modifiers:

Nonessential Modifiers

These subterms are listed immediately to the right of the main term and are enclosed in parentheses. They serve as examples to help translate written terminology into numeric codes and do not affect the selection of the procedure code.

> Amputation (cineplastic) (closed flap) (guillotine) (kineplasty) (open) 84.91

Essential Modifiers

These subterms are listed below the main terms and are indented two spaces. They are generally presented in alphabetical order, with the exceptions of "with" and "without," which appear before the alphabetized modifiers. Each additional essential modifier clarifies the previous one and is indented two additional spaces to the right. These descriptive terms affect code selection and describe essential differences in site, method, or type of procedure.

> Lysis
>> adhesions
>>> bladder (neck) (intraluminal) 57.12
>>>> external 59.11
>
> Ligation
>> fallopian tube (bilateral) (remaining) (solitary) 66.39
>>> by endoscopy (culdoscopy) (hysteroscopy) (laparoscopy) (peritoneoscopy) 66.29
>>> with
>>>> crushing 66.31
>>>>> by endoscopy (laparoscopy) 66.21
>>>> division 66.32
>>>>> by endoscopy (culdoscopy) (laparoscopy) (peritoneoscopy) 66.22
>>>> Falope ring 66.39
>>>>> by endoscopy (laparoscopy) 66.29

When a main term in the index has only one essential modifier, it appears on the same line as the main term separated by a comma.

> Litholapaxy, bladder 57.0

DEFINITIONS

Essential modifiers. Subterms listed below the main term and indented.

Nonessential modifiers. Subterms listed to the right of the main term and enclosed in parentheses.

Step 5: Cross-Reference the Index to Procedures in the Tabular Section of Volume 3

The tabular section is the authoritative ICD-9-CM volume 3 coding reference. It contains procedure codes, full descriptions, additional instructional notes, and examples of terms assigned to each code. These are intended to enhance the verification process and ensure proper code selection. There are times, however, when a descriptive term listed in the index is not found in the tabular section. In these instances, trust the index as the most often updated and use the number listed there.

USING SOFTWARE IN CODE ASSIGNMENT

Coding software products are available to facilitate a productive coding environment.

These software systems use the information the coder provides and translates it into codes and corresponding code descriptions. Virtually unseen by the coder, the software—called encoders and groupers—assign the DRGs. The software is faster at following the same steps as a coder performing a hard copy assignment of the DRG.

Encoders are based on book logic where the ICD-9-CM index and tabular chapters are accessed through key terms entered into the encoder system. The encoder then uses the information the coder provides and translates it into codes and corresponding code descriptions. Groupers contain the DRG logic that interfaces with the encoder to help assign the appropriate DRG based on codes entered through the encoding system. The grouper containing the DRG logic (unseen by the coder) assigns an MDC, the medical or surgical partitioning, and follows the tree through the decision-making process based on information the coder enters into the product, (e.g., age) to assign a DRG. Encoder and grouper software can be based on a boolean logic process demanding a yes or no answer. Information entered from the medical record leads the coder ultimately to assign the appropriate diagnoses and procedure codes. However, the coder still must go through the medical record, apply correct coding guidelines, and determine the principal diagnosis and the secondary diagnoses as well as any principal procedures performed. The coder must take into account complications and comorbidities, the principal procedure, and any applicable secondary procedures.

The sequencing of procedures is critical to appropriate reimbursement. Most encoder systems allow flexibility in the number of diagnosis and procedures codes allowed. However, for appropriate DRG assignment practices, pay attention to the sequencing of the first nine diagnosis and first six procedure codes. These fields must contain the key codes driving DRG reimbursement. Most encoder and grouper systems have an internal automatic sequencing function that will resequence codes higher when they appear below the ninth diagnosis and sixth procedure and affect the DRG.

ICD-10 CODING SYSTEM: THE POSSIBLE FUTURE OF CODING

ICD-10 is a revision to the International Classification of Diseases (ICD), and is currently in the stages of final development and approval. It will replace the ICD-9-CM coding system. The ICD-9-CM coding system has been the standard system for the United States since 1979. The evolution of ICD-10 began in 1994 as the World Health Organization (WHO), National Center for Health Statistics (NCHS), and the Centers for Medicare and Medicaid Services (CMS) cooperatively began work on the project. The intent of the revision is to address the limitations of the current ICD-9-CM system and enhance the classifications of mortality and morbidity data.

KEY POINT

Groupers contain the DRG logic that interfaces with the encoder to help assign the appropriate DRG based on codes entered through the encoding system.

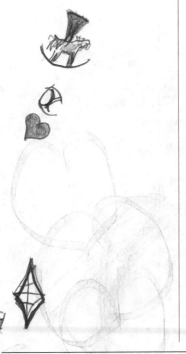

ICD-10-CM (clinical modification) was drafted to encompass the classification of diseases and related health problems as classified in the current ICD-9-CM volumes 1 and 2. ICD-10-PCS (procedure coding system) was drafted to report procedures as currently used in ICD-9-CM volume 3.

The ICD-10-PCS proposed draft is being considered as a long-term approach to assign a new technology coding system. The system provides great flexibility and capacity to accommodate temporary coding categories. In addition, the transition from ICD-9-CM to ICD-10 would drastically increase the number of procedural codes available to report. ICD-9-CM currently is limited to a maximum of 10,000 codes. The current draft of ICD-10-PCS contains 197,769 codes and could be expanded further.

SUMMARY

As you have learned from this chapter, while using diagnosis and procedure codes for inpatient cases may seem like a straightforward task, many factors are considered for appropriate code assignment. Selection of the principal diagnosis code and principal procedure for hospital can greatly affect the reimbursement a hospital receives for an inpatient admission.

The following discussion questions and issues are for your consideration upon completion of this chapter. A full series of test questions on this chapter are found on the accompanying CD-ROM and in the instructor's manual.

DISCUSSION QUESTIONS

- Compare the chapters of the procedural ICD-9-CM volume 3 with those of the procedural CPT code book. Notice that they mirror one another—the hospital codes begin with nervous system procedures and end with integumentary, while CPT is just the opposite. Do the two-digit categories of volume 3 compare favorably with the "thousands-style" approach of the CPT code book?

- Has training on ICD-9-CM volumes 1 and 2 helped you gain an understanding of the conventions of volume 3? Do you feel comfortable with the major concepts of inpatient coding? Can you mentally segregate a major procedure from minor procedures? Does the concept comorbidity and comortality factors during hospitalization seem logical to you? Can you see how CCs sometimes alter the admitting diagnosis so that the patient is discharged with a different diagnosis?

- Outline a few of the advantages that ICD-10 might offer as the replacement diagnosis and inpatient coding reference.

Chapter 8: Coding for Outpatient Facility Services— APCs and ASCs

INTRODUCTION

There is a direct relationship between coding and reimbursement in the outpatient facility environment. Codes identify an outpatient grouping for payment. Coding errors, such as the omission of HCPCS/CPT codes for all services provided, or incorrect code assignment. can lead to inaccurate outpatient payment. In this chapter, we examine these outpatient reimbursement systems and how coding affects payment.

OUTPATIENT SERVICES DEFINED

The evolution of technological advances over the last 20 has years shifted a focus from traditional inpatient care to outpatient or ambulatory care services. The trend for cost-effective delivery of heath care services, such as invasive surgical procedures, has prompted Medicare as well as other health care insurers to focus on cost containment and payment reform. Ambulatory surgeries do not require hospital admission and provide a cost-effective and convenient environment. These facilities may perform surgeries in a variety of specialties or dedicate their services to one specialty, such as eye care. Patients who elect to have surgery in an outpatient facility arrive on the day of the procedure, have the surgery in an operating room, and recover under the care of the nursing staff, all without a hospital admission.

The foundation of outpatient payment systems currently in place emphasizes the importance of reporting accurate financial information for all services, such as CPT codes or HCPCS codes for procedures. The coding and subsequent payment for outpatient services depends directly on the site of service (i.e., whether the service is delivered in an ambulatory hospital-based or free-standing setting). Outpatient services are typically classified according to the level of care required. For example, most hospital registration systems classify patients by the type of encounter as identified by the ordering physician:

- Single visits (example, radiology exams)
- Recurring or series visits (example, physician therapy visits weekly)
- Emergency department
- Observation unit

Generally, there are two primary elements in the total cost of performing a surgical procedure: The cost of the physician's professional services to perform the procedure, and the cost of services furnished by the facility where the procedure is performed (e.g., surgical supplies and equipment, and nursing services).

OBJECTIVES

In this chapter, you will learn:
- Basic concepts and history of outpatient payment systems
- How the service reported with HCPCS and CPT codes is paid
- Basic concepts behind packaging and bundling of services
- How modifiers affect multiple procedure payment

DEFINITIONS

The *Code of Federal Regulations,* sec. 410.2 contains the following definitions:

Encounter. A direct personal contact between a patient and a physician, or other person who is authorized by state licensure law and, if applicable, by hospital staff bylaws, to order or furnish hospital services for diagnosis or treatment of the patient.

Facility services. Services that are furnished in connection with covered surgical procedures performed in an ASC, or in a hospital on an outpatient basis.

Outpatient. A person who has not been admitted as an inpatient but who is registered on the hospital records as an outpatient and receives services (rather than supplies alone) directly from the hospital.

Currently there are primarily two outpatient reimbursement methodologies which apply the payment for costs incurred by a facility such as a hospital or other ambulatory facilities treating Medicare outpatients: ambulatory surgery center and ambulatory payment classification. In addition to Medicare coverage, some Medicaid programs as well as commercial insurers have adopted a similar payment schedule. These two payment systems and how each payment system defines the coding principles are discussed in this chapter. The definition and basic premise behind each payment system is defined as follows.

Ambulatory surgery center (ASC). An ASC, as defined by Medicare, is a distinct entity that operates exclusively for the purpose of furnishing outpatient surgical services to patients. It enters into an agreement with the Centers for Medicare and Medicaid Services (CMS) to do so and is either classified as independent (i.e., not a part of a provider of services or any other facility), or operated by a hospital (i.e., under the common ownership, licensure, or control of a hospital). A set payment rate is applied based on the facility's charge or the technical component of the services, such as supplies, materials, and nursing costs.

Ambulatory payment classification (APC). As applicable to hospital-based outpatient services, the outpatient prospective payment system classifies services into groups called ambulatory payment classifications. Services in each APC are similar clinically and in terms of the resources they require. A payment rate is established for each APC. A hospital may bill for a number of APC payments furnished to an individual patient on a single day. Each APC is assigned a relative weight that reflects the relative resources used in treating a patient. The higher the relative weight, the greater the payment.

CLAIMS PROCESSING

A federal directive requires hospitals to follow specific billing procedures, itemizing all services on a single claim. Freestanding facilities bill charges to Medicare and some other third-party payer claims using the 837p format or the CMS-1500 form, the same form used to bill professional services and durable medical equipment. Other third-party payers may require the freestanding facility bill charges using the 837i format or the UB-92 claim form, the form used by hospitals for inpatient billing. Hospital ASC and APC charges are billed using the 837i format or the UB-92 claim form.

In compliance with the Health Insurance Portability and Accountability Act (HIPAA) of 1996 legislation, the nationally approved formats 837i and 837p were designed for electronic submission of all claims. Containing all the information fields required by the UB-92 and CMS-1500 forms, Medicare and other payers for most health care claims now require the electronic format. The 837i and UB-92 include fields for three-digit revenue codes. A revenue code represents the cost center for services and supplies provided to a patient. Revenue codes are used for inpatient and outpatient services. Cost centers include pharmacy, room and bed, operating room, etc.

The bill type is a code indicating the specific type of bill (inpatient, outpatient, adjustments, cancels, late charges) for 837i and UB-92 reporting. This is a three-position field and is mandatory for all outpatient bills paid under the outpatient prospective payment system (OPPS).

The three-digit alphanumeric code gives three specific pieces of information. The first digit identifies the type of facility. The second classifies the type of care. The third indicates the sequence of this bill in this particular episode of care: it is referred to as the frequency code.

Data elements in the CMS uniform billing specifications are consistent with the UB-92.

The bill types affected by OPPS are:

12X Hospital—inpatient (Medicare Part B only)

13X Hospital—outpatient with condition code (CC) 41

13X Hospital—outpatient

14X Hospital—other

34X Home health—other

75X CORF

76X CMHC

APCs and the Outpatient Prospective Payment System (OPPS)

Effective for claims with dates of service on or after August 1, 2000, APCs were implemented for hospital outpatient services provided to Medicare beneficiaries. The OPPS applies to hospital outpatient departments, community mental health centers (CMHC), some services provided by comprehensive outpatient rehabilitation facilities (CORF), home health agencies (HHA), and services provided to hospice patients for the treatment of nonterminal illness. The OPPS does not apply to cancer centers, children's hospitals, the Indian Health Service, or critical access hospitals.

A transition period through January 1, 2004, allowed some hospitals to adjust to the new system without suffering substantial financial loss. Payments applied during this period were referred to as the transitional pass-throughs and cover certain medical devices, drugs, and biologicals. To qualify for this separate payment, hospitals reported all pass-through services using HCPCS codes, such as a C code category for devices. Therefore, accurate coding is extremely vital in generating additional revenue in addition to the APC payment rate for the surgical procedure. Special payment rules apply to these services such as special revenue codes and requirements for meeting eligibility.

What Is an APC?

The APC categorizes procedures and services according to similarities in costs and clinical characteristics, rather than according to CPT codes. The category or group determines the level of reimbursement for a specific service. The same concept is applied to the ASC payment group classification system. Variations among APC values depend on the site where the service or procedure is performed.

Status indicators identify how individual HCPCS or CPT codes are paid or not paid under the OPPS. The following are the payment status indicators and description of the particular services each indicator identifies:

 Definitions

APC. The APC categorizes procedures and services according to similarities in costs and clinical characteristics, rather than according to CPT codes. The category or group determines the level of reimbursement for a specific service.

Indicator	Service	Status
A	Pulmonary Rehabilitation Clinical Trial	Not Paid Under Outpatient PPS
A	Durable Medical Equipment, Prosthetics and Orthotics	DMEPOS Fee Schedule
A	Physical, Occupational and Speech Therapy	Physician Fee Schedule
A	Ambulance	Ambulance Fee Schedule
A	EPO for ESRD Patients	National Rate
A	Clinical Diagnostic Laboratory Services	Laboratory Fee Schedule
A	Physician Services for ESRD Patients	Physician Fee Schedule
A	Screening Mammography	Physician Fee Schedule
C	Inpatient Procedures	Admit Patient; Bill as Inpatient
D	Deleted Code	Codes are deleted effective with the beginning of the calendar year.
E	Non-Covered Items and Services	Not Paid Under Outpatient PPS
F	Acquisition of Corneal Tissue	Paid at Reasonable Cost
G	Drug/Biological Pass-Through	Additional Payment
H	Device Pass-Through	Additional Payment
K	Non Pass-Through Drug/Biological	Paid Under Outpatient PPS
N	Incidental Services, packaged into APC Rate	Packaged
P	Partial Hospitalization	Paid Per Diem APC
S	Significant Procedure, Not Discounted When Multiple	Paid Under Outpatient PPS
T	Significant Procedure, Multiple Procedure Reduction Applies	Paid Under Outpatient PPS
V	Visit to Clinic or Emergency Department	Paid Under Outpatient PPS
X	Ancillary Service	Paid Under Outpatient PPS

In determining payment, each APC is assigned a relative weight, For example, CPT code 11043 groups to APC 0016 Level V Debridement and Destruction, which has a relative weight of 3.53 under the Medicare APC system. The relative weight is then multiplied by the conversion factor, applicable to all APCs, for the APC payment rate. The proposed conversion factor for 2005 is $57.098.

APC Grouper Logic

APCs are defined by type, and there are four types as follows:

- Medical
- Significant procedures
- Surgical services
- Ancillary services

Medical APCs

Medical APCs are constructed using HCPCS Level II and/or CPT codes, providing consistency with the overall PPS grouping strategy and the approach followed in the establishment of payment groups for surgical and diagnostic services. In order to develop the medical APCs, CMS collapsed 31 CPT codes for clinic and emergency visits into six groups: three each for clinic visits, and three each for emergency department visits. The medical category includes all ambulatory visits to a clinician for conditions that do not involve a significant procedure. Incidental procedures such as venipunctures, which do not significantly increase the time and resources expended during a visit, are always bundled into the APCs and do not generate additional payment. Emergency department encounters and hospital-based clinic visits both result in medical APC groups when evaluation and management (E/M) codes from the CPT code book are reported.

Observation services are included in the medical APC category. The majority of observation is packaged or bundled into the payment for other diagnostic or therapeutic services provided in conjunction. However, the 2001 update to OPPS established a new APC 0339 to classify approximately 23 covered diagnosis codes for three conditions: chest pain, asthma, and congestive heart failure.

Significant Procedures

Surgical Service and Ancillary APCs

The APCs in these categories all consist of HCPCS Level II and/or CPT codes.

Surgical procedures and significant procedures include operating room, recovery room, anesthesia, medical/surgical supplies, pharmaceuticals, observation, blood, intraocular lenses, casts, splints, donor tissue, and various incidental services.

Significant procedures include normally scheduled procedures that are the reason for the visit and dominate the use of time and resources during the visit. It includes therapy such pulmonary therapy and stress tests.

Ancillary services include immunizations and tests (e.g., immunizations, radiological, laboratory, and pathology tests). Each test is paid separately. Medicare patients who receive services in ancillary areas of the hospital outpatient departments are reimbursed according to an ancillary visit group APC assignment.

SERVICES COVERED IN AN APC

The APC system lists covered and noncovered resources.

Covered Resources

The following resources are directly related to and are included in the performance of a procedure or service on an outpatient basis (for Medicare beneficiaries). This list of

KEY POINT

There are four kinds of APCs:
- Medical
- Significant procedures
- Surgical services
- Ancillary services

services/items are generally included in the APC group payment rate unless identified as paid separately:

- Operating suite, procedure room, or treatment room or area
- Recovery room
- Observation bed (with exception to current criteria)
- Anesthesia services
- Medical clinic visits (unless 25 modifier is met)
- Radiology procedures (some are paid separately)
- Diagnostic services and tests
- Surgical pathology
- Immunizations and allergy injections
- Specific dental procedures
- Hospital areas excluded from DRGs
- Anesthesia, drugs, biologicals, and other pharmaceuticals
- Blood (some are paid separately)
- Medical and surgical supplies and equipment
- Supplies and equipment used for administering and monitoring anesthesia or sedation
- Incidental procedures (e.g., venipuncture)
- Cancer hospitals excluded under the DRG payment system
- Partial hospitalization services provided in community mental health centers
- Specific services rendered to inpatients who have expended all of their Medicare Part A benefits or for services not covered during a hospital stay otherwise covered by Medicare Part A

Noncovered Services

Some services are paid under other payment systems, such as fee schedules and composite payments. These services are not paid as part of the APC amount and are considered "excluded" from the APC payment. These excluded services include:

- Physician services
- Certain nonphysician practitioner services
- Therapy services (physical, occupational, speech)
- Screening mammography
- Rehabilitation services
- Ambulance services
- Durable medical equipment supplied by the hospital for the patient's home use
- Prosthetics and prosthetic supplies implants (except IOLs) and orthotic devices
- Clinical diagnostic laboratory services (paid under the laboratory fee schedule)
- Dialysis services furnished to end-stage renal disease (ESRD) patients (paid under an ESRD composite rate)
- Procedures and/or services that are considered unsafe when performed or provided in the outpatient setting (inpatient only procedures)
- Services specific to other sites of service, such as inpatient and home health services
- Services provided to inpatients of a skilled nursing facility (SNF), subsequent to the assessment or creation of the comprehensive care plan but billable and covered under the SNF PPS

✓ **QUICK TIP**

Be clear about what constitutes covered and noncovered services in the APC group payment rate.

- Services otherwise not covered by Medicare, including those deemed unreasonable and/or unnecessary for diagnosing or treating an illness or disease (noncovered)

APC COST CONTROLS

To minimize upcoding and to control costs, not all services provided to a patient are used to compute payment. The areas that apply concepts for cost controls include:

- The bundling of related significant procedures
- Incidental services
- Ancillary packaging
- Discounting

Bundling

Under APCs it is possible to have more than one group; therefore, billing edits are in place to prohibit the unbundling of services. The Correct Coding Initiative (CCI) edits are incorporated in the payment for APCs. These edits rely on a comprehensive group of codes, rather than the component parts of a service reported by separate codes. Mutually exclusive codes are not billed simultaneously. For example, 93797 Cardiac rehabilitation without ECG monitoring, should not be billed in addition to 93798 Cardiac rehabilitation with ECG monitoring.

Incidental Services

Services classified with an N status indicator are considered incidental or packaged into other APCs. Therefore, if any incidental service is performed during an outpatient visit, the hospital is reimbursed for the incidental service through another APC group. Most HCPCS Level II J codes for drugs and pharmaceuticals are incidental.

Ancillary Packaging

Many HCPCS/CPT codes are packaged meaning that the payment for the service is included in the payment for another APC assigned service. For example, operating room, recovery room, anesthesia, medical/surgical supplies, and pharmaceuticals are all services included in the packaging concept. The fact that an item is packaged should not affect the coding and reporting of the service. While these services will not directly generate APC payment, the reporting of these services indirectly affect the calculation of outlier payments and transitional outpatient payments over time.

Discounting

There are two reasons a payment may be reduced or discounted:

- Multiple procedures
- Terminated procedures

Multiple Procedures

APC payments are discounted when more than one surgical service is performed during a single, operative session. The APC procedure with the highest payment amount will be reimbursed at full value. All other surgical services performed are reimbursed at 50 percent of the normal Medicare payment amount.

Payment for multiple procedures is reduced since the patient must be prepped only once for the surgery, which saves on the incremental costs related to anesthesia, use of rooms, and separate procedures such as incisions and sutures.

 KEY POINT

Cost controls in APCs are accomplished by considering the following factors:

- Bundling
- Incidental services
- Ancillary packaging
- Discounting

Terminated Procedures

A facility may use three modifiers when procedures are discontinued at the physician's discretion due to medical necessity or the patient's well-being. They are:

Modifier 52: Reduced services

Modifier 52 is used in those situations where modifier 73 or modifier 74 would have been appropriate, but since the use of anesthesia was not an inherent part of performing the procedure, modifier 52 is used to show that the procedure was discontinued.

Modifier 73: Discontinued outpatient hospital/ambulatory surgery center (ASC) procedure prior to the administration of anesthesia

Modifier 73 is used for procedures for which anesthesia (general, regional, or local) is planned.

Example: A patient is prepared for procedure 49590 repair spigelian hernia. Before anesthesia is administered, the physician decides the procedure should not be performed. This is billed as 49590-73.

Modifier 74: Discontinued outpatient hospital/ambulatory surgery center (ASC) procedure after administration of anesthesia

Modifier 74 is used for surgical procedures for which anesthesia (general, regional, or local) has been started.

Example: Anesthesia for procedure 33647 (repair of incomplete or partial atrio-ventricular canal with or without repair) is given and the procedure has been started, but the physician terminates the procedure before it is completed. This is billed as 33647-74.

APC Data Reporting Requirements

The primary elements for APC grouping are the assigned HCPCS codes. While the ICD-9-CM coding system is used in the assignment of diagnosis-related groups (DRGs), the coding systems used for APCs include the American Medical Association (AMA) CPT and CMS's HCPCS Level II codes. As a national industry standard, HCPCS coding comes from the charge description master 70 percent of the time and the remaining 30 percent comes from a qualified coding department such as a health information management (HIM) department. The majority of laboratory, radiology, and other diagnostic type services are coded through the charge master. Of the nearly 4,900 services that have payment values under the APC system, 3,200 of these, or roughly 65 percent are surgical codes taken from the range 10000–69999 of the CPT coding system. Qualified coders are typically responsible for the coding of these invasive type procedures, which are typically done in an operating or treatment room. Coordinating and communicating the responsibilities of coding accountability between the departments is extremely important to ensure the billing systems transmit the appropriate code or override the coding from the CDM when appropriately coded by a coder.

Numerous HCPCS or CPT codes are not reimbursed or are considered ungroupable under the APC system. The following are the reasons why codes may not be applicable for payment:

- Reimbursement will be made under another payment system
- The code represents a noncovered Medicare service
- The code represents an inpatient service
- The code is considered bundled or packaged

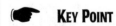

KEY POINT

The primary elements for APC grouping are the assigned HCPCS codes.

Modifier Reporting

CMS requires CPT and HCPCS Level II modifier reporting for accuracy in reimbursement, editing, and to capture payment data for constructing Medicare outpatient groups for the future APC system. The following CPT codes frequently require modifiers (when applicable) and are reported either through coding departments or utilize the charge description master (charge order entry system):

- Surgical procedures (CPT codes 10000–69999)
- Radiology (CPT codes 70010–79999)

Not all HCPCS/CPT modifiers are applicable to APCs. One high profile area of focus for accurate modifier reporting under APCs is evaluation and management services. E/M services are reported for hospital-based medical visits in the clinic(s) or emergency room through the use of HCPCS/CPT codes. In cases where a surgical procedure or services is performed as the immediate result of an outpatient visit (such as the removal of skin lesions following a visit to a dermatology clinic) or as a result of an emergency department visit, the visit is billed with modifier 25, indicating that a separately identifiable E/M service was furnished. Physician documentation is critical in assigning the modifier appropriately.

Units of Service

A unit of service is defined as the number of times the service or procedure being reported was performed according to the HCPCS/CPT code definition. It is imperative under the APC system that the code descriptions are reviewed to determine multiple reporting implications.

Annual APC Changes

In addition to annual revisions in the ICD-9-CM, HCPCS Level II, and CPT coding systems, facilities should anticipate changes in the procedure reimbursement classifications. CMS has stated that it will not routinely reclassify services and procedures from one payment group to another. However, CMS may revise a payment group based on evidence that reassignment improves the group clinically. A procedure also may be reclassified due to cost estimates.

New and revised CPT codes are assigned to an APC group. Reimbursement for the code stays the same unless charge history and associated data deem a different category than the group originally selected. It takes at least two years to create new APC groups from existing groups due to the time required for gathering and analyzing data.

New outpatient procedures and services will be added to the payment system as needed. CMS will review and update groups, relative payment weights, wages, and other adjustments required to take into account changes in medical practice, technology, services, cost data, and other factors.

AMBULATORY SURGERY CENTER

An ASC is a facility where physicians perform surgeries and procedures that do not require an overnight stay. The work is sometimes referred to as "day surgeries." An ASC may be categorized as one of the following:

- **Freestanding ambulatory surgery center.** A surgical center physically separate from a hospital campus. It may be a center of surgical and ancillary facilities without physicians' offices. Or it may be a space attached to a physician's office or clinic, part of which is dedicated to surgical procedures.

CODING AXIOM

Not all HCPCS/CPT modifiers are applicable to APCs.

- **Hospital ambulatory surgery center.** A surgical center owned and operated by a hospital. This type of ASC uses the hospital's resources for supplies, staff, claims submission, and overhead.

The basis for payment depends on where the services are furnished in a hospital outpatient department (APC payment) or freestanding ASC setting (ASC payment).

ASC payment is based on a prospectively determined rate. This rate covers the cost of services such as supplies, nursing services, equipment, etc. The rate does not cover physician services or other medical services (for example, x-ray services or laboratory services), which are not directly related to the performance of the surgical procedures. Those services may be billed separately and paid on a reasonable charge basis.

Single and multiple surgical procedure concept—If one covered surgical procedure is furnished to a beneficiary in an operative session, payment is based on the prospectively determined rate for that procedure.

If more than one surgical procedure is furnished in a single operative session, payment is based on both of the following:

- The full rate for the procedure with the highest prospectively determined rate
- One half of the prospectively determined rate for each of the other procedures

---

LEGISLATION AFFECTING REIMBURSEMENT

Federal legislation was enacted in 1986 to segregate and pay specific ambulatory surgical procedures performed at hospitals on an outpatient basis. The methodology, implemented in October 1987, requires Medicare to pay the same rates to hospitals and ASC facilities for all outpatient procedures approved for ASC coverage. ASCs that receive Medicare payments must meet the program's certification criteria and receive payments only for those procedures that have been approved by Medicare. Today, more 2,000 ASC procedures have been granted that approval.

ASC payments are based on blends of hospital costs and the rates paid in other ambulatory settings, such as separately certified ambulatory settings including ASCs or physician offices certified for certain surgery, radiology, and other diagnostic procedures. Freestanding ASCs are currently paid 80 percent of the ASC payment rate (20 percent is subject to coinsurance or deductible amounts). Payment to freestanding ASCs generally covers only the facility's charge or the technical component of the service, such as supplies, materials, and nursing costs.

Today, laws also regulate payment to ASC facilities, especially to reimburse Medicare beneficiaries. Private third party payers usually follow Medicare payment guidelines, although some do pay on a contract basis or a fee-for-service based on reasonable and customary costs.

Medicare pays ASCs for surgeries performed in ASCs. To receive reimbursement, ASCs must meet Medicare criteria.

Condition for Coverage—Surgical Services

Surgical procedures must be performed in a safe manner by qualified physicians who have been granted clinical privileges by the governing body of the ASC in accordance with approved policies and procedures of the ASC.

Standard: Anesthetic risk and evaluation. A physician must examine the patient immediately before surgery to evaluate the risk of anesthesia and of the procedure to

KEY POINT

ASC payment is based on a prospectively determined rate. This rate covers the cost of services such as supplies, nursing services, equipment, etc.

be performed. Before discharge from the ASC, each patient must be evaluated by a physician for proper anesthesia recovery.

Standard: Administration of anesthesia. Anesthetics must be administered by only one of the following:

- A qualified anesthesiologist
- A physician qualified to administer anesthesia, a Certified Registered Nurse Anesthetist (CRNA), or an anesthesiologist's assistant as defined by CMS, or a supervised trainee in an approved educational program. In those cases in which a nonphysician administers the anesthesia, unless exempted in accordance with regulations, the anesthetist must be under the supervision of the operating physician, and in the case of an anesthesiologist's assistant, under the supervision of an anesthesiologist.

Standard: Discharge. All patients are discharged in the company of a responsible adult, except those exempted by the attending physician.

ASC PAYMENT GROUPS

If an ASC is approved for Medicare participation, the ASC can only be reimbursed for procedures that are on a list of procedures that Medicare will reimburse to an ASC. Procedures on the list fall into one of eight groupings with a payment rate assigned to each group.

ASC procedures are classified into eight standard payment groups according to CPT code. Each procedure within the same group is reimbursed at a single rate, adjusted for geographical variations.

Medicare payment rates for ASCs effective October 1, 2004, are:

- Group 1—$333
- Group 2—$446
- Group 3—$510
- Group 4—$630
- Group 5—$717
- Group 6—$826 ($676 + $150 for intraocular lenses)
- Group 7—$995
- Group 8—$973 ($823 + $150 for intraocular lenses)
- Group 9—$1,339

Coding for ASCs

The same coding systems applied under APCs, HCPCS or CPT codes and modifiers, are applicable in the ASC setting. As in the APC system, codes are assigned status indicators for ASCs. These status indicators determine payment and cost control policies such as the CCI edits or noncovered procedures.

Example:

> ASC status indicator "2" indicates a procedure, item, or service for which Medicare does not allow a separate payment. Payment is always packaged into and subsumed within payment for other services. Some codes with a "2" indicator describe items or services that fall within the scope of ASC facility services, whose costs are taken into account within the ASC facility fee. Examples of these include CPT code 36000, introduction of needle or

 KEY POINT

ASC procedures are classified into eight standard payment groups according to CPT code.

intracatheter; or CPT code 81002 Urinalysis. When these services are furnished at an ASC, payment for them is included as part of the ASC facility fee.

Differences From OPPS

There is some variation between the freestanding ASC allowed surgery list and the services reimbursed for hospital outpatient departments under OPPS. Several surgeries are allowable in a freestanding ASC setting and are indicated as *inpatient only* in a hospital setting. Some of these surgeries include free muscle, skin, and fascia flap grafts with microvascular anastomosis and open treatment of palatal, malar and maxillary fractures. Additionally some services that are considered incidental and are packaged into the APC payment in a hospital outpatient setting are separately reimbursable procedures in an ASC. For example, the preoperative placement of needle localization wires in a breast. With the implementation of OPPS, CMS intended to extend the APC grouping payment concept to the freestanding ASC setting; however, free-standing ASCs were not addressed in the OPPS final regulation.

At this point, each list is independent and neither list affects the other. However when APCs are implemented for freestanding ASCs these facilities may face significant changes in reimbursement and allowed services if the hospital outpatient APC regulations and structures are applied unchanged to ASCs.

Covered and Noncovered Services

Each of the eight ASC payment groups cover the following:

- Nursing services, technical personnel, and others involved in patient care
- Use of the hospital or ASC facility by the patient
- Drugs and biologicals that cannot be self-administered
- Primary surgical dressings
- Supplies, splints, casts, appliances, and equipment directly related to the surgical procedures
- Intraocular lens (IOL) implants
- Blood, blood plasma, and components (except those to which the Medicare blood deductible applies)
- Anesthesia materials
- Administrative, record-keeping, and housekeeping services and supplies
- Diagnostic and therapeutic tests directly related to the surgical procedure

Performance of Listed Surgical Procedures on an Outpatient Hospital Basis

The inclusion of any procedure as a covered surgical procedure does not preclude its coverage in an inpatient hospital setting under Medicare.

Covered Surgical Procedures

General Standards

Covered surgical procedures are those surgical and other medical procedures that:

- Are commonly performed on an inpatient basis in hospitals, but may be safely performed in an ASC
- Are not of a type that are commonly performed, or that may be safely performed, in physicians' offices

- Are limited to those requiring a dedicated operating room (or suite), and generally requiring a post-operative recovery room or short-term (not overnight) convalescent room
- Are not otherwise excluded by regulation

Specific Standards

Covered surgical procedures are limited to those that do not generally exceed a total of 90 minutes operating time and a total of 4 hours recovery or convalescent time.

If the covered surgical procedures require anesthesia, the anesthesia must be local or regional anesthesia, or general anesthesia of 90 minutes or less duration.

Covered surgical procedures may not be of a type that:

- Generally result in extensive blood loss
- Require major or prolonged invasion of body cavities
- Directly involve major blood vessels
- Are generally emergency or life-threatening in nature

Noncovered Services

Payment groups do not include coverage for the following:

- Physician services
- Sale, lease, or rental of durable medical equipment (DME) for surgery patients to use in their homes
- Prosthetic devices (except IOL implants)
- Ambulance services
- Leg, arm, back, and neck braces
- Laboratory, x-rays, or diagnostic procedures not directly related to performance of the surgical procedures
- Anesthetist services furnished on or after January 1, 1989

Excluded Services

Not all CPT codes are included in the payment groups. Services excluded by CPT code are not reimbursed through Medicare for ASC services, although there are exceptions for "out-of-scope" services. A procedure that does not fall into one of the eight ASC payment groups, though incorporated into an ASC payment rate, is called an out-of-scope procedure. A procedure that does not fall into any of the ASC payment groups but is generally incorporated in the ASC payment rate is considered an out-of-scope procedure.

Hospitals are required to report out-of-scope procedures using HCPCS codes. Out-of-scope data are gathered for statistical purposes to identify procedures that typically are performed in an outpatient setting. When an out-of-scope procedure appears alone on the claim or with a non-ASC procedure, it may be reimbursed on a cost or charge basis using the HCPCS code.

Clinical Documentation Impact on Outpatient Payment

Coding is often affected by the documentation available. Major outpatient payment issues occur when there is insufficient documentation to support an appropriate HCPCS/CPT procedure code assignment or an ICD-9-CM diagnosis code assignment. Insufficient documentation is also the absence of documents that are critical for appropriate code assignments, such as operative reports, history and physicals, laboratory reports, pathology reports, and radiology reports. Coding staff

 KEY POINT

Not all CPT codes are included in the payment groups. Services excluded by CPT code are not reimbursed through Medicare for ASC services, although there are exceptions for "out-of-scope" services.

personnel are responsible for communicating documentation deficiencies and ensuring that the coding process is complete with the appropriate documentation.

SUMMARY

One of the most significant developments in health care over the past 20 years is the trend toward outpatient services. Procedures once offered only in hospitals are now routinely performed in outpatient settings.

Numerous incentives have driven this migration of services away from hospital settings. Better medical technologies and services rates high on the list—the procedures only recently became safe to perform in outpatient settings. A marketplace incentive has also been at work. Many physician groups understood early on that certain procedures could be technically and economically performed on an outpatient basis. Setting up surgical centers allowed these groups to capture facility and equipment dollars that previously went to hospitals. For their part, hospitals moved to set up their own satellite outpatient facilities.

This is how the ASC and APC system came to fill such a major role in medical services. Not surprisingly, coding issues surrounding these types of facilities soon surfaced. In this primer on outpatient coding issues, we hope that you have grasped the important role and duties that coders possess in this arena of health care.

The following discussion questions and issues are for your consideration upon completion of this chapter. A full series of test questions on this chapter are found on the accompanying CD-ROM, and in the instructor's manual.

DISCUSSION QUESTIONS

- Think about how outpatient services are operated, either from your own experiences, or those of family and friends. Do you know of anyone who has had an intraocular lens inserted in an outpatient clinic? How about vascular catheterization procedures? Both are now commonly performed in these types of settings.
- Do you understand the differences and similarities among the APC model and ASCs? Think about possible reasons for the two systems.
- Do you see similarities between APCs and DRGs? Can you define differences and similarities between aa hospital-based ASC and a freestanding ASC? What is meant by an "out-of-scope" procedure? What does it mean to you?

Appendix A: Insurance Commissioners

Alabama Dept of Insurance
201 Monroe St, Ste 1700
Montgomery, AL 36104
(334) 269-3550
www.aldoi.org/

Alaska Division of Insurance
Juneau Office
9th Fl State Office Bldg
333 Willoughby Ave
Juneau, AK 99811-0805
(907) 465-2515
Fax: (907) 465-3422
Anchorage Office
Robert B. Atwood Bldg
550 W 7th Ave, Ste 1560
Anchorage, AK 99501-3567
(907) 269-7900
Fax: (907) 269-7910
www.dced.state.ak.us/insurance/

American Samoa Government
Insurance Commissioner
Pago Pago, AS 96799 USA
(011) (684) 633-4116
Fax: (011) (684) 633-2269
www.samoanet.com

Arizona Dept of Insurance
2910 N 44th St, Ste 210
Phoenix, AZ 85018
(602) 912-8400
www.state.az.us/id/

Arkansas Insurance Dept
1200 W Third St
Little Rock, AR 72201
(501) 371-2600 or (800) 282-9134
www.state.ar.us/insurance/

California Dept of Insurance
Consumer Communications Bureau
300 S Spring St South Tower
Los Angeles, CA 90013
Los Angeles Area and Outside
California: (213) 897-8921
Within California only: (800) 927-4357
San Francisco Office: (415) 904–6072
TDD – (800) 485-4833
www.insurance.ca.gov

Colorado Division of Insurance
1560 Broadway, Ste 850
Denver, CO 80202
(303) 894-7499 or (800) 930-3745
Fax: (303) 894-7455
www.dora.state.co.us/insurance/

Connecticut Insurance Dept
153 Market St, 7th Fl
Hartford, CT 06103
Mailing address:
PO Box 816
Hartford, CT 06142-0816
(860) 297-3800
Within CT only: (800) 203-3447
Fax: (860) 566-7410
www.state.ct.us/cid/

Delaware Insurance Dept
841 Silver Lake Blvd
Dover, DE 19904
(302) 739-4251
www.state.de.us/inscom/

District of Columbia
DC Dept of Insurance and Securities
Regulation
810 First St NE, Ste 701
Washington, DC 20002
(202) 727-8000
www.disr.washingtondc.gov/main.shtm

Florida Dept of Insurance
200 E Gaines St
Tallahassee, FL 32399-0300
(850) 413-3100
www.doi.state.fl.us/

Georgia Insurance and Safety Fire Commission
Two Martin Luther King, Jr. Drive
West Tower, Ste 704
Atlanta, GA 30334
(404) 656-2070 or (800) 656-2298
Fax: (404) 651-8719
www.inscomm.state.ga.us/

Government of Guam
Dept of Revenue & Taxation
Insurance Branch
Building 13-1 Mariner Ave
Tiyan, Barrigada, GU 96913
Mailing Address:
PO Box 23607
GMF, GU 96921
(671) 475-5000
Fax: (671) 472-2643
www.gov.gu/government.html

Hawaii Dept of Commerce and Consumer Affairs
Hawaii Insurance Division
250 S King St, 5th Fl
Honolulu, HI 96813
Mailing Address:
PO Box 3614
Honolulu, HI 96811
(808) 586-2790
www.state.hi.us/dcca/ins/

Idaho Dept of Insurance
700 W State St, 3rd Fl
PO Box 83720
Boise, ID 83720-0043
(208) 334-4250
Fax: (208) 334-4398
www.doi.state.id.us/

Illinois Dept of Insurance
320 W Washington St
Springfield, IL 62767-0001
(217) 782-4515
Fax: (217) 782-5020
TDD: (217) 524-4872
www.state.il.us/ins/default.htm

Indiana Dept of Insurance
311 W Washington St, Ste 300
Indianapolis, IN 46204-2787
(317) 232-2385
Fax: (317) 232-5251
www.ai.org/idoi/index.html

Iowa Insurance Division
330 Maple St
Des Moines, IA 50319-0065
(515) 281-5705 or (877) 955-1212
Fax: (515) 281-3059
www.iid.state.ia.us/

Kansas Insurance Dept
420 SW 9th St
Topeka, KS 66612
(785) 296-3071 or (800) 342-2484
Fax: (785) 296-2283
www.ksinsurance.org/

Kentucky Dept of Insurance
215 W Main St
Frankfort, KY 40601
(502) 564-3630 or (800) 595-6053
TTY: (800) 462-2081
www.doi.state.ky.us/

Louisiana Dept of Insurance
950 N 5th St
PO Box 94214
Baton Rouge, LA 70804-9214
(225) 342-0895 or (800) 259-5300
Within LA only: (800) 259-5301
www.ldi.la.gov/

Maine Bureau of Insurance
Dept of Professional and Financial
Regulation
124 Northern Ave
Gardiner, ME 04345
Mailing address:
34 State House Station
Augusta, ME 04333-0034
(207) 624-8475
Within ME only: (800) 300-5000
Fax: (207) 624-8599
www.state.me.us/pfr/ins/inshome2.htm

Maryland Insurance Administration
525 St Paul Place
Baltimore, MD 21202-2272
(410) 468-2000 or (800) 492-6116
TTY: (800) 735-2258
www.mdinsurance.state.md.us/

Massachusetts Division of Insurance
One S Station, 5th Fl
Boston, MA 02110-2208
(617) 521-7794
TTD/TDD: (617) 521-7490
www.state.ma.us/doi/

Michigan Office of Financial and Insurance Services
Ottawa Building, 2nd Floor
611 W Ottawa
Lansing, MI 48933-1070
Mailing Address:
PO Box 30220
Lansing, MI 48909-7720
(517) 373-0220 or (877) 999-6442
Fax: (517) 335-4978
www.cis.state.mi.us/ofis/

Minnesota Dept of Commerce
85 7th Place E, Ste 500
St. Paul, MN 55101
(651) 296-6025
www.commerce.state.mn.us/

Mississippi Insurance Dept
1001 Woolfolk State Office Bldg
501 N West St
Jackson, MS 39201
Mailing Address:
PO Box 79
Jackson, MS 39205
(601) 359-3569
Within MS only: (800) 562-2957
www.doi.state.ms.us/

Missouri Dept of Insurance
301 W High St
PO Box 690
Jefferson City, Missouri 65102
(573) 751-4126
www.insurance.state.mo.us/

Montana State Auditor's Office
Insurance Division
840 Helena Ave
Helena, MT 59601
(406) 444-2040
Within MT only: (800) 332-6148
www.state.mt.us/sao/index.html

Nebraska Dept of Insurance
Terminal Bldg
941 "O" St, Ste 400
Lincoln, NE 68508-3639
(402) 471-2201
TDD: (800) 833-7352
www.nol.org/home/NDOI/

Nevada Division of Insurance
Carson City:
788 Fairview Dr, Ste 300
Carson City, NV 89701-5491
(775) 687-4270
Fax: (775) 687-3937
Las Vegas:
2501 E Sahara Ave, Ste 302
Las Vegas, NV 89104
(702) 486-4009
Fax: (702) 486-4007
www.doi.state.nv.us/

New Hampshire Insurance Dept
56 Old Suncook Rd
Concord, NH 03301-7317
(603) 271-2261
Fax: (603) 271-1406
www.state.nh.us/insurance/

New Jersey Dept of Banking and Insurance
20 W State St
PO Box 325
Trenton, NJ 08625
(609) 292-5360 or (800) 838-0935
Fax: (609) 292-2431
www.njdobi.org

New Mexico Insurance Division
PERA Bldg, Rm 428
1120 Paseo de Peralta
Santa Fe, NM 87501
Mailing Address:
PO Drawer 1269
Santa Fe, NM 87504-1269
(505) 827-4601
Fax: (505) 827-4734
www.nmprc.state.nm.us/inshm.htm

New York State Insurance Dept
New York City
25 Beaver St
New York, NY 10004
(212) 480-6400 or (800) 342-3736
Albany:
Empire State Plaza
Agency Bldg No 1
Albany, NY 12257
(518) 474-6272
Buffalo:
Walter Mahoney Office Bldg
65 Court St
Buffalo, NY 14202
(716) 847-7619
Long Island:
200 Old Country Rd
Mineola, NY 11501
(516) 248-5886
www.ins.state.ny.us/

North Carolina Dept of Insurance
PO Box 26387
Raleigh, NC 27611
(919) 733-2032 or (800) 546-5664
Eastern:
233 Middle St
PO Box 1691
New Bern, NC 28563
(252) 514-4813
Western:
537 College St
PO Box 1688
Asheville, NC 28802
(828) 251-6483
www.ncdoi.com/

North Dakota Dept of Insurance
600 E Blvd, Dept 401
Bismarck, ND 58505-0320
(701) 328-2440
Fax: (701) 328-4880
www.state.nd.us/ndins/

Ohio Dept of Insurance
2100 Stella Ct
Columbus, OH 43215-1067
(614) 644-2658
Fax: (614) 644-3743
www.ohioinsurance.gov/

Oklahoma Insurance Dept
2401 NW 23rd, Ste 28
PO Box 53408
Oklahoma City, OK 73152-3408
(405) 521-2828 or (800) 522-0071
Fax: (405) 522-3642
www.oid.state.ok.us/

Oregon Dept of Consumer and Business Services
Oregon Insurance Division
350 Winter St NE, Rm 440
Salem, OR 97301-3883
(503) 947-7980
Fax: (503) 378-4351
www.cbs.state.or.us/external/ins/index.html

Pennsylvania Insurance Dept
1326 Strawberry Sq
Harrisburg, PA 17120
(717) 783-0442 or (877) 881-6388
Fax: (717) 787-8585
TTY/TDD: (717) 783-3898
www.insurance.state.pa.us/

Puerto Rico Dept of Insurance
Cobian's Plaza Bldg
1607 Ponce de Leon Ave
Santurce, PR 00909
Mailing address:
PO Box 8330
Fernandez Juncos Station
Santurce, PR 00910-8330
(787) 722-8686
Fax: (787) 722-4400
www.ocs.gobierno.pr

Rhode Island Insurance Division
Dept of Business Regulation
233 Richmond St, Ste 233
Providence, RI 02903-4233
(401) 222-2223
Fax: (401) 222-5475
www.dbr.state.ri.us/

South Carolina Dept of Insurance
300 Arbor Lake Dr, Ste 1200
Columbia, SC 29223
Mailing address:
PO Box 100105
Columbia, SC 29202-3105
(803) 737-6212
Fax: (803) 737-6229
www.state.sc.us/doi/

South Dakota Division of Insurance
Dept of Commerce and Regulation
118 W Capitol
Pierre, SD 57501-2000
(605) 773-4104
Fax: (605) 773-5369
www.state.sd.us/dcr/insurance/

Tennessee Dept of Commerce and Insurance
Davy Crocket Tower
500 James Robertson Parkway, 4th Fl
Nashville, TN 37243-0565
(615) 741-2241
www.state.tn.us/commerce/

Texas Dept of Insurance
333 Guadalupe
Austin, TX 78701
Mailing address:
PO Box 149104
Austin, TX 78714-9104
(512) 463-6169 or (800) 578-4677
TDD: (512) 322-4238
www.tdi.state.tx.us/

Utah Dept of Insurance
State Office Bldg, Rm 3110
Salt Lake City, UT 84114-6901
(801) 538-3800
Fax: (801) 538-3829
TDD: (801) 538-3826
www.insurance.state.ut.us/

Vermont Dept of Banking, Insurance, Securities & Health Care Administration
Insurance Division
89 Main St, Drawer 20
Montpelier, VT 05620-3101
(802) 828-3301
www.bishca.state.vt.us/

Virgin Islands Dept of Finance
No 76 Kronprindsens Gade
GERS Bldg, 2nd Fl
St. Thomas, USVI 00802
(340) 774-4750
Fax: (340) 776-4028
www.usvi.org/

Virginia Bureau of Insurance
Tyler Bldg, 9th FL
1300 E Main St
Richmond, VA 23219
Mailing address:
PO Box 1157
Richmond, VA 23218
(804) 371-9741
Within VA only: (800) 552-7345
TDD: (804) 371-9206
www.state.va.us/scc/division/boi/index.htm

Washington State Insurance Commission
Insurance Bldg
5000 Capitol Blvd
Tumwater, WA 98501
Mailing address:
PO Box 40255
Olympia, WA 98504-0255
(360) 753-7300
Fax: (360) 586-3535
TDD: (360) 664-3154
www.insurance.wa.gov/

West Virginia Insurance Commission
Administrative Division
1124 Smith St
Charleston, WV 25301
Mailing address:
PO Box 50540
Charleston, WV 25305-0540
(304) 558-3707 or (304) 558-3725
Fax: (304) 558-4967
www.state.wv.us/insurance/

Wisconsin Office of the Commissioner of Insurance
121 E Wilson St
Madison, WI 53702
(608) 266-3585 or (800) 947-3529
Within WI only: (800) 236-8517
Fax: (608) 266-9935
TDD: (800) 947-3529 ask for (608) 266-3586
www.oci.wi.gov/oci_home.htm

Wyoming Insurance Dept
Herschler Bldg 3rd Fl East
122 W 25th St
Cheyenne, WY 82002
(307) 777-7401
Within WY only: (800) 438-5768
Fax: (307) 777-5895
http://insurance.state.wy.us/index.htm

Appendix B: Valid Three-Digit ICD-9-CM Codes

Three-digit ICD-9-CM codes are used to identify a condition or disease only when a fourth or fifth digit is not available. The following are the only ICD-9-CM codes that are valid without further specificity.

024	Glanders
025	Melioidosis
035	Erysipelas
037	Tetanus
042	Human Immunodeficiency Virus (HIV) Infection
048	Other enterovirus diseases of central nervous system
061	Dengue
064	Viral encephalitis transmitted by other and unspecified arthropods
071	Rabies
075	Infectious mononucleosis
080	Louse-borne [epidemic] typhus
096	Late syphilis, latent
101	Vincent's angina
118	Opportunistic mycoses
124	Trichinosis
129	Intestinal parasitism, unspecified
135	Sarcoidosis
138	Late effects of acute poliomyelitis
179	Malignant neoplasm of uterus, part unspecified
181	Malignant neoplasm of placenta
185	Malignant neoplasm of prostate
193	Malignant neoplasm of thyroid gland
217	Benign neoplasm of breast
220	Benign neoplasm of ovary
226	Benign neoplasm of thyroid gland
243	Congenital hypothyroidism
260	Kwashiorkor
261	Nutritional marasmus
262	Other severe protein-calorie malnutrition
267	Ascorbic acid deficiency
311	Depressive disorder, not elsewhere classified
316	Psychic factors associated with diseases classified elsewhere
317	Mild mental retardation
319	Unspecified mental retardation
325	Phlebitis and thrombophlebitis of intracranial venous sinuses
326	Late effects of intracranial abscess or pyogenic infection
340	Multiple sclerosis
347	Cataplexy and narcolepsy
390	Rheumatic fever without mention of heart involvement
393	Chronic rheumatic pericarditis
412	Old myocardial infarction
430	Subarachnoid hemorrhage
431	Intracerebral hemorrhage
436	Acute, but ill-defined, cerebrovascular disease
438	Late effects of cerebrovascular disease
452	Portal vein thrombosis
460	Acute nasopharyngitis [common cold]
462	Acute pharyngitis
463	Acute tonsillitis
470	Deflected nasal septum
475	Peritonsillar abscess
481	Pneumococcal pneumonia
485	Bronchopneumonia, organism unspecified
486	Pneumonia, organism unspecified
490	Bronchitis, not specified as acute or chronic
494	Bronchiectasis
496	Chronic airway obstruction, not elsewhere classified
500	Coal workers' pneumoconiosis
501	Asbestosis
502	Pneumoconiosis due to other silica or silicates
503	Pneumoconiosis due to other inorganic dust

504	Pneumoconopathy due to inhalation of other dust	605	Redundant prepuce and phimosis	920	Contusion of face, scalp, and neck except eye(s)
505	Pneumoconiosis, unspecified	630	Hydatidiform mole	931	Foreign body in ear
		631	Other abnormal product of conception	932	Foreign body in nose
514	Pulmonary congestion and hypostasis			936	Foreign body in intestine and colon
		632	Missed abortion		
515	Postinflammatory pulmonary fibrosis	650	Delivery in a completely normal case	937	Foreign body in anus and rectum
541	Appendicitis, unqualified	677	Late effect of complication of pregnancy, childbirth, and the puerperium	938	Foreign body in digestive system, unspecified
542	Other appendicitis			981	Toxic effect of petroleum products
566	Abscess of anal and rectal regions				
		683	Acute lymphadenitis	986	Toxic effect of carbon monoxide
570	Acute and subacute necrosis of liver	684	Impetigo		
		700	Corns and callosities	990	Effects of radiation, unspecified
585	Chronic renal failure	725	Polymyalgia rheumatica		
586	Renal failure, unspecified	734	Flat foot	V51	Aftercare involving the use of plastic surgery
587	Renal sclerosis, unspecified	769	Respiratory distress syndrome		
591	Hydronephrosis				
600	Hyperplasia of prostate	797	Senility without mention of psychosis		

Appendix C: The Office of Inspector General 2005 Work Plan for Medicare Physicians and Other Health Professionals

BILLING SERVICE COMPANIES

We will identify and review the relationships among billing companies and the physicians and other Medicare providers who use their services. We will also identify the various types of arrangements physicians and other Medicare providers have with billing services and determine the impact of these arrangements on the physicians' billings.

(OAS; W-00-05-35162; various reviews; expected issue date: FY 2005; new start)

MEDICARE PAYMENTS TO VA PHYSICIANS

We will assess the validity of Medicare reimbursement for services billed by physicians who receive remuneration from the Department of Veterans Affairs (VA) for the time the physicians reported as being on duty at a VA hospital. Physicians employed by VA may not bill Medicare for services rendered at other hospitals during the times they were on duty at a VA hospital. Our preliminary work has identified a number of VA physicians who received Medicare reimbursements totaling approximately $105 million for services rendered between January 1, 2001 and June 30, 2003. Using time reporting and payroll documentation from the VA, we will identify the services rendered while the physicians were reported as on duty at the VA hospitals and remunerated for such duty.

(OAS; W-00-04-35155; A-00-00-0000; expected issue date: FY 2005; work in progress)

CARE PLAN OVERSIGHT

We will evaluate the efficacy of controls over Medicare payments for care plan oversight claims submitted by physicians. Under the Medicare home health and hospice benefits, care plan oversight is physician supervision of beneficiaries who need complex or multidisciplinary care requiring ongoing physician involvement. Reimbursement for care plan oversight increased from $15 million in 2000 to $41 million in 2001. We will assess whether these services were provided in accordance with Medicare regulations.

(OAS; W-00-04-35114; A-02-00-00000; expected issue date: FY 2005; work in progress)

ORDERING PHYSICIANS EXCLUDED FROM MEDICARE

This review will quantify the extent of services, if any, ordered by physicians excluded from Federal health care programs and the amount paid by Medicare Part B. Under Federal regulation, physicians who are excluded from Federal health care programs generally are precluded from ordering or performing services for Medicare beneficiaries. During a current review, we identified a significant number of services that had been ordered by excluded physicians.

(OAS; W-00-04-35116; various reviews; expected issue date: FY 2005; work in progress)

PHYSICIAN SERVICES AT SKILLED NURSING FACILITIES

We will examine Medicare Part A and Part B claims with overlapping services for skilled nursing facility patients and determine whether duplicate payments were made to either the physicians or the nursing homes for the same patient services. Physicians may bill Medicare only for the professional component of a service on behalf of skilled nursing facility patients. The technical component of physicians' services is covered under the patient's Medicare Part B stay in the skilled nursing facilities and should not be billed separately by the nursing home. Under an exception to this rule, nursing homes may receive Part B payments for both the professional and technical components of physicians' services if both parties have an agreement under which only the nursing home may bill and receive these Part B payments.

(OAS; W-00-05-35163; various reviews; expected issue date: FY 2005; new start)

PHYSICIAN PATHOLOGY SERVICES

Our review will focus on pathology services performed in physicians' offices. Pathology services include the examination of cells or tissue samples by a physician who prepares a report of his findings. Medicare pays over $1 billion annually to physicians for pathology services. We will identify and review the relationships between physicians who furnish pathology services in their offices and outside pathology companies.

(OAS; W-00-05-35164; various reviews; expected issue date: FY 2005; new start)

CARDIOGRAPHY AND ECHOCARDIOGRAPHY SERVICES

We will review Medicare payments for cardiography and echocardiography services to determine whether physicians billed appropriately for the professional and the technical components of the services. Like many physician services, cardiography and echocardiography include both technical and professional components. When a physician performs the interpretation separately, the modifier 26 should be used to bill Medicare for professional services.

(OAS; W-00-05-35165; various reviews; expected issue date: FY 2005; new start)

PHYSICAL AND OCCUPATIONAL THERAPY SERVICES

We will review Medicare claims for therapy services provided by physical and occupational therapists to determine whether the services were reasonable and medically necessary, adequately documented, and certified by physician certification statements. Physical and occupational therapies are medically prescribed treatments concerned with improving or restoring functions, preventing further disability, and relieving symptoms.

(OAS; W-00-04-35141; various reviews; expected issue date: FY 2005; work in progress)

PART B MENTAL HEALTH SERVICES

We will determine whether Medicare Part B mental health services provided in physicians' offices were medically necessary and billed in accordance with Medicare requirements. Payments for mental health services provided in the physician's office setting accounted for approximately 55 percent of the $1.3 billion in Medicare payments for Part B mental health services in 2002. In a prior report, we found that Medicare allowed $185 million for inappropriate mental health services in the outpatient setting. We will also determine the financial impact of claims that do not meet Medicare requirements.

(OEI; 09-04-00220; expected issue date: FY 2005; work in progress)

WOUND CARE SERVICES

We will determine whether claims for wound care services were medically necessary and billed in accordance with Medicare requirements. Medicare-allowed amounts for certain wound care services billed by physicians increased from approximately $98 million in 1998 to $147 million in 2002. We will also examine the adequacy of controls to prevent inappropriate payments for wound care services.

(OEI; 02-04-00410; expected issue date: FY 2006; work in progress)

CODING OF EVALUATION AND MANAGEMENT SERVICES

We will examine patterns of physician coding of evaluation and management services and determine whether these services were coded accurately. In 2003, Medicare allowed over $29 billion for evaluation and management services. In prior work, we found that a significant portion of certain categories of these services is billed with incorrect codes resulting in large overpayments. We will also assess the adequacy of controls to identify physicians with aberrant coding patterns.

(OEI; 00-00-00000; expected issue date: FY 2005; new start)

USE OF MODIFIER 25

We will determine whether providers used modifier –25 appropriately. In general, a provider should not bill evaluation and management codes on the same day as a procedure or other service unless the evaluation and management service is a significant, separately identifiable service from such procedure or service. A provider reports such a circumstance by using modifier –25. In 2001, Medicare allowed over $23 billion for evaluation and management services. Of that amount, approximately $1.7 billion was for evaluation and management services billed with modifier –25. We will determine whether these claims were billed and reimbursed appropriately.

(OEI; 07-03-00470; expected issue date: FY 2005; work in progress)

USE OF MODIFIERS WITH NATIONAL CORRECT CODING INITIATIVE EDITS

We will determine whether claims were paid appropriately when modifiers were used to bypass National Correct Coding Initiative edits. The initiative, one of CMS's tools for detecting and correcting improper billing, is designed to provide Medicare Part B carriers with code pair edits for use in reviewing claims. A provider may include a modifier to allow payment for both services within the code pair under certain circumstances. In 2001, Medicare paid $565 million to providers who included the modifier with code pairs within the National Correct Coding Initiative. We will determine whether modifiers were used appropriately.

(OEI; 03-02-00771; expected issue date: FY 2005; work in progress)

LONG DISTANCE PHYSICIAN CLAIMS

We will review Medicare claims for face-to-face physician encounters where the practice setting and the beneficiary's location were separated by a significant distance. While all beneficiaries may seek professional services for specialized consultation during leisure travel, those with ongoing illnesses requiring skilled care would be unlikely to travel long distances from home. We will examine these claims to confirm that services were provided and accurately reported. If warranted, we will recommend enhancements to existing program integrity controls.

(OEI; 00-00-00000; expected issue date: FY 2006; new start)

PROVIDER-BASED ENTITIES

We will determine the extent to which health care entities that have been designated as "provider based" are in compliance with requirements for receiving this designation. In prior work, we found that hospital ownership of physician practices is widespread and that fiscal intermediaries are frequently unaware whether these hospitals are being treated as provider based or freestanding. Medicare and its beneficiaries may be paying excessive amounts for services inappropriately billed as provider based. We will also determine the impact on Medicare reimbursements of entities billing as provider based instead of freestanding.

(OEI; 00-00-00000; expected issue date: FY 2006; new start)

Glossary

Abstractor. A person who selects and extracts specific data from the medical record and enters the information into computer files.

Abuse. As defined by Medicare, an incident that is inconsistent with accepted sound medical, business or fiscal practices and directly or indirectly results in unnecessary costs to the Medicare program, improper reimbursement, or reimbursement for services that do not meet professionally recognized standards of care or which are medically unnecessary. Examples of abuse include excessive charges, improper billing practices, billing Medicare as primary instead of other third-party payers that are primary, and increasing charges for Medicare beneficiaries but not to other patients.

Accredited record technician (ART). A former certification describing medical records practitioners; now known as a registered health information technician (RHIT).

Actual charge. The charge a physician or supplier bills for a service rendered or a supply item.

Acute care facility. A health care facility that provides continuous professional medical care to patients in an acute phase of illness or injury.

Acute. Sudden, severe.

ADA. See American Dental Association.

Add-on codes. A procedure performed in addition to the primary procedure and designated with a + in the CPT book. Add-on codes are never reported for stand-alone services but are reported secondarily in addition to the primary procedure.

Adjudication (claims). The completion of a processed claim that results in a payment, rejection, or denial.

Administrative services only (ASO). A contract stipulation between a self-funded plan and an insurance company in which the insurance company assumes no risk and provides administrative services only.

Admission date. The date the patient was admitted to the health care facility for inpatient care, outpatient service, or the start of care.

Admission. Registration of a patient for services in a health care facility.

Against medical advice. The discharge status of patients who leave the hospital after signing a form that releases the hospital from responsibility, or who leave the hospital premises without notifying hospital personnel.

AHA. See American Hospital Association.

AHIMA. See American Health Information Management Association.

Allowable charge (also called approved charge). Fee schedule amount for a medical service as determined by the physician fee schedule methodology as published annually by CMS.

ALOS. See Average length of stay.

Altering patient records. The practice of inappropriately changing or amending patient records, usually to obtain reimbursement or because of pending audits and legal review of records.

AMA. See American Medical Association.

Ambulance fee schedule. The final rule published on February 27, 2002, established a fee schedule for the payment of ambulance services under the Medicare program effective on or after April 1, 2002. The rule established a five-year transition during which payment is based on a blended amount-part fee schedule and part provider reasonable cost or suppliers' reasonable charge.

Ambulatory patient group. A reimbursement methodology developed for the Centers for Medicare and Medicaid Services.

Ambulatory payment classification (APC). A cost-containment tool developed by CMS and the basis for the outpatient prospective payment system (OPPS). Outpatient services are grouped into multiple payment classifications based on resource utilization. Facilities are paid a fixed rate dependent on the service classification.

Ambulatory surgery center (ASC). Any distinct entity that operates exclusively for the purpose of providing surgical services to patients not requiring inpatient hospitalization.

Ambulatory surgery. A surgical procedure in which the patient is admitted, treated, and released on the same day.

Amendment. See Amendments and corrections.

Amendments and corrections. In the final privacy rule, an amendment to a record would indicate that the data are in dispute while retaining the original information, while a correction to a record would alter or replace the original record.

American Academy of Orthopaedic Surgeons (AAOS). A nonprofit organization for orthopaedic surgeons and allied health professionals.

American Academy of Professional Coders (AAPC). A national organization for coders and billers offering certification based upon physician- or facility-specific guidelines.

American Dental Association (ADA). A professional organization for dentists. The ADA maintains a hardcopy dental claim form and the associated claim submission specifications, and also maintains the Current Dental Terminology (CDT-4) medical code set. The ADA and the Dental Content Committee (DeCC), which it hosts, have formal consultative roles under HIPAA.

American Health Information Management Association (AHIMA). An association of health information management professionals. AHIMA sponsors some HIPAA educational seminars.

American Hospital Association (AHA) Central Office. The central office of the AHA works in partnership with the National Center for Health Statistics (NCHS), American Health Information Management Association (AHIMA), and Centers for Medicare and Medicaid Services (CMS) to maintain the integrity of and develop education regarding the ICD-9-CM coding system.

American Hospital Association (AHA). A health care industry association that represents the concerns of institutional providers. The AHA hosts the NUBC, which has a formal consultative role under HIPAA.

American Medical Association (AMA). A professional organization for physicians. The AMA is the secretariat of the NUCC, which has a formal consultative role under HIPAA. The AMA also maintains the Physician's Current Procedural Terminology (CPT) coding system.

American National Standards Institute (ANSI). An organization that accredits various standards-setting committees and monitors their compliance with the open rule-making process that they must follow to qualify for ANSI accreditation. HIPAA prescribes that the standards mandated under it be developed by ANSI-accredited bodies whenever practical.

American Society of Anesthesiologists (ASA). A national organization for anesthesiology that maintains and publishes the guidelines and relative values for anesthesia coding.

Analgesia. Absence of a normal sense of pain without loss of consciousness.

Analgesic. An agent that relieves pain without causing loss of consciousness.

Ancillary services. Services, other than routine room and board charges, which are incidental to the hospital stay. These services include operating room; anesthesia; blood administration; pharmacy; radiology; laboratory; medical, surgical, and central supplies; physical, occupational, speech pathology, and inhalation therapies; and other diagnostic services.

Anesthesia formula. Reimbursement formula consisting of base units plus time units plus modifying units (e.g., physical status and qualifying circumstances) plus other allowed unit/charges that is multiplied by a conversion factor.

Anesthesia. A loss of feeling or sensation, usually induced to permit the performance of surgery or other painful procedures.

Antikickback Act. Prohibits knowing or willful solicitation or receipt of remuneration in return for referring, recommending, or arranging for the purchase, lease, or ordering of items or services for which payment will be made from any federal or state health care program.

Any willing provider. Statutes requiring a provider network to accept any provider who meets the network's usual selection criteria.

AOA. American Osteopathic Association.

APA. American Psychiatric Association.

APC. See Ambulatory payment classification.

APG. See Ambulatory patient group.

Appeal. A specific request made to a payer for reconsideration of a denial or adverse coverage or payment decision and potential restriction of benefit reimbursement.

Appropriateness of care. Term often used to denote the proper setting of medical care that best meets the patient's care or diagnosis.

ASC (facility). See Ambulatory surgery center and Accredited Standards Committee.

ASC payment group rate. The facility payment received by an ASC when a covered surgical procedure is performed on a Medicare beneficiary. This rate is adjusted for geo-economic variation. Covered ASC surgical procedures are grouped into eight payment categories for reimbursement purposes.

Assessment. The process of collecting and studying information and data, such as test values, signs, and symptoms.

Assigned claim. A claim from a physician or supplier who has agreed to accept the Medicare allowable amount as payment in full for the services rendered. Reimbursement is made directly to the provider of the service.

Assignment of benefits. An authorization from the patient allowing the third-party payer to pay the provider directly for medical services. Under Medicare, an assignment is an agreement by the hospital or physician to accept Medicare's payment as the full payment and not to bill the patient for any amounts over the DRG or allowance amount, except for deductible and/or coinsurance amounts or noncovered services. Payment is made directly to the provider accepting assignment.

Assignment. An arrangement in which the provider submits the claim on behalf of the patient and is reimbursed directly by the patient's plan and agrees to accept what the plan pays.

Assistant-at-surgery. A physician or other appropriate health care provider who assists another provider during performance of a surgery.

Audit. An examination or review that establishes the extent to which performance or a process conforms to predetermined standards or criteria. An audit may target utilization, quality of care, or reimbursement.

Auditing and monitoring. Auditing an organization's practices involves regularly reviewing an organization's claim development and submission process from the point where a service for a patient is initiated to the submission of a claim for payment. Monitoring involves a system of checks of and controls over, as well as a method of reporting, all areas of compliance, including regulations and audits.

Auditor. A professional who evaluates a provider's utilization, quality of care, or level of reimbursement.

Authorization (services). Approval to provide a service to a member or beneficiary.

AWP (insurance). Any willing provider.

AWP (pharmaceutical). Average wholesale price.

Backlog. The queue of claims that have not been adjudicated.

Balance billing. An arrangement prohibited by government regulations and some payer contracts whereby a provider bills the patient for charges not reimbursed by the payer.

Base rate. A number assigned to a hospital used to calculate DRG reimbursement. Base rates vary from hospital to hospital. The base rate adjusts reimbursement to allow for such individual characteristics of the hospital as geographic location, status (urban/rural, teaching), and local labor costs.

Baseline. A starting point or place of reference from which to base progression or treatment of a condition.

Basic value or base unit (anesthesia services). A relative weighted value based upon the usual anesthesia services and the relative work or cost of the specific anesthesia service assigned to each anesthesia-specific procedure code.

BBA. See Balanced Budget Act of 1997.

BCBSA. See Blue Cross and Blue Shield Association.

Beneficiary. A person entitled to receive Medicare or other payer benefits who maintains a health insurance policy claim number.

Benefit. Services an insurance program agrees to cover under a contractual arrangement.

Biller. A person who submits claims for services provided by a health care provider or supplier to payers.

Blue Cross and Blue Shield Association (BCBSA). An association that represents the common interests of Blue Cross and Blue Shield health plans. The BCBSA serves as the administrator for the Health Care Code Maintenance and also helps maintain the HCPCS Level II coding system.

Board certification. A certification in a particular specialty based on the physician's demonstration of expertise and experience.

Bundled (codes). The inclusive grouping of codes related to a procedure when submitting a claim.

Care plan oversight services. A physician's ongoing review and revision of a patient's care plan involving complex or multidisciplinary care modalities.

Carrier (CMS). An organization that contracts with CMS to process Medicare claims under Part B, the supplemental medical insurance program.

Carrier (insurance). An insurer or health plan that may underwrite, administer, or sell a range of health benefit programs.

Case management. The ongoing review of cases by professionals to ensure the most appropriate utilization of services.

Cash deductible. The dollar amount assumed by the hospital to be applied to the patient's deductible for a particular insurance benefit program. The Medicare cash deductible is the amount the patient must pay each benefit period for inpatient hospital (Part A) services. Under Part B, it is an annual deductible amount that the patient is responsible for paying before Medicare payment can be made.

CCI. See Correct Coding Initiative.

CDC. See Centers for Disease Control and Prevention.

CDT-4. See Current Dental Terminology.

Centers for Disease Control and Prevention (CDC). An organization that maintains several code sets included in the HIPAA standards, including the ICD-9-CM codes. The ICD-9-CM codes are created by the World Health Organization. The clinical modifications that occur in the United States. are made by the CM committee. The CDC participates in the committee.

Centers for Medicare and Medicaid Services (CMS). CMS is charged with the responsibility of maintaining, controlling, and enforcing the Health Insurance Portability and Accountability Act (HIPAA) transaction standards. References in this book to CMS refer to its function as overseer of HIPAA and not its administration of the Medicare and Medicaid programs.

Certified nurse midwife. A registered nurse who has successfully completed a program of study and clinical experience or has been certified by a recognized organization to practice as a maternity health care provider.

CFR. Code of Federal Regulations.

CHAMPUS. See Civilian Health and Medical Program of the Uniformed Services.

CHAMPVA. See Civilian Health and Medical Program of the Veteran's Administration.

Charges. The dollar amount assigned to a service or procedure by a provider and reported to a payer.

Charts. A compilation of documents maintained by the provider for each patient that includes treatment/progress notes, test orders and results, correspondence from other health care providers, and other documents pertinent to the patient's care.

Chief complaint. A disease, condition, illness, injury, symptom, sign, finding, complaint, or other reason for the patient encounter.

CHIP. Child Health Insurance Program.

CIM. See Coverage Issues Manual.

Civil monetary penalty. Financial payment or remuneration as punishment for violating the civil laws that protect the rights of individuals or the general public, including violations of HIPAA legislation and regulations governing federally funded health care programs.

Civilian Health and Medical Program of the Uniformed Services (CHAMPUS). A federal program that covered the health benefits for families of all uniformed service employees. The program has been replaced by TRICARE.

Civilian Health and Medical Program of the Veteran's Administration (CHAMPVA). Program similar to TRICARE under which the insured must be a disabled veteran's spouse or dependent or a survivor of someone who died of service-related causes.

Claim attachment. Any of a variety of hardcopy forms or electronic records needed to process a claim in addition to the claim itself.

Claim denial. Denial of an entire claim. The provider cannot resubmit the claim but can appeal the claim denial.

Claim. Statement of medical services rendered requesting payment from an insurance company or government entity.

Clean claim. A claim that is complete and error free that passes through the payer's edit programs without need for adjudication before reimbursement.

Clearinghouse. See Health Care clearinghouse.

CLIA. See Clinical Laboratory Improvement Amendments.

Clinic. Outpatient facility that provides scheduled diagnostic, curative, rehabilitative, and educational services for walk-in (ambulatory) patients.

Clinical Laboratory Improvement Amendments (CLIA). Requirements set in 1988, CLIA imposes varying levels of federal regulations on clinical procedures. Few laboratories, including those in physician offices, are exempt. Adopted by Medicare and Medicaid, CLIA regulations redefine laboratory testing in regard to laboratory certification and accreditation, proficiency testing, quality assurance, personnel standards, and program administration.

Closed claim. A claim for which all apparent benefits have been paid.

CMS manual system. A system of Web-based manuals organized by functional area that contains all program instructions in the National Coverage Determinations Manual, the Medicare Benefit Policy Manual, Pub 100, one-time notifications, and manual revision notices.

CMS-1450. CMS's name for the institutional uniform claim form, or UB-92. Previously named the HCFA-1450.

CMS-1500. A standard paper claim form used by Medicare and commercial payers for physician and other outpatient service claims in limited circumstances when the claims are not being submitted electronically. Also known as the UCF-1500. Previously named the HCFA-1500.

CMS. See Centers for Medicare and Medicaid Services.

COB. See Coordination of benefits.

COBRA. See Consolidated Omnibus Reconciliation Act.

Coder. A trained professional who translates written or transcribed oral diagnoses and procedures into numeric and alphanumeric medical codes for reimbursement and/or statistical purposes.

Coding conventions. Each space, typeface, indentation, and punctuation mark determining how ICD-9-CM codes are interpreted when the diagnoses and procedures performed are reported.

Coding guidelines. Official guidelines that specify how procedure, diagnosis, or durable medical equipment codes are to be translated and listed for various purposes.

Coding rules. Official rules and coding conventions used for diagnosis and procedure coding.

Coding specificity. The codes assigned are the most specific available; i.e., a three-digit disease code is assigned only when there are no four-digit codes within that category, a four-digit code is assigned only when there is no fifth-digit subclassification within that category, or a fifth digit is assigned for any category for which a fifth-digit subclassification is provided.

Coinsurance. A portion of the balance of covered medical expenses for which a beneficiary is responsible after the payment of a deductible amount. Under Medicare Part B, the coinsurance amount is 20 percent of allowed charges. Under Medicare's outpatient prospective payment system, the copayment for a single procedure or service effective for claims with dates of service on or after January 1, 2004, cannot exceed the inpatient hospital deductible amount of $876.

Commercial carriers. For-profit insurance companies issuing health coverage.

Commercial plan. A health benefit coverage package offered by a commercial carrier.

Common Working File (CWF). A system of local databases containing total beneficiary histories developed by CMS to improve Medicare claims processing. Medicare fiscal intermediaries and carriers interact with these databases to obtain data on eligibility, utilization, Medicare secondary payer (MSP), and other detailed claims information. The CWF is authorized to deny payment on claims on a prepayment basis. There are nine CWF regionally based sectors.

Community mental health center. A facility providing outpatient mental health day treatment, assessments, and education as appropriate to community members.

Comparative performance report (CPR). Report that provides an annual comparison of a physician's services and procedures with those of another physician in the same specialty and geographic area.

Complete procedure (diagnostic services). The entire service when the procedure can be separated into a professional component that must be performed by a physician and a technical component that includes technical staff, equipment, overhead, and supplies.

Complex. A composite or collection of related things, such as symptoms, anatomical parts, or surgical procedures.

Compliance audits. Internal or external monitoring and review of activities to ensure compliance with all laws, regulations, and guidelines related to health care.

Compliance committee. Individuals assigned to help the compliance officer teach and comply with all laws, regulations, and guidelines related to health care.

Compliance officer. Individual with authority, funding, and staff to perform all necessary compliance activities, including planning, implementing, and monitoring the compliance program.

Compliance plan. A plan of established methods to eliminate errors in coding, billing, and other issues through auditing and monitoring, training, or other corrective actions. Such a plan also provides an avenue for employees and others to report problems.

Compliance program. A set of written policies and procedures related to the delivery of services and developed and monitored internally to ensure that the facility/business is providing high-quality services, while at the same time eliminating waste, fraud, and abuse.

Compliance. Active monitoring of all services to ensure that services are being provided and reported according to applicable laws, regulations, and guidelines related to health care.

Component code, column II. In the Corrective Coding Initiative (CCI) edits, the code following the column I code that cannot be charged when the more comprehensive code is charged.

Component coding. Standardizes the reporting of interventional radiology services. Component coding allows a physician, regardless of specialty, to specifically identify and report those aspects of the service he or she provided, whether the procedural component, the radiological component, or both.

Comprehensive code, column I. In the Corrective Coding Initiative (CCI) edits, a column I, comprehensive code, that represents the major procedure or service when reported with another code.

Comprehensive codes. In the Corrective Coding Initiative (CCI) edits, a column I, comprehensive code that represents the major procedure or service when reported with another code. See also Correct Coding Initiative.

Comprehensive outpatient rehabilitation facility (CORF). A facility that provides services that include physician's services related to administrative functions; physical, occupational, speech and respiratory therapies; social and psychological services; and prosthetic and orthotic devices. A service is covered as a CORF service if it is also covered as an inpatient hospital service provided to a hospital patient. CORF services require a plan of treatment within a maximum of 60-day intervals for rereviews.

Concomitant operations. Accompanying procedures that are completed during the same surgical session.

Concomitant. Occurring at the same time, accompanying.

Conversion factor. 1) The dollar value for each relative value unit. When this dollar amount is multiplied by the total relative value units, it yields the reimbursement rate for the service; 2) a national multiplier that converts the geographically adjusted relative value units into Medicare fee schedule dollar amounts that applies to all services paid under the MFS.

Coordinated care. A system of health care delivery that influences utilization, quality of care, and cost of services. Managed care integrates financing and management with an employed or contracted organized provider network that delivers services to an enrolled population.

Coordination of benefits (COB). A method of integrating benefits payable when there is more than one group insurance plan so that the insured's benefits and the payment of insurance benefits from all sources do not exceed 100 percent of the allowed medical expenses.

Copayment. A cost-sharing arrangement in which a covered person pays a specified charge for a specified type of service, usually at the time the health care is rendered.

CORF. See Comprehensive outpatient rehabilitation facility.

Correct Coding Council. The Centers for Medicare and Medicaid Services (CMS) established the national Correct Coding Council to develop coding methodologies based on established coding conventions to control improper coding that leads to inappropriate and increased payment of Part B claims.

Correct Coding Initiative (CCI). An official list of codes from the Centers for Medicare and Medicaid Services' (CMS) National Correct Coding Policy Manual for Part B Medicare Carriers that identifies services considered either an integral part of a comprehensive code or mutually exclusive of it.

Coverage Issues Manual (CIM). Revised and renamed the National Coverage Determination Manual in the CMS manual system, it contains national coverage decisions and specific medical items, services, treatment procedures, or technologies paid for under the Medicare program.

Covered charges. Charges for medical care and supplies that the insurance plan will pay.

Covered person. Any person entitled to benefits under the policy, whether a member or dependent.

Covered services. Diagnostic or therapeutic services considered medically necessary and that are payable by the health care plan.

CPR (health information). See Computerized patient record.

CPT code. See Current Procedural Terminology coding system.

CPT modifier. A two-character code used to indicate that a service was altered in some way from the stated CPT or HCPCS description but not enough to change the basic definition of the service.

CPT. See Current Procedural Terminology.

Credentialing. Reviewing the medical degrees, licensure, malpractice, and any disciplinary record of medical providers for panel and quality assurance purposes and to grant hospital privileges.

Critical care. The care of critically ill or injured patients in various medical emergencies that requires the constant attendance of the physician (e.g., cardiac arrest, shock, bleeding, respiratory failure, postoperative complications, critically ill neonate).

CRNA. Certified registered nurse anesthetist.

Cross-over. See Coordination of benefits.

Current Dental Terminology (CDT-4). A medical code set, maintained and copyrighted by the American Dental Association, that has been selected for use in the HIPAA transactions.

Current Procedural Terminology. The definitive procedural coding system developed by the American Medical Association that lists descriptive terms and identifying codes to provide a uniform language that describes medical, surgical, and diagnostic services for nationwide communication among physicians, patients, and third parties.

Customary, prevailing, and reasonable charge (CPR). The basis for Medicare's reimbursement rates before the resource-based relative value scale (RBRVS) was implemented. CPR reimbursement rates were based on historical physician charges rather than relative values, which caused wide variation in Medicare payments among physicians and specialties.

CWF. See Common Working File.

Date of service (DOS). The DOS is noted on the medical chart as the day the encounter or procedure is performed or the day a supply is issued.

DC. Doctor of chiropractic medicine.

Deductible. A predetermined dollar amount of covered billed charges that the patient must pay towards the cost of his or her care.

Denial (Medicare). The status of a claim that is returned without payment because the service is noncovered, is deemed not medically

Department of Health and Human Services (HHS or DHHS). The cabinet department that oversees the operating divisions of the federal government responsible for health and welfare. HHS oversees the Centers for Medicare and Medicaid Services, Food and Drug Administration, Public Health Service, and other such entities.

Diagnosis code. An ICD-9-CM code that describes the patient's medical condition, symptoms, or the reason for the encounter as documented in the patient record.

Diagnosis-related group (DRG). The inpatient classification scheme used for Medicare's hospital inpatient reimbursement system. Currently, 506 DRGs make up the inpatient classification system. The DRG system classifies patients based on principal diagnosis, surgical procedure, age, presence of comorbidities or complications and other pertinent data.

Diagnosis. Determination or confirmation of a condition, disease, or syndrome and its implications.

Diagnostic and Statistical Manual of Mental Disorders, Fourth Edition (DSM-IV). The manual used by mental health workers as the diagnosis coding system for substance abuse and mental health patients.

Diagnostic laboratory services. Laboratory services that are required to diagnose a disease or injury, regardless of where the services are rendered. These services include certain mechanical or machine tests such as EKGs and EEGs. For Medicare purposes, these services are paid under a fee schedule.

Diagnostic procedures. A procedure performed on a patient to obtain information to assess the medical condition of the patient or to identify a disease and to determine the nature and severity of an illness or injury.

Diagnostic services. An examination or procedure performed on a patient to obtain information to assess the medical condition of the patient or to identify a disease and to determine the nature and severity of an illness or injury (e.g., diagnostic laboratory tests, x-rays, EKGs, pulmonary function tests, or psychological tests).

Diagnostic x-ray services. X-ray and other related services performed for diagnostic purposes, including portable x-ray services.

Dialysis. Artificial filtering of the blood to remove contaminating waste elements and restore normal balance.

Disabled beneficiary. A person who is eligible for Medicare benefits because he or she is totally and permanently disabled. Individuals under age 65 who have been entitled to disability benefits under Social Security or the Railroad Retirement System for at least two years are classified as disabled for Medicare purposes.

Discharge date. The date the patient is formally released, dies, or is transferred from the hospital or skilled nursing facility (SNF).

Discharge plan. A treatment plan by the provider for continued patient care after discharge that may include home care, the services of case managers or other health care providers, or transfer to another facility.

Discharge status. Disposition of the patient at discharge (for example, left against medical advice, discharged home, transferred to an acute care hospital, expired).

Discharge transfer. Discharge of a patient from one facility to another.

Discharge. To release from care by a health care provider at the completion of the prescribed treatment in an inpatient or outpatient setting.

DME. See Durable medical equipment.

DMEPOS. Durable medical equipment, prosthetics, orthotics, and supplies. See also Durable medical equipment.

DMERC. See Medicare durable medical equipment regional carrier.

DO. Doctor of osteopathy.

DOS. See Date of service.

Downcoding (provider). Reporting a lower-level code for a service so that an additional code may be used rather than using one higher-level and more comprehensive code.

DPM. Doctor of podiatric medicine.

DRG. See Diagnosis-related group.

DSM-IV. See Diagnostic and Statistical Manual of Mental Disorders, fourth edition.

Durable medical equipment (DME). Medical equipment that can withstand repeated use, is not disposable, is used to serve a medical purpose, is generally not useful to a person in the absence of a sickness or injury, and is appropriate for use in the home. Examples of durable medical equipment include hospital beds, wheelchairs, and oxygen equipment.

E code. A diagnosis code that describes the circumstance that caused an injury, not the nature of the injury. E codes are used to classify external causes of injury, poisoning, or other adverse effects. An E code should not be used as a principal diagnosis because the intermediary will reject the claim. FL 77 is for reporting E codes on the UB-92 form.

E/M codes. See Evaluation and management codes.

E/M. See Evaluation and management.

EDI. See Electronic data interchange.

Electronic claim. Claim submitted by a provider or electronic media claim (EMC) vendor via central processing unit (CPU) transmission, tape, diskette, direct data entry, direct wire, dial-in telephone, digital fax, or personal computer upload or download. Effective October 1, 1993, clean claims submitted to Medicare electronically are paid 13 days after the claim is received.

Electronic commerce (EC). The exchange of business information by electronic means.

Electronic data interchange (EDI). Usually means X12 and similar variable-length formats for the electronic exchange of structured data. It is sometimes used more broadly to mean any electronic exchange of formatted data.

Electronic media claim (EMC). Automated claims processing method that uses a data storage tool to transfer claims data to the payer. Has been replaced by electronic data interchange (EDI).

Eligibility. Refers to individuals and services that are qualified for coverage under a specific health care plan.

Emergency department. An on-site hospital department that is open 24 hours a day to provide medical attention for unscheduled patients requiring immediate medical care.

Emergency. A serious medical condition or symptom (including severe pain) resulting from injury, sickness, or mental illness that arises suddenly and requires immediate care and treatment, generally received within 24 hours of onset, to avoid jeopardy to the life, limb, or health of a covered person.

Emergent care. Treatment for a medical condition or symptom (including severe pain) that arises suddenly and requires immediate care and treatment.

Employee Retirement Income Security Act (ERISA). An act with several provisions protecting both payer and member, including requiring that payers send the member an explanation of benefits when a claim is denied.

EMR. Electronic medical record.

Encounter (or visit). A face-to-face meeting between a covered person and a health care provider that includes diagnosis and treatment of an illness or injury.

End-stage renal disease (ESRD). Chronic kidney disease requiring renal dialysis or a kidney transplant.

Enrollee. An individual who is enrolled for coverage under a health plan contract and is eligible on his/her own behalf (not by virtue of being an eligible dependent) to receive the health services provided under the contract; also known as a subscriber.

EOB. See Explanation of benefits.

EOMB. Explanation of Medicare benefits, explanation of Medicaid benefits, or explanation of member benefits.

Episode of care. One or more health care services received during a period of relatively continuous care by a hospital or health care provider.

EPSDT. Early and periodic screening, diagnosis, and treatment.

ERA. See Electronic remittance advice.

ERISA. The Employee Retirement Income Security Act of 1974.

ESRD. See End-stage renal disease.

Established patient. Evaluation and management guidelines define an established patient as one who has received professional services in a face-to-face setting within the last three years from the same physician or another physician of the same specialty who belongs to the same group practice.

Evaluation and management (E/M) codes. Describe the assessment and management of a patient's health care using the 99000 series of CPT codes.

Evaluation and management service components. The components of history, examination, and medical decision-making, which are key to selecting the correct E/M codes.

Examination. A comprehensive visual and tactile screening and specific testing leading to diagnosis or, as appropriate, to a referral to another practitioner.

Excluded services. Services not covered by Medicare, including routine physical check-ups, eye exams, foot care, eyeglasses, hearing aids, immunizations not related to injury or immediate risk of infection, cosmetic surgery not related to an illness or injury, items and services not reasonable and necessary for diagnosing and treating an illness or injury, custodial care, personal comfort items, and others.

Exclusions. Specific conditions or circumstances listed in the contract or employee benefit plan for which the policy or plan will not provide coverage; also known as exceptions.

Exclusive provider organization (EPO). Similar to an HMO, but the member must remain within the provider network to receive benefits. EPOs are regulated under insurance statutes rather than HMO legislation.

Explanation of benefits (EOB). A statement mailed to the member and provider explaining claim adjudication and payment.

Explanation of Medicare benefits (EOMB). A Medicare statement mailed to the member and provider explaining claim adjudication and payment.

Extended care facility. An institution that provides any type of long-term care. Usually refers to a skilled nursing facility, but may be used in reference to other types of long-term care institutions.

Facility practice expense. One of the three components used to determine the relative value of physician services paid under the resource-based relative value scale (RBRVS). Facility practice expense represents the physician's direct and indirect costs related to each service provided in a hospital, ambulatory surgery center (ASC), or skilled nursing facility (SNF).

Facility. A building, house, or a place of patient care, including inpatient and outpatient, for acute or long-term care.

False Claims Act. Governs civil actions for filing false claims. Liability under this act pertains to any person who knowingly presents or causes to be presented a false or fraudulent claim to the government for payment or approval.

Federal Register. A government publication listing changes in regulations and federally mandated standards, including coding standards such as HCPCS Level II and ICD-9-CM.

Fee for service. 1) Payment for services, usually physician services, on a service-by-service basis rather than an alternative payment system like capitation. Fee-for-service arrangements may be discounted or undiscounted rates; 2) situation in which payer pays full charges for medical services.

Fee schedule. A list of codes and related services with pre-established billing amounts by a provider, or payment amounts by a payer that could be percentages of billed charges, flat rates, or maximum allowable amounts established by third-party payers. Medicare fee schedules apply to clinical laboratory, radiology, and durable medical equipment services.

FI. See Fiscal intermediary.

Fiscal intermediary (FI). A federally designated contractor that processes Medicare claims for Part A benefits and some Part B claims.

Fiscal year (FY). Twelve-month period that an organization designates and uses to denote an accounting period or during which it plans to use funds. Fiscal years are referred to by the calendar year in which they end. The federal government's fiscal year runs from October 1 to September 30.

FR. See Federal Register.

Fraud and abuse. A method of obtaining unauthorized benefits, fraud is an intentional deception or misrepresentation or statement that is known to be false, and abuse is a practice that is inconsistent with accepted medical, business, or fiscal practice.

Fraud. An intentional deception or misrepresentation or statement that is known to be false and could result in unauthorized benefit to patient, provider, or other persons.

Frequency. The number of times a given service is provided during a specified time period.

Gatekeeper. The practice whereby a member's care must be provided by a primary care physician unless the physician refers the member to a specialist or approves the care provided by a specialist.

General anesthesia. A state of unconsciousness produced by an anesthetic agent or agents in which the patient is unable to control protective reflexes, such as breathing.

Global surgery package. A code denoting a normal surgical procedure with no complications that includes all of the elements needed to perform the procedure and includes routine follow-up care.

Government mandates. Services mandated by state or federal law such as the correct use of ICD-9-CM codes.

Group practice. A group of providers that shares facilities, resources, and staff and who may represent a single unit in a managed care network.

Guidelines. Recommendations or information providing definitions, explanations of terms, and factors relevant to the correct assignment of procedure or diagnosis codes and modifiers.

HCFA. See Centers for Medicare and Medicaid Services. Also see 45 CFR, part II, 160.103.

HCPCS Level I. See Healthcare Common Procedure Coding System Level I.

HCPCS Level II. See Healthcare Common Procedure Coding System Level II.

HCPCS modifiers. See Healthcare Common Procedure Coding System modifiers.

HCPCS. See Healthcare Common Procedure Coding System.

Health and Human Services (HHS). See Department of Health and Human Services.

Health Care Code Maintenance Committee. An organization administered by the Blue Cross and Blue Shield Association that maintains certain coding schemes used in the X12 transactions and elsewhere. These include the claim adjustment reason codes, the claim status category codes, and the claim status codes.

Health Care Financing Administration (HCFA). The former name of the federal agency that oversees the administration of the public health programs (e.g., Medicare, Medicaid, State Children's Insurance Program), now known as the Centers for Medicare and Medicaid Services.

Health care provider. According to HIPAA privacy standards (160.103, a person or entity that provides care to a patient such as a hospital, skilled nursing facility, inpatient/outpatient rehabilitation facility, home health agency, hospice program, physician, diagnostic department, outpatient physical or occupational therapy, rural clinics, or home dialysis supplier. See 45 CFR, part II, 160.103.

Health care. See 45 CFR, part II, 160.103.

Health information. According to HIPAA, any information, whether oral or recorded in any form or medium, that is created or received by a covered entity; relates to the past, present, or future physical or mental health or condition of an individual; the provision of health care to an individual; or the past, present, or future payment for the provision of health care to an individual. See 45 CFR, part II, 160.103.

Health insurance claim number (HICN). A number issued by the Social Security Administration to individuals or beneficiaries entitled to Medicare benefits. The HICN and card provide the beneficiary information that is necessary for processing Medicare claims.

Health Insurance Portability and Accountability Act of 1996 (HIPAA). A federal law that allows persons to qualify immediately for comparable health insurance coverage when they change their employment relationships. Title II, subtitle F, of HIPAA gives the Department of Health and Human Services the authority to mandate the use of standards for the electronic exchange of health care data; to specify what medical and administrative code sets should be used within those standards; to require the use of national identification systems for health care patients, providers, payers (or plans), and employers (or sponsors); and to specify the types of measures required to protect the security and privacy of personally identifiable health care information. Also known as the Kennedy-Kassenbaum Bill, the Kassenbaum-Kennedy Bill, K2, or Public Law 104-191.

Health maintenance organization (HMO). A form of medical health insurance coverage that pays claims based on a provider cost, per diem or charge basis. Hospitals contract with an HMO to provide care at a contractually reduced price. HMO members pay a set monthly amount for coverage and are treated without additional cost, except for a copayment or deductible amount, payable by the patient. Like all managed care organizations, HMOs use a variety of mechanisms to control costs, including utilization management, discounted provider fee schedules, and financial incentives. HMOs use primary care physicians as gatekeepers and tend to emphasize preventive care. See 45 CFR, part II, 160.103.

Healthcare Common Procedure Coding System (HCPCS) Level I. A numeric coding system used by facility outpatient departments and ambulatory surgery centers (ASCs) to code ambulatory, laboratory, radiology, and other diagnostic services for Medicare billing. This coding system contains only the American Medical Association's Physicians' Current Procedural Terminology (CPT) codes. The AMA updates codes annually. See Physicians' Current Procedural Terminology (CPT).

Healthcare Common Procedure Coding System (HCPCS) Level II. A national coding system, developed by CMS, that contains alphanumeric codes for physician and nonphysician services not included in the CPT coding system. HCPCS Level II covers such things as ambulance services, durable medical equipment, and orthotic and prosthetic devices.

Healthcare Common Procedure Coding System (HCPCS). Two levels of codes used by Medicare and other payers to describe procedures and supplies. Level I includes of all of the codes listed in CPT, and Level II are alphanumeric supply and procedure codes.

Hemodialysis. Cleansing of wastes and contaminating elements from the blood by virtue of different diffusion rates through a semipermeable membrane, which separates blood from a filtration solution that diffuses other elements out of the blood.

HHS. See Department of Health and Human Services. Also see 45 CFR, part II, 160.103.

HIPAA. See Health Insurance Portability and Accountability Act of 1996.

HMO. See Health maintenance organization.

Home health agency (HHA). A health care provider, licensed under state or local law, that provides skilled nursing and other therapeutic services. HHAs include visiting nurse associations and hospital-based home care programs. To participate in Medicare, an HHA must meet health and safety standards established by the U.S. Department of Health and Human Services (HHS). Home health services usually are provided in the patient's home, although some outpatient services performed in a hospital, SNF or rehabilitation center may be covered under home health if the equipment is required and cannot be used in the patient's home.

Home health services. Services furnished to patients in their homes under the care of physicians. These services include part-time or intermittent skilled nursing care, physical therapy, medical social services, medical supplies and some rehabilitation equipment. Home health supplies and services must be prescribed by a physician, and the beneficiary must be confined at home in order for Medicare to pay the benefits in full.

Home health. Palliative and therapeutic care and assistance in the activities of daily life to homebound Medicare and private plan members.

HPSA. Health professional shortage area.

ICD-10-CM. See International Classification of Diseases, Tenth Edition, Clinical Modification.

ICD-10-PCS. See International Classification of Diseases, Tenth Edition, Procedure Coding System.

ICD-9-CM. See International Classification of Diseases, Ninth Edition, Clinical Modification.

ICF. See Intermediate care facility.

ID card. The wallet card carried by a plan member providing name, member and group numbers, effective dates, deductibles, and other information.

Imaging. Radiologic means of producing pictures for clinical study of the internal structures and functions of the body, such as x-ray, ultrasound, magnetic resonance, or positron emission tomography.

In plan. Services chosen from a network provider.

Indemnification. A type of hold-harmless clause that requires the responsible party in a liability claim to compensate the second party should the responsible party's actions result in a liability to the second party.

Independent medical evaluation (IME). An examination carried out by an impartial health care provider, generally board certified, to resolve a dispute related to the nature and extent of an illness or injury.

Indirect costs. Practice costs not directly associated with the physician service being provided. Examples include general office supplies, rent, utilities, and other office overhead.

Individual practice association (IPA). An organization made up of providers who, along with the rest of a group, contract with payers at a discounted fee-for-service or capitated rate.

© 2004 Ingenix, Inc.

Individual practice organization (IPO). An organization made up of providers who, along with the rest of a group, contract with payers at a discounted fee-for-service or capitated rate.

Information services (IS). The internal administrators of the computer systems used by an organization or institution.

Inpatient hospitalization. A period in which a patient is housed in a single hospital, usually without interruption.

Inpatient reimbursement. The payment to a hospital for the costs incurred to treat a patient for the time the patient was considered an inpatient.

Inpatient services. Items and services furnished to an inpatient, including room and board, nursing care and related services, diagnostic and therapeutic services, and medical and surgical services. An inpatient service requires the beneficiary to reside in a specific institutional setting during treatment (Medicare Pub. 100-04, trans #25, October 31, 2003).

Integrated delivery systems. A health care delivery system that joins the various parts of the health care system, including facilities, physicians, and ancillary service providers, into a cohesive group to provide a complete network of health care services for a given patient population or geographic area.

Intermediate care facility (ICF). A health care facility that furnishes services to patients who do not require the degree of care provided by a hospital or skilled nursing facility or a step-down facility for patients who are leaving the hospital but who cannot be discharged to home because of continuing medical needs.

International Classification of Diseases (ICD). A medical code set maintained by the World Health Organization (WHO). The primary purpose was to classify causes of death. A U.S. extension, maintained by the National Center for Health Statistics within the Centers for Disease Control and Prevention, identifies morbidity factors, or diagnoses. The ICD-9-CM codes have been selected for use in the HIPAA transactions.

International Classification of Diseases, Ninth Edition, Clinical Modification (ICD-9-CM). A clinical modification of the international statistical coding system used to report, compile, and compare health care data, using numeric and alphanumeric codes to help plan, deliver, reimburse, and quantify medical care in the United States.

International Classification of Diseases, Tenth Edition (ICD-10). Classification of diseases by alphanumeric code, used by the World Health Organization but not yet adopted in the United States.

International Classification of Diseases, Tenth Edition, Clinical Modification (ICD-10-CM). Clinical modification of ICD-10 developed for use in the United States.

International Classification of Diseases, Tenth Edition, Procedure Coding System (ICD-10-PCS). A procedure coding system developed by 3M HIS under contract with the Centers for Medicare and Medicaid Services.

Invalid ICD-9-CM code. A diagnosis code that is incorrect or not specific because one or more digits are missing, numbers have been transposed, or numbers presented are not listed in the ICD-9-CM listing.

IPA. See Individual practice association.

IPO. Individual practice organization. See Individual practice association.

Itemized statement. A detailed statement of each item or service the patient received from the physician, hospital, or other health care supplier or professional. The BBA of 1997 gives Medicare beneficiaries the right to submit a written request for an itemized statement from their provider or supplier for any Medicare item or service. Providers and suppliers are required to furnish the itemized statement within 30 days of the request or be subject to a civil monetary penalty of up to $100 for each offense. Recommended information to be included on the itemized statement are: date(s) of service, description of services provided, number of services provided, benefit days used, noncovered charges, deductible and coinsurance amounts, amount charged, beneficiary liability, total paid by Medicare, referring physician, provider/supplier submitting the claim, and the Medicare claim number.

J codes. A subset of the HCPCS Level II code set with a high-order value of "J" that has been used to identify certain drugs and other items.

JCAHO. See Joint Commission on Accreditation of Healthcare Organizations.

Joint Commission on Accreditation of Healthcare Organizations (JCAHO). An organization that accredits health care organizations. In the future, the JCAHO may play a role in certifying these organizations' compliance with the HIPAA A/S requirements. Previously known as the Joint Commission for the Accreditation of Hospitals.

Late effect. A residual, long-term, or chronic condition occurring after the acute phase of an illness or injury has terminated or the injury has healed.

LCSW. Licensed clinical social worker.

Length of stay. The number of inpatient bed days for a single patient during a single admission.

Level of specificity. Refers to diagnosis coding specificity; i.e., a three-digit disease code is assigned only when there are no four-digit codes within that category, a four-digit code is assigned only when there is no fifth-digit subclassification within that category, or a fifth digit is assigned for any category for which a fifth-digit subclassification is provided.

Liability insurance. Insurance, including self-insured plans, that provides payment based on legal liability for injuries, illness, or damage to property such as automobile, uninsured and underinsured motorist, homeowner's, malpractice, product liability, and general casualty insurance.

Limiting charge. The maximum amount a nonparticipating physician or provider can charge for services to a Medicare patient.

Limits. The ceiling for benefits payable under a plan.

Linking codes. To establish medical necessity, CPT and HCPCS Level II codes must be supported by the ICD-9-CM diagnosis and injury codes submitted on the claim form and supported by the documentation.

Local anesthesia. An induced loss of feeling or sensation restricted to a certain area of the body, including topical, local tissue infiltration, field block, or nerve block methods.

Local medical review policy (LMRP). A carrier-specific policy applied in the absence of a national coverage policy to make local Medicare medical coverage decisions, including the development of a draft policy based on a review of medical literature, an understanding of local practice, and the solicitation of comments from the medical community and Carrier Advisory Committee; also known as local carrier decisions.

Long-term care facility. A nursing home or, more specifically, a facility offering extended, nonacute care to a resident patient whose illness does not require acute care.

LPN. Licensed practical nurse.

LTC. Long-term care.

LVN. Licensed vocational nurse/licensed visiting nurse.

M+CO. See Medicare+Choice organization.

MA. Master of arts degree/medical assistant.

Malpractice costs. One of three components used to develop relative value units (RVUs) under the resource-based relative value scale. This portion represents the cost of professional liability insurance for each procedure.

Managed care organization. A generic term for various health benefit plans that provide coverage for health care services in conjunction with management and review of services provided to ensure that services are medically necessary and appropriate.

Managed care organized (MCO). Term covers health care businesses such as HMOs, preferred provider arrangements (PPAs), or preferred provider organizations (PPOs).

Managed health care. 1) The concept of managing active cases to ensure care is the most appropriate, efficient, and effective; 2) a system of health care meant to manage overall cost; 3) a method of health care whereby contracted physicians participate in managing health care costs.

Management information system. A system incorporating hardware and software to facilitate claims management.

Mandated benefits. Services mandated by state or federal law such as in cases of child abuse or rape, not necessarily covered by insurers.

Mandated providers. Providers of medical care, such as psychologists, optometrists, podiatrists, and chiropractors, whose licensed services must, under state or federal law, be included in coverage offered by a health plan.

Mandatory assignment. Although not in effect nationally, this alternative system stipulates that only those services for which the physician agrees to accept the Medicare payment as payment in full are fully reimbursable.

Mandatory exclusion provisions. Stipulations that any individual or entity that has been convicted of a health care felony that involves controlled substances, will be excluded from Medicare participation by the provider for 10 years for the first offense or permanently if convicted on two or more previous occasions.

Maximum allowable charge (MAC). The amount set by the insurer as the highest amount that can be charged for a particular medical service or by a pharmacy vendor.

Maximum out-of-pocket costs. The limit on total member copayments, deductibles, and coinsurance under a benefit contract.

MCM. See Medicare Carriers Manual.

MCO. See Managed care organization.

MD. See Medical doctor.

Medicaid fiscal agent (FA). The organization responsible for administering claims for a state Medicaid program.

Medicaid state agency. The state agency responsible for overseeing the state's Medicaid program.

Medicaid. A joint federal and state program that covers medical expense for some people with low incomes and limited resources with variations from state to state.

Medical and other health services. Any of the services provided to a patient to diagnose, treat, or maintain health status, including services of health care providers and professionals; rural, inpatient, outpatient, and diagnostic services; physical/occupational/speech/sports therapy; dialysis; immunization and vaccines; blood products; drugs; nutritional and diagnosis instruction; equipment; supplies; and ambulance services.

Medical consultation. Advice or an opinion rendered by a physician at the request of the primary care provider.

Medical doctor (MD). An allopathic, or traditional, physician.

Medical documentation. Patient care records, including operative notes; physical, occupational, and speech-language pathology notes; progress notes; physician certification and recertifications; emergency room records; or the patient's medical record in its entirety.

Medical necessity. The evaluation of health care services to determine if they are medically appropriate and necessary to meet basic health needs; consistent with the diagnosis or condition and rendered in a cost-effective manner; and consistent with national medical practice guidelines regarding type, frequency, and duration of treatment.

Medical Records Institute (MRI). An organization that promotes the development and acceptance of electronic health care record systems.

Medical review. Review by a Medicare fiscal intermediary, carrier, and/or quality improvement organization (QIO) of services and items provided by physicians, other health care practitioners, and providers of health care services under Medicare. The review determines if the items and services are reasonable and necessary and meet Medicare coverage requirements, whether the quality meets professionally recognized standards of health care, and whether the services are medically appropriate in an inpatient, outpatient, or other setting as supported by documentation.

Medicare carrier. An organization that contracts with the Centers for Medicare and Medicaid Services to process Medicare claims for eligible beneficiaries under Part B, the supplemental medical insurance program, and are responsible for daily claims processing, utilization review, records maintenance, and dissemination of information based on CMS regulations.

Medicare Carriers Manual (MCM). The manual the Centers for Medicare and Medicaid Services provides to Medicare carriers containing instructions for processing and paying Medicare claims, preparing reimbursement forms, billing procedures, and adhering to Medicare regulations. This has been replaced by the Medicare manual system.

Medicare contractor. A Medicare Part A fiscal intermediary, a Medicare Part B carrier, or a Medicare durable medical equipment regional carrier (DMERC).

Medicare durable medical equipment regional carrier (DMERC). A Medicare contractor that administers durable medical equipment (DME) benefits for a region.

Medicare fee schedule (MFS). A fee schedule based upon physician work, expense, and malpractice designed to slow the rise in cost for services and standardize payment to physicians regardless of specialty or location of service with geographic adjustments.

Medicare Part A fiscal intermediary (FI). A Medicare contractor that administers the Medicare Part A (institutional) benefits for a given region.

Medicare Part A. Administered by fiscal intermediaries, coverage includes hospital, nursing home, hospice, home health, and other inpatient care.

Medicare Part B carrier. A Medicare contractor that administers the Medicare Part B (professional) benefits for a given region.

Medicare Part B. Administered by carriers, coverage provides payment for physician and outpatient services.

Medicare remittance advice remark codes. A national administrative code set for providing either claim-level or service-level Medicare-related messages that cannot be expressed with a claim adjustment reason code. This code set is used in the X12 835 Claim Payment & Remittance Advice transaction, and is maintained by the Centers for Medicare and Medicaid Services.

Medicare secondary payer (MSP). Specified circumstances when other third-party payers cover beneficiaries and Medicare is the secondary payer such as for workers' compensation, automobile, medical no-fault, and liability insurance as well as employer group health plans, and certain employer health plans covering aged and disabled beneficiaries.

Medicare supplement. Private insurance coverage that pays costs of services not covered by Medicare; also known as Medigap coverage.

Medicare. A federally funded program authorized as part of the Social Security Act that provides for health care services for people age 65 or older, people with disabilities, and people with end-stage renal disease (ESRD).

Medicare+Choice organization. Created in 1997 as part of the Balanced Budget Act (BBA), which allows managed care plans, such as health maintenance organizations (HMOs) and preferred provider organizations (PPOs) to join the Medicare system.

Medigap policy. A health insurance or other health benefit plan offered by a private company to those entitled to Medicare benefits. The policy covers charges not payable by Medicare because of deductibles, coinsurance amounts, or other Medicare-imposed limitations.

Member. A subscriber of a health plan.

MFS. See Medicare fee schedule.

MGMA. Medical Group Management Association.

Midlevel practitioners (MLPs). Professionals such as nurse practitioners, nurse midwives, physical therapists, physician assistants, and others who provide medical care but do so with physician input.

Minor procedure. A self-limited procedure, usually with an assignment of 0 or 10 follow-up days. May be considered by many payers to be part of the global package for a primary surgical service.

Miscoding. Any type of incorrect coding.

MLP. See Midlevel practitioners.

MLT. Medical laboratory technician.

Modifier. A descriptive two-character code attached to a CPT or HCPCS code as a suffix that changes the procedure description or

Monitored anesthesia care. Sedation, with or without analgesia, used to achieve a medically controlled state of depressed consciousness while maintaining the patient's airway, protective reflexes, and ability to respond to stimulation or verbal commands. In dental conscious sedation, the patient is rendered free of fear, apprehension, and anxiety through the use of pharmacological agents.

Monitoring (compliance). To keep track, regulate, or control the compliance process.

Most-favored-nation clauses. Contract provision requiring the provider to bill the third-party payer the lowest fee charged to any other person or entity.

MSA. Medical savings account.

National Coverage Determination Manual (NCD). Part of the Centers for Medicare and Medicaid Services manual system, it contains national coverage decisions and specific medical items, services, treatment procedures, or technologies paid for under the Medicare program and was revised from the Coverage Issues Manual (CIM).

National coverage determinations (NCDs). National policy statements granting, eliminating, or excluding Medicare coverage for a service, item, or test. NCDs state the Centers for Medicare and Medicaid Services' policy regarding the circumstances under which the service, item, or test is considered reasonable and necessary and not screening or otherwise not covered for Medicare purposes. These polices apply nationwide.

National coverage policy. Policy outlining Medicare coverage decisions that apply to all states and regions indicating whether and under what circumstances items/services are covered and are published in Centers for Medicare and Medicaid Services regulations in the Federal Register, contained in CMS rulings, or issued as program memorandums or manual issuances to the CMS manual system.

National Drug Codes (NDCs). A medical code set that identifies prescription drugs and some over-the-counter products and that has been selected for use in the HIPAA transactions.

NDC. See National Drug Codes.

Nebulizer. A device pressurized by an oxygen tank for converting a liquid medication into a fine mist that can be inhaled.

New patient. Patient who, for the first time in three years, is receiving face-to-face care from the provider or another physician of the same specialty who belongs to the same group practice.

Newborn admission. An infant born in the facility.

Newborn intensive care unit (NICU/NBICU). A special care unit for premature and seriously ill infants.

NOC. Not otherwise classified or nursing outcomes classification.

Nomenclature. The assignment of a name or the description of a term or procedure such as a HCPCS code description.

Noncovered procedure. A procedure that is not reimbursable by the Medicare program and for which the fiscal intermediary will deny the claim.

Nonfacility practice expense. The physician's direct and indirect practice costs related to each service when that service is provided in the physician's office, patient's home, or other nonhospital setting, such as a residential care facility.

Nonoperating room procedure. A procedure that does not normally require the use of the operating room and that can affect DRG assignment.

Nonspecific code. A catchall code that specifies the diagnosis as ill defined, other, or unspecified and may be a valid choice if no other code closely describes the diagnosis.

Not Elsewhere Classifiable (NEC). The condition or diagnosis is not provided with its own specified code in ICD-9-CM, but included in a more broadly defined code for other specified conditions.

Not Otherwise Specified (NOS). The condition or diagnosis remains ill defined and is unspecified without the necessary information for selecting a more specific code.

NP. Nurse practitioner.

Nurse practitioner. A specially trained, degreed nurse who assesses, treats, and prescribes medication.

Observation patient. A patient who needs to be monitored and assessed for inpatient admission or referral to another site for care.

Observation services. According to the Medicare Pub. 100-02, chap. 6, sec. 70.4, those services "furnished on a hospital's premises, including use of a bed and periodic monitoring by a hospital's nursing or other staff, which are reasonable and necessary to evaluate an outpatient's condition or determine the need for a possible admission to the hospital as an inpatient. Such services are covered only when provided by the order of a physician or another individual authorized by state license laws and hospital staff bylaws to admit patients to the hospital or to order outpatient tests." Observation services normally do not extend beyond 23 hours. They are reported using RC 0762. New requirements for reporting observation services have been implemented as the result of the APC final rule issued November 30, 2001.

Occupational therapy. Therapy meant to help someone who is recovering from a serious illness or injury to retain the ability to perform activities of daily life.

Occurrence code. A two-digit number and date used to report specific circumstances that are relevant to the claim being submitted.

OCE. See Outpatient Code Editor (OCE).

Off-site. A place other than the provider's usual place of practice.

Office of Inspector General (OIG). An agency within the Department of Health and Human Services that is ultimately responsible for investigating instances of fraud and abuse in the Medicare and Medicaid and other government health care programs.

OIG work plan. An annual plan released by the Office of Inspector General that details the areas of focus for fraud and abuse investigations.

OIG. See Office of Inspector General.

On-site. Regular place of practice of the provider; his or her primary clinic or department location.

Open enrollment period. A time during which subscribers in a health benefit program have an opportunity to re-enroll or select an alternative health plan being offered to them, usually without evidence of insurability or waiting periods.

Open panel. An arrangement in which a managed care organization that contracts with providers on an exclusive basis is still seeking providers.

Operating room (OR) procedure. A procedure that falls into a defined group of procedures that normally requires the use of an operating room.

Other specified. A term in ICD-9-CM referring to codes reported when a diagnosis has been made and there is no code identifying it more specifically as with NEC, or not elsewhere classified.

OTR. Occupational therapist registered.

Out of plan. Services of a provider who is not a member of the preferred provider network.

Out of service area. Medical care received out of the geographic area that may or may not be covered, depending on the plan.

Outpatient code editor (OCE). The Centers for Medicare and Medicaid Services' outpatient software program that analyzes hospital outpatient claims to detect incorrect billing and coding data, assign an ambulatory payment classification for covered services, determine if ambulatory surgery center payment limitations apply to the claim, and determine the appropriate payment.

Outpatient physical therapy services. The physical therapy services provided to an outpatient of a clinic, rehabilitation agency, or public health agency. The attending physician must establish a plan of physical therapy or periodically review a plan developed by a qualified physical therapist. A group of professional personnel, including one or more physicians (associated with the clinic or rehabilitation agency) and one or more qualified physical therapists, must govern services and maintain clinical records of all patients. Outpatient clinics must provide a surety bond of $50,000 to guarantee the efficiency and effectiveness of programs. The term outpatient physical therapy services also includes physical therapy services provided by a physical therapist in office or at the patient's home and speech-language pathology services.

Outpatient services. Medical and other services provided by the hospital or other qualified supplier that are either diagnostic or help the physician treat the patient.

Outpatient surgery list. A list of surgical procedures that can be performed on an outpatient basis without adversely affecting the quality of care.

Outpatient visit. An encounter in a recognized outpatient facility.

Outpatient. A patient who receives care without being admitted for inpatient or residential care.

Overutilization. Services rendered by providers more frequently than usual, performed by peers or desired by payers.

PA. 1) Physician assistant; 2) physician association.

Paper claim. A claim that is submitted on paper, including optical character recognition (OCR) claims and claims that are converted to electronic format by Medicare.

Participating provider. A provider who has contracted with the health plan to deliver medical services to covered persons; also known as network or in-network provider.

Patient problem. A disease, condition, illness, injury, symptom, sign, finding, complaint, or other reason for an encounter, with or without a diagnosis being established at the time of the encounter.

Payer. An organization, such as a health plan, self-insured employer, HMO, or uninsured patient, that assumes risk by paying for health care expenses.

Payment floor. Minimum number of calendar days that must pass before the Medicare Part B carrier can pay a claim, established by the Omnibus Budget Reconciliation Act of 1987 for Medicare claims.

Payment rate. The amount that is to be paid to the provider for health care services rendered to a plan member.

PE. See Practice expense.

PhD. Doctor of philosophy.

PHI. See Protected health information.

Physical status modifiers (anesthesia services). An alphanumeric modifier used to identify the patient's health status as it affects the work related to providing the anesthesia service.

Physical therapy modality. A therapeutic agent or regiment applied or used to provide appropriate treatment of the musculoskeletal system.

Physician services. Professional services performed by physicians, including surgery; consultation; and home, office, and institutional calls.

Physician work. One of three components used to develop relative value units (RVUs) under the resource-based relative value scale. Physician work represents the value of the skill and time required to perform a service.

Physician-directed clinic. A clinic where 1) a physician (or a number of physicians) is present to perform medical (rather than administrative) services at all times; 2) each patient is under the care of a clinic physician; and 3) the nonphysician services are under medical supervision.

Physician. The following legally authorized practitioners: a doctor of medicine or osteopathy; a doctor of dental surgery or of dental medicine; a doctor of podiatric medicine; a doctor of optometry; a chiropractor and only with respect to treatment by means of manual manipulation of the spine (to correct a subluxation).

Physician's assistant (PA). A medical professional who receives additional training and can assess, treat, and prescribe medications under a physician's review.

Physicians' Current Procedural Terminology (CPT). A definitive procedural coding system developed and owned by the American Medical Association that is a listing of descriptive terms and identifying codes used for reporting medical services and procedures.

Place of Service. The location where the service was provided and identified by a two digit number assigned by CMS.

PIN. Physician identification number.

Point of service (POS) plan. A health benefit plan allowing the covered person to choose to receive a service from a participating or nonparticipating provider, with different benefit levels associated with the use of participating providers.

Posting date. The date a charge is posted to a patient account by the provider, frequently not the same as the actual date of service, but usually within five days of the actual date of service.

PPO. See Preferred provider organization.

PPS. See Prospective payment system.

Practice expense. One of three components used to develop relative value units under the resource-based relative value scale. Practice expense represents the physician's direct and indirect costs associated with providing a service.

Preauthorization. A requirement that approval for requested services be obtained before providing those services.

Precertification. Preadmission certification. The approval in advance of a procedure or hospital stay by a payer employee, who considers the diagnosis, the planned treatment, and expected length of stay.

Preferred provider arrangement (PPA). Similar to a PPO. See Preferred provider organization.

Preferred provider organization (PPO). A program that establishes contracts with providers of medical care. Usually the benefit contract provides significantly better benefits and lower member cost for services received from preferred providers, encouraging covered persons to use these providers, who may be reimbursed on a discounted basis.

Primary care physician (PCP). The physician who makes an initial diagnosis and referral and retains control over the patient and utilization of services both in and outside the plan.

Primary care. Basic or general health care, including diagnosis and treatment, traditionally provided by family practice, pediatrics, and internal medicine practitioners.

Primary diagnosis. The current, most significant reason for the services or procedures provided.

Primary payer. The insurance company or governmental agency that has the first and greatest responsibility for reimbursing providers and suppliers of service.

Primary. Principal or first in the order of occurrence or importance.

Principal diagnosis code. The code that identifies the condition established after study to be chiefly responsible for occasioning the admission of the patient to the hospital for care.

Principal procedure. A procedure performed for definitive treatment rather than for diagnostic or exploratory purposes, or that was necessary to treat a complication. Usually related to the principal diagnosis.

Procedure. A diagnostic or therapeutic service provided for the care and treatment of a patient, usually conforming to a specific set of steps or instructions.

Professional component. The portion of a charge for healthcare services that represents the physician's (or other practitioner's) work in providing the service, including interpretation and report of the procedure.

Provider identification number (PIN). Also known as unique provider identification number (UPIN), PIN is a number assigned by the Centers for Medicare and Medicaid Services that identifies the provider (an institution, individual physician, clinic, or organization) of health care services.

Provider number. A number assigned by a payer or government agency that identifies a specific provider.

Provider of services. An institution, individual, or organization that provides health care.

Provider. An institution, entity, organization, or person that administers health care services.

PT. Physical therapy; physical therapist.

RA. See Remittance advice.

Radioelement. Any element that emits particle or electromagnetic radiations from nuclear disintegration, occurring naturally in any element with an atomic number above 83.

Radiograph. Image made by an x-ray.

Radiology services. Services that include diagnostic and therapeutic radiology, nuclear medicine, CT scan procedures, magnetic resonance imaging services, ultrasound and other imaging procedures. HCPCS codes are required for billing outpatient radiology procedures.

Radiotherapy. An external source of high-energy rays (x-rays or gamma rays) or internally implanted radioactive substances used in destroying tissue and stopping the growth of malignant cells.

Range of motion. Action of a body part throughout its extent of natural movement, measured in degrees of a circle.

RBRVS. Resource-based relative value study. A relative value scale originally developed by Harvard for use in Medicare. The scale assigns value to procedures based on the related resources rather than on historical data.

Reasonable and customary. Fees charged for medical services that are considered normal, common, and in line with the prevailing fees in the provider's geographical area.

Refer. Recommendation to another source.

Referenced diagnostic laboratory services. Laboratory services such as tests performed on samples that are referred to the hospital laboratory for diagnostic work.

Referral. An approval from the primary care physician to see a specialist or receive certain services. May be required for coverage purposes before a patient receives care from anyone except the primary physician.

Referred outpatient. A patient who is sent to a special diagnostic or therapeutic facility or to a hospital service department for the diagnosis and treatment of an illness or injury on an outpatient basis.

Registered health information administrator (RHIA). An accreditation for medical record administrators, previously known as a registered records administrator (RRA).

Registered health information technician (RHIT). An accreditation for medical records practitioners, previously known as accredited records technician (ART).

Regulation. An authoritative ruling or law put forth by an executive authority of the law.

Rehabilitation hospital. An inpatient institution that provides intensive rehabilitative services for the treatment of certain conditions (e.g., stroke, amputation, brain or spinal cord injuries, and neurological disorders).

Rehabilitation. Physical and mental restoration of disabled patients.

Reimbursement. Payment of actual charges or allowable incurred as a result of accident or illness.

rs existing between two parties' problems and issues.

Relative value scale (RVS). A numeric ranking of physician and ancillary services based on the intensity of the procedure or service being performed.

Relative value study (RVS). A guide that shows the relationship between the time, resources, competency, experience, severity, and other factors necessary to perform procedures that is multiplied by a dollar conversion factor to determine a monetary value for the procedure.

Relative value unit. A value assigned a procedure based on difficulty and time consumed. Used for computing reimbursement under a relative value study.

Release of information. An authorization from the patient that allows the hospital to release to the insurer or other payer the medical and billing information for determining coverage eligibility, medical necessity, the final diagnosis, and any procedures performed or as needed to process a claim for reimbursement.

Remittance advice. A statement, voucher, or notice that a provider of services receives from a payer that reflects adjudicated claims, either paid or denied; also known as explanation of Medicare benefits (EOMB).

Revenue code. A four-digit code that identifies a specific accommodation or ancillary charge on the bill.

RPT. Registered physical therapist.

Rural health clinic. A clinic in an area where there is a shortage of health services staffed by a nurse practitioner, physician assistant, or certified nurse midwife under physician direction that provides routine diagnostic services, including clinical laboratory services, drugs, and biologicals and that has prompt access to additional diagnostic services from facilities meeting federal requirements.

RVS. See Relative value study.

RVU. See Relative value unit.

Second opinion. A medical opinion obtained from another health care professional, relevant to clinical evaluation, before the performance of a medical service or surgical procedure. Includes patient education regarding treatment alternatives and/or to determine medical necessity.

Secondary care. Services provided by medical specialists, such as cardiologists, urologists, and dermatologists, who generally do not have first contact with patients.

Secondary insurer. In a coordination of benefits arrangement, the insurer that reimburses for benefits pending after payment by the primary insurer.

Secondary payer. An organization that pays, according to its coverage guidelines, any residual balance remaining after another insurer pays the claim.

Self-insured. An individual or organization that assumes the financial risk of paying for health care.

Self-pay patients. Patients who pay for medical care out of pocket.

Self-referral. A patient who was not referred to the outpatient clinic, emergency room, or hospital outpatient department, but who chose that facility on his or her own.

Separate procedures. Services that are commonly carried out as a fundamental part of a total service, and as such do not warrant a separate identification and are noted in the CPT book with the parenthetical phrase (separate procedure) at the end of the description.

Service-oriented V codes. ICD-9-CM codes that identify or define examinations, aftercare, ancillary services, or therapy; or the patient who is not currently ill but seeks medical services for some specific purpose such as follow-up or screening visits.

Signature. The signature of the physician acknowledges that he/she has performed or supervised the service or procedure and that the transcription has been read and corrections made before signing. Signed or initialed laboratory and x-ray results show auditors that the physician has reviewed the information.

Skilled nursing care. Daily care and other, related services for inpatients who require medical or nursing care or rehabilitation services for injuries, disabilities, or sickness, based on a written physician order certifying the need for such care.

Skilled nursing facility (SNF). A facility that cares for long-term patients with acute medical needs.

SNF. See Skilled nursing facility.

SNOMED. Systematized nomenclature of medicine.

SOAP. When documenting patients' visits, the SOAP approach (subjective, objective, assessment, plan) has been used historically as it standardizes physician documentation and easily adapts to history, exam, and medical decision making. The steps are defined as follows: • Subjective-The information the patient tells the physician; • Objective-The physician's observed, objective overview, including the patient's vital signs and the findings of the physical exam and any diagnostic tests; • Assessment-A list the physician prepares in response to the patient's condition, including the problem, diagnoses, and reasons leading the physician to the diagnoses; • Plan-The physician's workup or treatment planned for each problem in the assessment.

SSN. Social Security number.

Standard anesthesia formula. Reimbursement formula that consists of base units plus time units plus modifying units (e.g., physical status and qualifying circumstances) plus other allowed unit/charges that is multiplied by a conversion factor.

State insurance commission. The state group that approves insurance certificates for each state and that regulates the industry based on statutes.

Statute. A law enacted by a legislative branch of the government.

Subrogation. Recovery of monies or benefits from a third party who is liable for the payment.

Subsidiary "in addition to" codes. Services that are not included as part of the primary procedure but that are not performed alone and may be identified as each additional, or list-in-addition-to services.

Superbill. A multipurpose sheet used for all patient encounters that typically contains a check-off list of ICD-9-CM diagnosis codes, evaluation and management codes, and procedure and HCPCS Level II codes in the outpatient setting.

Supervision and interpretation. Radiology services that usually contain an invasive component and are reported by the radiologist for supervision of the procedure and the personnel involved with performing the examination, reading the film, and preparing the written report.

Surgical hierarchy. Ordering of surgical cases from most to least resource intensive. Application of this decision rule is necessary when patient stays involve multiple surgical procedures, each of which, occurring by itself, could result in the assignment to a different DRG. All patients must be assigned to only one DRG per admission.

Surgical package. A normal, uncomplicated performance of specific surgical services, with the assumption that, on average, all surgical procedures of a given type are similar with respect to skill level, duration, and length of normal follow-up care.

Swing bed. A bed used for acute or long-term care, depending on the patient's need and the hospital's level of occupancy. Swing beds typically are available in small and rural hospitals. A swing-bed patient may be admitted and discharged from acute care and readmitted to a swing bed to receive skilled or intermediate levels of care. At times, the patient may remain in the same bed while changes occur in his/her care, charges, and payment.

TCC. See Transitional care center.

Technical component. A portion of a health care service that identifies the provision of the equipment, supplies, technical personnel, and costs attendant to the performance of the procedure other than the professional services.

Technique. A manner of performance.

Therapeutic procedures. Treatment of a pathological or traumatic condition through the use of activities performed to treat or heal the cause or to effect change through the application of clinical skills or services that attempt to improve function.

Therapeutic treatment. The medical or surgical management of a patient.

Therapeutic. An act meant to alleviate a medical or mental condition.

Third-party administrator (TPA). An entity that processes health care claims and performs related business functions for a health plan.

Third-party payer. A public or private organization that pays for or underwrites coverage for health care expenses for another entity, usually an employer or employee.

Three-digit diagnosis codes. One of approximately 100 diagnosis codes used alone (without zero filler) only when no fourth or fifth digit is available.

Time limit. Set number of days in which a claim can be filed according to the payer or state insurance commission.

Total value. Under the resource-based relative value scale, total value is the sum of the three components used to determine the value of each service. These include physician work, practice expense, and malpractice costs.

TPA. See Third-party administrator or Trading partner agreement.

Transitional care center (TCC). Used in lieu of an extended care facility or before discharge to an extended care facility.

Transitional pass-through payment. Certain drugs, biologicals, and devices are eligible for payments in addition to the ambulatory payment classification payment under the outpatient prospective payment system. The drugs are identified with a HCPCS Level II code reported with RC 0636. Devices are reported with the new C codes under RC 0272, 0275, or 0278.

Treatment planning. The projected series and sequences of procedures necessary to restore the health of the patient, based on a problem or specific diagnosis and a complete evaluation of the patient.

UB-92. The common claim form used by facilities to bill for services.

UCR. See Usual, customary, and reasonable.

Ultrasound. Imaging using ultra-high sound frequency bounced off body structures.

Unbundling. Breaking a single service into its multiple components, usually so as to increase total billing charges.

Undocumented services. A billed service for which the supporting documentation has not been recorded or is unavailable to substantiate the service.

Unique physician identification number (UPIN). A six-character, unique, alphanumeric identification number assigned by the Centers for Medicare and Medicaid Services to each physician.

Unlisted procedures. Procedural descriptions in each section of the CPT book used when the overall procedure and outcome of the surgery are not adequately described by an existing CPT code. Such codes are used as a last resort and only when there is not a more appropriate CPT code.

Unspecified. A diagnostic description when more information is necessary to code the term more specifically.

Unusual circumstances. Any unusual or aberrant conditions affecting a patient encounter that should be documented.

Unusual service. A procedure or service that is unusual or unique, or an aberrant finding, result, response, procedure, method, or behavior that affects the patient's treatment.

Upcoding. The practice of billing for a procedure with higher reimbursement than that for the procedure actually performed.

UPIN. See Unique physician identification number.

Usual, customary, and reasonable (UCR). Fees charged for medical services that are considered normal, common, and in line with the prevailing fees in the provider's area.

V codes. Codes that describe circumstances that influence a patient's health status and identify reasons for medical encounters resulting from circumstances other than a disease or injury already classified in the main part of ICD-9-CM; also known as supplementary classification of factors influencing health status and contact with health services.

Visit (or encounter). See Encounter (or visit).

WEDI. See Workgroup for Electronic Data Interchange.

Weighting. The practice of assigning more worth to a fee based on the number of times it is charged, weighting the resource-based relative value fees for an area.

Well-baby care. Medical services, immunizations, and regular provider visits considered routine for an infant.

WHO. See World Health Organization.

Workgroup for Electronic Data Interchange (WEDI). A health care industry group that lobbied for HIPAA A/S, and that has a formal consultative role under the HIPAA legislation. WEDI also sponsors the strategic national implementation process (SNIP).

World Health Organization (WHO). International agency comprising UN members to promote the physical, mental, and emotional health of the people of the world and to track morbidity and mortality statistics worldwide. Maintains the International Classification of Diseases (ICD) medical code set.

Index

A

abdomen 43
abuse 74, 165
accident codes 123
add-on codes 83, 104
Administrative Services Organization (ASO) 68
admission 73
Ambulatory Payment Classification (APC) 72, 188, 189,
    190, 191, 193, 194, 195, 198, 200
    grouper logic 191
Ambulatory Surgery Center (ASC) 188, 195, 196, 197,
    198, 199, 200
American Academy of Professional Coders (AAPC) 3, 165
American Health Information Management Association
    (AHIMA) 3, 119, 165
American Hospital Association (AHA) 4, 119
    coding clinic 119
American Medical Association (AMA) 75, 87, 104, 165
    Physicians' Current Procedural Terminology (CPT)
        137
    surgical package guidelines 104
analyte 111
anatomy 8
ancillary
    packaging 193
    services 106, 191
anesthesia 98, 99
articular system 9
Association of Registered Medical Coders 4
auditory system 10, 57, 60
    cochlea 60
    malleus 60

B

Blue Cross/Blue Shield 65, 66, 72
brain 55, 56
bundled services 100
burns
    rule of nines 11

C

capitation 72
cardiovascular system 9, 27
    arterial 28
    atria 27
    carotid artery 30
    coronary
        arteries 29

    veins
        portal 29
    heart 27, 30
        aorta 30
        arteries 30
        atrium 30
        endocardium 27
        interatrial septum 27
        interventricular septum 27
        myocardium 27
        pericardium 27
        pulmonary valve 30
        superior vena cava 30
        vein 30
    portal vein 29, 30
    pulmonary artery 27
    trachea 26
    vein 30
    venous 29
    venous blood 27
    ventricles 27
    vessels 31
carrier discretion 140
case management services 96
case mix 154, 155
Category III codes 76, 79, 84
Centers for Medicare and Medicaid Services (CMS) 4, 68,
    73, 87, 101, 117, 119, 137, 164, 165, 184, 188
central office
    HCPCS 4
    ICD-9-CM 4
certificate of medical necessity (CMN) 145
Certified Coding Associate (CCA) 3
Certified coding Specialist (CCS) 3
Certified Coding Specialist Physician (CCS-P) 3
Certified Professional Coder (CPC) 3
Certified Professional Coder Hospital (CPC-H) 3
Certified Registered Nurse Anesthetist (CRNA) 197
charge description master (CDM) 167
chargemaster 152
chief complaint (CC) 91
circulatory system 9
    coronary artery 29
clean claims 140, 150
CMS-1500 claim form 73, 75, 188
codes
    accident 123
    add-on 83, 104

Physicians' Current Procedural Terminology (CPT) 75
planes 61
    coronal 61
    horizontal 61
    median 61
    sagittal 61
point of service (POS) 67
postitional terms
    distal 61
    exterior 61
    interior 61
    proximal 61
    superficial 61
practice management 147
preauthorization 148
    form 149
precertification 148
preferred provider organization (PPO) 67
presenting problem 91
principal diagnosis 168
principal procedure 177
procedure codes
    sequencing 176
professional component 106
professional services 90
progress notes 162
prolonged services 96
prospective payment system (PPS) 153, 154
prosthesis 144
Public Health Service Act 67
pulmonary valve 30

R

radiology 107, 164
    services 108
reasonable charge 66, 152
Registered Medical Coder (RMC) 4
registration 147, 148
relationship terms
    anterior 61
    inferior 61
    lateral 61
    medial 61
    posterior 61
    superior 61
relative value scale (RVS) 72
relative value units (RVU) 71, 152
relative values 71
renal system 47
reproductive system 9
resource based relative value scale (RBRVS) 71, 152, 153
respiratory system 9, 22, 26
    alveoli sacks 22, 26
    bronchi 22, 24, 26

bronchus 25
diaphragm 26, 34, 44
larynx 22, 24, 25
lung 22, 23, 25, 26
maxilla 22
mediastrinum 26
myocardium 26
nasal cavity 24
nose 22

        alae (ala) 22
      external 22
      internal 23
        nasolacrimal ducts 23
        paranasal sinuses 23
      nares 22
paranasal sinuses 24
pharynx 22, 24
pleura 25
sinuses 24
thorax 22
trachea 24
vocal cords 24

S

secondary payer 69
separate procedures 104
significant procedure 191
skilled nursing facility (SNF) 69, 95, 192
SOAP 90
    assessment 90
    objective 90
    plan 90
    subjective 90
Social Security Act 68
special coverage instructions 140
specificity 180
stapes 60
summary sheet 160, 161
surgery section 103

T

Table of Drugs and Chemicals 123
tabular list 123
    of diseases (volume 1) 119
technical component 75, 106
terminated procedures 194
third-party administrator (TPA) 68
transfusion medicine 112
TRICARE 70

U

UB-92 claim form 73, 75, 154, 188
UCR system 71

unbundle prevention
    charge ticket **101**
    routing sheet **101**
unbundling **74, 100**
uniform hospital discharge data set (UHDDS) **176**
unlisted procedures **84, 105**
urinary system **9, 45**
    bladder **45**
        sphincter **45**
    kidney **45**
    peritoneum **45**
    prostate **46**
    renal **47**
    ureter **45**
    urethra **46**
    urogenital tract **46**

V

V codes **125, 126**
Veterans Administration **69, 70**
visit code **89**
vocal cords **24, 25, 37**

W

word root **62, 63**
workers' compensation **69, 70, 127, 138**
World Health Organization (WHO) **117, 118, 184**